The Breast Cancer Book

A Johns Hopkins Press Health Book

THE
BREAST
CANCER
BOOK

A Trusted Guide for You and Your Loved Ones

Kenneth D. Miller, MD
Melissa Camp, MD, MPH
With Kathy Steligo

JOHNS HOPKINS UNIVERSITY PRESS
Baltimore

Note to the Reader: This book is not meant to substitute for medical care, and treatment should not be based solely on its contents. Instead, treatment must be developed in a dialogue between the individual and his or her physician. The book has been written to help with that dialogue.

Drug dosage: The authors and publisher have made reasonable efforts to determine that the selection of drugs discussed in this text conform to the practices of the general medical community. In view of ongoing research, changes in governmental regulation, and the constant flow of information relating to drug therapy and drug reactions, the reader is urged to check the package insert of each drug for any change in indications and dosage and for warnings and precautions. This is particularly important when the recommended agent is a new and/or an infrequently used drug.

© 2021 Johns Hopkins University Press
All rights reserved. Published 2021
Printed in the United States of America on acid-free paper
9 8 7 6 5 4 3 2 1

Johns Hopkins University Press
2715 North Charles Street
Baltimore, Maryland 21218-4363
www.press.jhu.edu

Library of Congress Cataloging-in-Publication Data

Names: Miller, Kenneth D., 1956– author. | Camp, Melissa, 1978– author. |
    Steligo, Kathy, author.
Title: The breast cancer book : a trusted guide for you and your loved ones /
    Kenneth D. Miller, MD, Melissa Camp, MD, MPH, with Kathy Steligo.
Description: Baltimore : Johns Hopkins University Press, 2021. |
    Series: A Johns Hopkins Press health book | Includes index.
Identifiers: LCCN 2020052701 | ISBN 9781421441900 (hardcover) |
    ISBN 9781421441917 (paperback) | ISBN 9781421441924 (ebook)
Subjects: LCSH: Breast—Cancer—Popular works.
Classification: LCC RC280.B8 M535 2021 | DDC 616.99/449—dc23
LC record available at https://lccn.loc.gov/2020052701

A catalog record for this book is available from the British Library.

Special discounts are available for bulk purchases of this book. For more information, please contact Special Sales at specialsales@jh.edu.

Johns Hopkins University Press uses environmentally friendly book materials, including recycled text paper that is composed of at least 30 percent post-consumer waste, whenever possible.

Contents

PART THREE
Understanding Treatment Choices and Making Decisions

PART FIVE

Moving On

Tables

The Breast Cancer Book

Introduction

A MESSAGE OF HOPE

The most important thing to know about breast cancer is that it can be treated, and in most cases, it can be cured.

When women are newly diagnosed with breast cancer, the first question they often ask is, Why me? or What did I do to cause this? Before you begin this book, know that breast cancer isn't your fault. It didn't develop from something you did or didn't do, and you shouldn't blame yourself for it.

A diagnosis of breast cancer, even if you suspect it, is a shock. You might be thinking that this must be a mistake. You're probably stunned and afraid, and because you don't know what's going to happen, you fear the worst. The most important thing to know about breast cancer is that it can be treated, and in most cases, it can be cured. Better screening technologies more often find breast cancers early, when they're easier to treat. And with the explosion of discoveries from genetic and genomic sciences, we can now identify the unique characteristics of each woman's tumor. As a result, today's treatments are smarter, more focused, and less toxic. They're also more effective: most breast cancer survivors live decades past their diagnosis.

If you're newly diagnosed, you probably have plenty of unanswered questions. Will I survive? Will I lose my breasts or my hair? What do all the medical terms and risk statistics mean? How will I get through something so frightening and overwhelming? You're not the first person to have these concerns or to ask these questions. More than 3.5 million women in the United States have found themselves in the same unwanted and unexpected situation. Just like you, each of them experienced that terrifying moment when they felt a lump or learned that they had an abnormal mammogram. Stunned by a diagnosis that confirmed they had breast cancer, they were uncertain about what might lie ahead, as you probably are. One day they were fine; the next day they found themselves on an unfamiliar and uncertain path. These women have walked in your shoes. Most importantly, they've also been treated, left breast cancer behind, and moved on with their lives.

We often hear that breast cancer is a journey, and in a way that's true. It's an experience that requires physical, emotional, and even spiritual strength. Like any journey, you have two choices as you set out: you can make your way through from start to finish not knowing what you'll encounter, or you can choose to learn what to expect and plan for what lies ahead. This book is your road map to understanding each step of the way, so that you'll have fewer surprises and detours. Learning about breast cancer is the most powerful way to regain control and restore order in a situation that probably feels chaotic and disruptive. It will also equip you to interact confidently with your medical team and make the numerous decisions that breast cancer requires.

The book you now hold in your hands is educational, inspirational, and most importantly informative. No matter where you are in your breast cancer experience, the information on these pages will help you understand your diagnosis and explain your treatment options so that you can become an engaged participant with your doctors and make the best possible decisions about your care.

We've organized the information into five parts to make it easy to find answers quickly.

1. Part One, "Understanding Breast Cancer," gives you a foundation of knowledge on which the remainder of the book builds. Here you'll learn about breast cancer basics, risks that affect the odds of being diagnosed, prevention strategies, and information on hereditary breast cancers.

2. Part Two, "Finding Breast Cancer and Dealing with a Diagnosis," explains various scans and tests that are used to diagnose

breast cancer, what all those confusing terms on the pathology report mean, and important steps to help you move forward after a diagnosis.

3. Part Three, "Understanding Treatment Choices and Making Decisions" includes the nine chapters that describe various treatment options. This is the core of the book's knowledge base. It will likely be the section that you'll return to again and again as you seek to learn more about treatment options and weigh the advantages and disadvantages of each alternative. These chapters are full of information to help you understand your alternatives before you decide what's best for you.

4. Part Four, "Finding Answers," is a section of practical answers to questions that just about all breast cancer patients have. You'll find helpful guidance about dealing with side effects as well as coping with the emotional ups and downs you may experience and what to do about them. This section also provides practical information about financial and insurance matters and support for dealing with family issues that can arise as a result of your diagnosis.

5. Part Five, "Moving On," contains just two chapters, but they're very important. In chapter 24, "Living Well beyond Cancer," you'll find information that aims to help soften your reentry into life beyond breast cancer, which can be a bit more difficult than you might expect. If you or someone you know is living with metastatic breast cancer, chapter 23 will help you understand two essential types of supportive care that can make life easier for you and your family.

We've supplemented several chapters with "An Expert's View," input from experienced medical experts who specialize in breast cancer. You'll also find stories from women who have been where you are now. They generously share their experiences to encourage, inform, and inspire you as you make your way through your own breast cancer journey.

The breast cancer experience isn't always quick and it isn't always easy, but knowledge can be both empowering and comforting. Enduring the disruption, side effects, and unsettling nature of dealing with breast cancer can be difficult. Some days you'll feel up; some days you may feel down. Even when you feel that you're in control and doing well, setbacks can occur. When that happens, take a deep breath and tell yourself, "I will beat this. I will survive." And then believe it.

Breast Cancer Survivors Look Back

"Looking back, I know that my faith, my sense of humor, and the support from my family and friends got me through. I am thankful to have had breast cancer when I did, because it made me reevaluate my life."
—Nancy, 1 year after diagnosis

"Five years have passed, and I have never once looked back. I tell others that my surgery was the best thing I have ever done, and I truly mean that."
—Debbie, 5 years after diagnosis

"If I had to do it all over again, I would. Would it be difficult? Yes. You just push yourself. I think ultimately it makes you a stronger person, and it makes you realize that you can do things that you never thought you'd be able to do, and that you could make decisions that you never thought you would have to make. It pushes you to a new level of maturity, and without a doubt it just makes you a more compassionate person."
—Susan, 12 years after diagnosis

"I feel good about the decisions that were made regarding my treatment plan eight years ago, and I wouldn't do anything differently."
—Joyce, 14 years after diagnosis

PART ONE

Understanding Breast Cancer

CHAPTER 1

What Is Cancer?

Cancer is incredibly complex. It's many different diseases, and no single cure works for all of them. The good news is that researchers continue to learn more about cancer every day, resulting in more effective screening, prevention, and lifesaving treatments. The outlook for people who are diagnosed with cancer has never been more positive and continues to improve, and many live well beyond their cancer diagnosis.

Increasingly, cancer is a treatable and curable disease. Nevertheless, *cancer* is a word we fear, and it's one that has become an all too common part of our lives. No matter what is going on in your life, a diagnosis of cancer immediately changes everything, as you face confusing new terms, unanswered questions, and so many decisions that must be made. We don't know why some people develop cancer or why others don't. Nor can we predict when cancer will develop.

According to the National Cancer Institute, an estimated 38 percent of men and women living in the United States will develop cancer during their lifetimes. Yet, thankfully, the death rate from cancer in the US has declined 26 percent since its highest point in 1991 and continues to do so, primarily resulting from early detection, improved treatment, and fewer smokers. Researchers continue to make strides in cancer treatment and improved survival—the number of cancer survivors in the United States is expected to exceed 20 million by 2026. The majority of these survivors were treated years or decades earlier and remember cancer as part of their past medical history.

CANCER BASICS

Cancer isn't contagious—you can't catch it from someone else. It develops when genetic damage occurs that the body can't repair. Acquired abnormalities develop after we grow older, as the wear and tear of living takes its toll on our recuperative abilities and our genetic repair mechanisms don't work as effectively as they used to. Although a small number of cancers are inherited, most are caused by abnormal cellular changes that are acquired by random events or environmental exposures that damage DNA.

Carcinogens, substances that can damage healthy tissue, are cancer catalysts. We're exposed to them every day: chemicals in the workplace and home, viruses such as hepatitis or human papillomavirus (HPV), pollution, the sun's ultraviolet rays, and some medical treatments, including radiation, chemotherapy, and other medications that suppress the immune system. Numerous behavioral choices are also cancer culprits in varying degrees, including poor nutrition, alcohol, smoking, obesity, and physical inactivity. In fact, the American Cancer Society estimates that about 40 percent of cancers and half of all cancer deaths are preventable by modifying behavioral risk factors. (Chapter 3 describes risk factors for breast cancer.)

All cancers have one thing in common: they develop from abnormal cells that grow uncontrollably. How and why this happens can be explained by *genetics*, the science of genes and how they relate to different diseases. Few areas of science have changed the world of medicine—and expanded our knowledge of cancer, including breast cancer—more in the past 50 years than genetics. More than 100 different cancers have been identified; some are rare while others are common (figure 1.1).

There are several different categories of cancers:

- Adenocarcinomas—including breast, colon, prostate, gastric, and pancreatic cancer—begin in the glands that line the inside of organs.
- Squamous cell carcinomas begin in the cells that cover internal and external body surfaces.

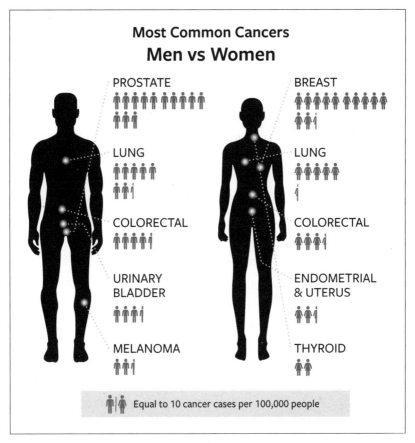

Figure 1.1. Common cancers in men and women

- Sarcomas develop in bone, fat, muscle, and other supporting tissues of the body.
- Leukemias develop in blood cells and grow in bone marrow.
- Lymphomas occur primarily in white blood cells and lymph nodes.

INSIDE A HEALTHY BODY

All living organisms, including plants, animals, and people, have fundamental microscopic cells that keep us operating. Cells are the smallest unit of all living things. Humans have trillions of microscopic cells, harmoniously growing, dividing, and joining to create tissue and organs. All cells have a similar basic structure, yet individually, they're programmed for specific tasks like breathing, converting food into energy, or sending messages to and from the brain. We have an almost unimaginable assortment of cells; most of them contain a complete set of genetic material sufficient to create an exact copy of ourselves.

With the exception of red blood cells, all other cells have a genetic control center called the *nucleus* (figure 1.2). Each nucleus stores 23 pairs of *chromosomes*, which are long strands of *deoxyribonucleic acid* (DNA) that carry all of the genetic information needed to build and maintain the human body. One set of each pair comes from your mother; the other set is from your father. (Egg and sperm cells are the exception; they have only one set of 23 chromosomes.) DNA acts like coded recipes that tell cells how to function. To use a computer analogy, cells operate as the body's hardware, while DNA is more like software, issuing instructions that tell cells what to do. *Genes*, bits of DNA code on chromosomes, issue blueprints for the thousands of proteins that support the body's elaborate operations: moving muscles, digesting food, and repairing damage in bones, muscles, cartilage, skin, and blood. Proteins are the chemical building blocks of life. Every cellular function depends on them.

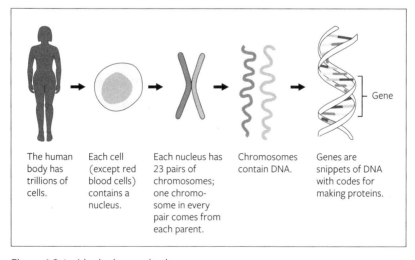

The human body has trillions of cells.

Each cell (except red blood cells) contains a nucleus.

Each nucleus has 23 pairs of chromosomes; one chromo-some in every pair comes from each parent.

Chromosomes contain DNA.

Genes are snippets of DNA with codes for making proteins.

Figure 1.2. Inside the human body

We all begin life as a single cell that grows and divides. One cell rapidly becomes two, two cells become four, and so on. This defined life cycle is normally carried out in a precise and orderly process: genes form, conduct their assigned functions, divide to create their own carbon-copy replacements—new cells are identical to the old—and then die. Genes instruct cells when to divide and when to stop. Once we reach adulthood, cells divide primarily to replace others that are worn out, damaged, or dying. Every day, our bodies shed billions of cells and create healthy new replacements. When you cut your skin, for example, your body produces only enough new cells to replace the missing tissue. Most often, this cellular division occurs perfectly every time. But mishaps during any of these divisions can create flawed cells. When that happens, some of these may survive and evolve into cancer cells.

It's in Your Genes

All humans share about 99.9 percent of our DNA. Yet, except for identical twins, no two people are exactly alike. The one-tenth of a percent of DNA that does vary determines characteristics like eye color and hair texture that pass from one generation to the next. Although you and your sister inherited most of the same genes, your own variation of those genes gives you brown eyes while hers are hazel. DNA contains all of the genetic instructions that make each living organism unique: that's why it can link suspects to crime scenes, prove someone's paternity, and screen for genetic defects that lead to disease.

CHAOS IN AN ORDERLY SYSTEM

Why do well-behaved, healthy cells turn into life-threatening renegades? Cancer occurs when abnormalities called *mutations* cause chemical or structural malfunctions in genes. Mutations can be acquired, developing during a patient's lifetime, or inherited, passed on from one generation to another. Most mutations are harmless. Some play an important evolutionary role, like changing an animal's appearance or behavior in ways that better adapt it to its surroundings. The end result of some mutations is disease. Sickle cell anemia, for instance, is an inherited disease that occurs when a gene mutation causes sticky, irregularly shaped red blood cells that become stuck in blood vessels and block the flow of oxygen to parts of the body. Down syndrome, cystic fibrosis, and Tay-Sachs disease are other examples of inherited diseases that are caused by genetic mutations.

Genes come in pairs; if one gene can't repair the damage, the other one can. Experts believe that cancer is more likely to develop when both copies of a gene become damaged and can't carry out their normal functions. Damaged cells often divide rapidly, creating damaged clones of themselves, and every subsequent division of these unhealthy cells perpetuates the errors that have already occurred. In some cases, one primary error or mutation to the DNA leads to cancer. In other cases, the normal cells in a part of the body accumulate multiple types of damage to their genes over time until they become *malignant* (cancerous). In cancer care, this transformation from healthy cell to cancer cell is referred to as the "multi-hit" hypothesis, meaning that many different types of cellular damage must occur before a cancer develops (figure 1.3).

By the time a cancerous tumor is diagnosed, it holds billions of "bad" cells that:

- grow when they don't need to
- disregard instructions to stop growing and die
- evade signals from other cells
- lose the "stickiness" that normal cells produce to stay together, allowing cancer cells to clump together and form tumors
- may be able to break away from the primary tumor and spread to other areas of the body

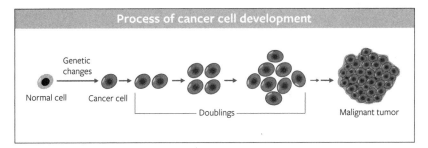

Figure 1.3. Cancer develops only after a series of cellular changes occur

Mutations That Increase the Likelihood of Cancer

Cancers are more likely when irreversible mutations occur in certain types of genes.

Acquired mutations

- Oncogenes regulate normal cellular growth and division. When damaged, oncogenes instruct cells to make proteins that stimulate abnormal cell growth. Mutations that develop in the HER2 gene, for instance, cause uncontrolled growth in breast cells.
- A DNA change can cause genes that are involved in normal cell growth to become *oncogenes*. Unlike normal genes, oncogenes cannot be turned off, so they cause uncontrolled cell growth.

Acquired or inherited mutations

- Tumor suppressor genes stop or slow the cycle of cellular growth and division and repair damaged DNA. Abnormalities in these genes disable this braking mechanism, allowing cells to divide and grow uncontrollably. Mutations in the BRCA1 or BRCA2 genes, which are tumor suppressor genes, greatly increase the risk of breast and ovarian cancer.
- DNA repair genes (also known as mismatch repair genes) impede cancer by fixing errors that occur when cells duplicate, so that newly replicated genes function normally. Mutations in these genes disable that repair function. If DNA damage overwhelms the repair capability, the accumulation of cellular errors can eventually result in cancer.

What Happens after a Tumor Develops?

Once a tumor develops, unchecked cancer cells create havoc. They grow into the surrounding tissue, enter the blood or lymphatic system, and then *metastasis* occurs, meaning that they spread into healthy tissue in other parts of the body. (*Benign* or noncancerous tumors don't spread to other tissues.) If not treated successfully, metastasis overpopulates the body with cancer cells that compete with healthy cells for space and nutrients. Cancer kills by invading and destroying healthy cells in the lungs, brain, liver, or other organs until they can no longer function.

Cancer develops in three stages:

1. *Initiation:* Damage occurs to a cell's DNA, which allows the cell to reproduce abnormal, damaged copies of itself.
2. *Promotion:* New cancer cells adapt to become larger and stronger with their own circulatory system that provides them with oxygen and nutrients.
3. *Progression:* Metastasis occurs as cancer cells spread beyond their point of origin to invade other parts of the body.

Cancer cells can be surprisingly adaptable (table 1.1). They adapt and acquire new characteristics to take advantage of other cells and to survive and spread. Cancer cells recruit healthy cells to create blood vessels that provide tumors with oxygen and nutrients. Tumors create a more hospitable environment for themselves, paving the way for metastasis. Malignant cells can also evade the immune system, the army of cells that protect the body from infection and illness. Malignant cells sometimes seem to disappear after treatment, only to reappear later.

Table 1.1. Cellular Bad Behavior

Normal Cells	Cancer Cells
Are of uniform shape and size	Have irregular shapes and sizes
Adhere to DNA rules that govern normal cell behavior	Ignore DNA rules
Grow in an orderly fashion	Grow faster and uncontrollably
Exist harmoniously with other cells	Attack healthy cells; compete for space and nutrients
Are destroyed by the immune system when damaged	Can evade the immune system
Have specific functions	Have no specific functions
Self-destruct after they mature and serve their purpose	Never "grow up"; ignore cellular signals to die

FINDING ANSWERS WITH RESEARCH

Cancer has been acknowledged for thousands of years, but only in the modern era has treatment progressed beyond surgical removal of diseased tissue. It was only a few years ago that scientists knew little about how genes influence the development and growth of cancer. Now, because of research, we know far more about the nature of many cancers and how to target a cancer's unique weaknesses to stop it from growing and spreading.

Many treatment approaches are being studied in the laboratory and in clinical trials. Some are investigating methods of editing genes, while others are exploring how to inactivate proteins that may cause or promote the growth of cancer or to prevent cancer cells from being able to spread. Researchers continue to search for a deeper understanding of cancer behavior, so that preventive measures and effective treatments can be developed.

State-of-the-art treatment for many cancers now includes *targeted drugs or therapies* that attack cancer cells without affecting healthy cells, and *immunotherapy*, which stimulates a patient's own immune system to destroy cancer cells. Other approaches destroy cancer cells by inhibiting their ability to create new blood supply. These and other new tools in the fight against cancer are helping more patients to survive the cancer experience.

A GLIMPSE INTO THE FUTURE

When cars malfunction, we fix them. When hips wear out, we replace them. Can we do the same with rogue genes? That's the focus of *gene editing*, a way of manipulating genes to change an organism's DNA and influence cellular behavior. Scientists are already editing genes in cells and animal models in the lab environment. CRISPR is a group of gene-editing technologies that could eventually enable scientists to fix or remove disease-causing genes or insert new genes that could cure cancers. If the technology is found to be reliable and safe, it could be beneficial in numerous ways. Foods could be engineered to be more nutritious, more resistant to disease, or better tasting. Editing genes of mosquitos and other insects might eradicate the danger of malaria, dengue fever, and other insect-borne diseases. One exciting but controversial use for gene editing might be to repair a person's faulty genes or to override a gene's cancer-causing ways. At some point in the future, mutated genes that cause cancer and other diseases might be repaired or swapped for healthy replacements. Ultimately, gene editing may provide a way to prevent and treat cancers, heart disease, and eradicate viruses like human immunodeficiency virus (HIV) or herpes and other serious or life-threatening conditions.

CHAPTER 2

Breast Cancer Basics

One thing that every woman with newly diagnosed breast cancer should hear is, "You didn't cause this, and you couldn't have prevented it." Breast cancer doesn't occur because you've done anything wrong or because you didn't do something right. To the best of our knowledge, it is not caused by working too hard, using a cell phone, coloring your hair, or not getting enough sleep.

For many women, the emotional attachment to their breasts is significant. Breasts enhance the feminine form, provide sensual pleasure, and help women forge close maternal bonds as they nourish their infants. Other women, however, do not feel as emotionally attached to their breasts. Designed to make and deliver milk, breasts comprise milk glands, milk ducts, fatty tissue, and the supporting tissues that provide shape. Microscopic *lobules* in the breast produce and deliver milk to a fan of multiple *ducts* that spread throughout the breast and carry milk to the nipple (figure 2.1). The remainder of the breast is primarily fatty tissue. Breasts contain no muscle—that's why no amount of exercise makes them bigger. They're a unique part of the human anatomy, although like other parts of the body, they can be ground zero for cancer development. But what exactly is breast cancer?

WHAT IS BREAST CANCER?

Breast cancer is the second most common cancer (after skin cancer) and the second most frequent cause of death (after lung cancer)

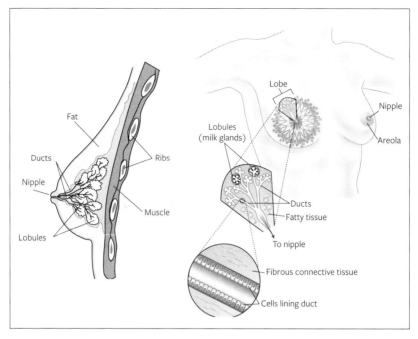

Figure 2.1. Inside the breast

among women in the United States—approximately 40,000 women die each year from breast cancer. The rate of new diagnoses increased during the 1980s as more women began to have routine mammograms. Then new cases began to drop in the early 2000s as women stopped using hormone replacement therapy for menopausal side effects when it was found to increase the risk of breast cancer. Incidence has again been trending upward since 2012, mainly because of our aging population and increasing rates of obesity. Approximately 245,000 women in the United States are diagnosed with breast cancer every year (figure 2.2). Fortunately, fewer women are dying from breast cancer: death rates declined 40 percent from 1989 to 2016, mainly as a result of improved methods of early detection and more effective treatments.

Cancer in the breast develops over time—usually in the ducts or the lobules—as multiple genetic, hereditary, or environmental events transform healthy cells into malignant cells. The insides of ducts

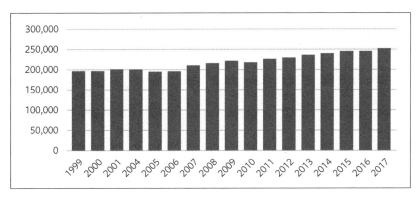

Figure 2.2. Annual number of new breast cancers in the United States. Data from "United States Cancer Statistics: Data Visualizations," Centers for Disease Control and Prevention and National Cancer Institute, released in June 2020, https://gis.cdc .gov/Cancer/USCS/DataViz.html

and lobules are lined with cells that grow and divide in a controlled manner; every day, millions of these cells are shed and replaced by new, healthy cells. All cells have controls that issue instructions for when to divide and when to stop. If these controls don't work well, the normal process of cellular replication gets carried away, as described in chapter 1. When this happens, the breast ducts or lobules can fill up with too many abnormal cells, which is the defining characteristic of cancer, and a tumor then forms. It may grow in place, often destroying the tissue around it, or cancer cells may break away from the tumor and metastasize to other parts of the body.

Signs and Symptoms

Breast cancer often develops without signs or symptoms. Some changes, however, can be early indications of the disease. Symptoms may appear as cancer progresses: a lump or thickening in the breast, a change in breast size or shape, tenderness, or a nipple that turns inward or discharges fluid. The most common symptom of breast cancer is a new lump or mass that is usually firm and may or may not be painful or tender. Mammograms and other screening procedures often identify breast cancer before symptoms appear; these screening methods provide more information about a lump than what is found on a physical examination, because even an exam by the most experienced physician can't determine with certainty whether a lump is cancerous. Having a baseline understanding of the way your breasts look and feel will help you to identify any changes that develop, which should then be examined by a physician as soon as possible.

Most women know that a breast lump is the most common symptom of breast cancer. So, finding a lump in your breast can be frightening, even though 80 percent of lumps aren't cancerous. Aside from lumps, breast cancer may show other symptoms. Having one or more of the following symptoms doesn't necessarily signal breast cancer, because these same changes can develop from other noncancerous conditions. It's important to recognize these signs, however, and to follow up to identify any abnormalities as early as possible (figure 2.3).

- Swelling of part or all of the breast.
- A change in the size of one breast compared to the other.
- A bump or growing vein on the breast skin.
- Breast or nipple pain that doesn't go away.
- A bloody or clear nipple discharge.
- A nipple or breast skin that becomes red, crusty, or thickened.
- Skin irritation or dimpling of the skin, like the texture of an orange peel.
- A nipple that turns inward (if this is a new development).
- Enlarged lymph nodes in the armpit or above the collarbone.

NOT EVERY CHANGE IS CANCER

Benign Breast Conditions

Numerous benign changes can develop in the breast, causing unusual thickening, masses, or texture (figure 2.4). Any lumps or other changes in the breast should be evaluated by your doctor to determine

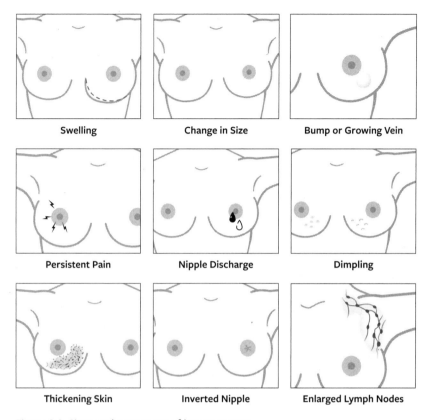

Figure 2.3. Signs and symptoms of breast cancer

whether the area needs careful monitoring or warrants further tests. Some changes can mimic breast cancer and may require a biopsy to determine their true nature. (Most biopsies don't find cancer.) Some benign changes also increase the risk of developing breast cancer.

Calcifications. Mineral deposits called *calcifications* in the breast often show up in mammograms. These may be caused by breast cysts or other benign breast conditions (they don't develop from high levels of dietary calcium). *Macrocalcifications* are large white dots that are almost always benign and don't need further follow-up. *Microcalcifications*, smaller specks that look like grains of salt, are most often noncancerous; however, their size, shape, and pattern can indicate tumor growth or a *precancerous* change in breast tissue.

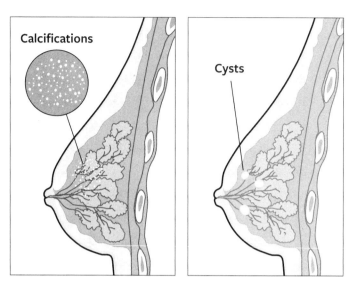

Figure 2.4. Two of the benign conditions often found in breasts

Mastitis. Women who breastfeed can develop *mastitis*, a blockage in a milk duct. The infected breast may become red or tender and feel lumpy or warm to the touch. If antibiotics don't clear the infection, the duct may need to be drained. Limited data suggest that women who have a long history of mastitis may have slightly increased risk for breast cancer.

Sclerosing adenosis. Adenosis is an excess of enlarged lobules. It's often identified by a biopsy in women who have breast cysts or fibrosis. A sclerosing adenosis occurs when the enlarged lobules become distorted by scar-like tissue and may form a lump or cause pain. Sclerosing adenosis may slightly raise breast cancer risk.

Papillomas. A papilloma is a small, benign, wartlike growth that develops in one or more of the ducts, often close to the nipple. These growths may cause nipple pain or discharge; if necessary, they can be surgically removed. A single papilloma is associated with a risk of invasive breast cancer when it contains areas of atypical ductal hyperplasia or when it's located close to ductal carcinoma in situ (a type of precancer that develops in the milk ducts). Having multiple papillomas may also increase breast cancer risk.

Radial scars. Also called complex sclerosing lesions, radial scars are not true scars, but under a microscope, these growths resemble scars. They're typically identified from a breast biopsy that is performed for some other purpose. In most cases, they don't cause symptoms. If they grow large enough, radial scars can distort breast tissue and may look like cancer on a mammogram or biopsy. Some physicians recommend careful monitoring; others recommend surgical removal. Radial scars slightly increase the risk of breast cancer.

Gynecomastia. Men or boys who have elevated estrogen levels can develop gynecomastia, or enlarged breasts that may be tender. This condition often occurs at birth or during puberty, and it can also develop from being obese or taking certain medications. Although breast reduction surgery can be performed, it isn't often recommended unless the individual is experiencing severe pain or extreme embarrassment. Gynecomastia slightly increases a man's risk for breast cancer.

Conditions That Do Not Increase Breast Cancer Risk

Fibrocystic changes. Half of all women experience *fibrocystic breast changes* during their lives. This umbrella term encompasses numerous noncancerous breast changes that are particularly common in premenopausal women. Fibrocystic symptoms include swelling, a ropelike texture in the breast, benign lumps, and pain or tenderness, especially before a menstrual period.

Fibroadenomas. *Fibroadenomas* are solid, rounded tumors that are made up of normal breast cells and move easily beneath the skin when touched. Although they aren't cancerous, fibroadenomas can grow and may need to be removed if they become painful or too large. These are the most common type of breast mass, especially in young women ages 15 to 35.

Cysts. Breast cysts are usually benign, fluid-filled sacs within the tissue. Most cysts are round or oval lumps that move easily and feel firm or soft. They may be very small or as large as an egg. Cysts can be painful, especially just prior to a menstrual cycle. Large and painful cysts can be drained; otherwise, no treatment is needed. Women of all ages develop breast cysts, most often between ages 35 and 50. Postmenopausal women who take hormone replacement therapy may also be more susceptible to developing breast cysts.

Phyllodes tumors. Phyllodes tumors develop outside the ducts and lobules in the ligaments and fatty tissue of the breast. Most, but not all, of these rare breast tumors are benign. They generally don't venture beyond the breast and are typically removed with a short surgical procedure.

Fat necrosis. When the breast suffers an injury or blunt trauma, portions of the damaged cells can die and form a round, hard ball. This *necrosis* (tissue death) can occur as a result of a fall, when something bumps into your breast, or after breast surgery or radiation. If you're obese, you're more susceptible to developing necrosis in your breast. Necrosis is benign, but it can look like cancer on a mammogram, and a biopsy may be required to determine its true nature.

Duct ectasia. When breast ducts thicken and become blocked with fluid, duct ectasia causes reddened, tender, or inverted nipples that may have a greenish discharge. A lump may be felt beneath the nipple if the blocked duct becomes infected. Antibiotics, pain medication, or application of moist heat can relieve symptoms, and often no further treatment is required.

Trauma. Being hit in the chest or falling may bruise the breast and cause painful swelling, but it doesn't cause breast cancer or increase the risk of developing breast cancer.

Conditions That Increase Breast Cancer Risk

Hyperplasia. If the normal process of cellular replication gets carried away, *hyperplasia*—an excessive number of normal-looking cells—can form in the ducts or the lobules. In *usual hyperplasia* (the most common form of hyperplasia), the dividing cells look normal under a microscope. They're benign and don't affect cancer risk, but if they continue to divide and become more abnormal, these cells can transform into breast cancer. *Atypical hyperplasia*, which can occur in the milk ducts or in the lobules, is less common. It's characterized by dividing cells that have an abnormal shape or unusual internal features (figure 2.5). Although hyperplasia isn't cancerous, it can signal development of early-stage breast cancer. Women with this condition have about four times the breast cancer risk in either breast than women who don't have the condition. The risk is greater for someone who has hyperplasia and a strong family history of breast cancer.

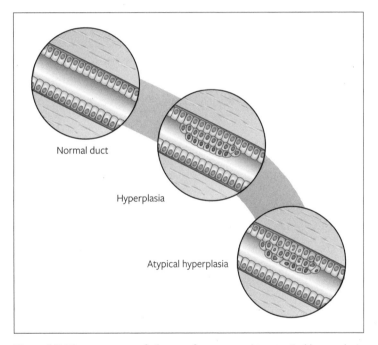

Normal duct

Hyperplasia

Atypical hyperplasia

Figure 2.5. The spectrum of changes from normal to atypical hyperplasia

Atypical hyperplasia and lobular carcinoma in situ. Two other abnormalities in the breast, atypical hyperplasia and *lobular carcinoma in situ* (LCIS), are benign, but both are red flags for developing breast cancer. These conditions are types of *lobular neoplasia*, an overarching term that describes the formation of irregular cells in the lobules. In both cases, the normal process of cellular replication gets carried away, and the lobules fill up with too many abnormally shaped cells. Neither condition has symptoms, and neither usually shows up on a mammogram. Both conditions are most often discovered by chance, often during a breast biopsy that is performed for another reason.

Because atypical hyperplasia isn't a true cancer, treatment isn't normally necessary, although some doctors recommend having the affected and nearby tissues removed. A second opinion can be helpful to confirm the diagnosis and to ensure that the atypical cells aren't an early type of breast cancer. If you develop atypical hyperplasia while you're taking replacement hormones for the symptoms of menopause, your doctor may recommend that you stop the medication, because it can stimulate some breast cancers.

Lobular carcinoma in situ is a greater expansion of abnormal cells in the lobules (figure 2.6). In the 1980s, it was considered to be a noninvasive cancer that was treated with lumpectomy and radiation

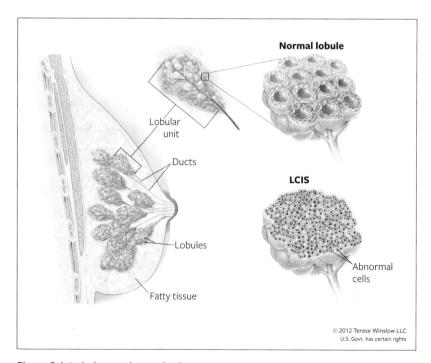

Figure 2.6. Lobular carcinoma in situ

or mastectomy. We've learned, however, that LCIS isn't malignant. It remains within the lobules and doesn't form a tumor or spread to surrounding tissue as breast cancer often does, although it may be associated with neighboring invasive cancer that may be treated with surgery and/or radiation. LCIS is more concerning than atypical hyperplasia because it increases the likelihood of developing invasive breast cancer in the ducts or lobules of both breasts.

Preventive medication (tamoxifen or raloxifene) is often recommended for women with LCIS or atypical hyperplasia to lower the risk of both noninvasive and invasive breast cancers. Both the affected breast and the healthy breast should then be monitored closely, so that any cancer that develops can be treated as soon as possible. Recommended surveillance includes monthly self-exams of your breast, a clinical breast exam every 6 to 12 months, and an annual mammogram beginning at age 30. For some women, an annual breast MRI (*magnetic resonance imaging*) may also be advised. Some doctors recommend removing the area of LCIS. If you're diagnosed with atypical hyperplasia, LCIS, and/or you have a strong family history of breast cancer or an inherited mutation in a BRCA gene, your doctor may advise that you take tamoxifen, raloxifene, or an aromatase inhibitor (described in chapter 13), or less commonly to remove both breasts to decrease your high risk of a future invasive breast cancer.

TYPES OF BREAST CANCER

Breast cancer is many diseases (figure 2.7). *Noninvasive breast cancers* are said to be in situ (in place); the cancer cells are contained within the ducts or lobules and haven't spread beyond their point of origin into the fatty tissue of the breast. *Invasive breast cancers* are more worrisome, because they have penetrated the walls of ducts or lobules and infiltrated nearby tissues. If these cancers enter the lymphatic channels or blood vessels, they can then metastasize to other parts of the body. Treatment is then more involved, and remission or cure is less likely. Most breasts cancers are invasive. For the majority of women who are diagnosed, breast cancer is a treatable and curable disease when it's confined to the breast or surrounding lymph nodes, and millions of survivors in the United States now live well beyond their breast cancer diagnosis.

Noninvasive Breast Cancers

Cancer cells that are confined within the ducts are referred to as *ductal carcinoma in situ* (DCIS). About one in five breast cancers is DCIS, the earliest stage of breast cancer that is often considered to be a type of precancer. DCIS doesn't normally show any signs or symptoms, although some women may develop a breast lump or a bloody discharge from the nipple. Too small to be felt, about 80 percent of DCIS is found by mammography; it's sometimes also identified by MRI. DCIS is discussed extensively in chapter 12.

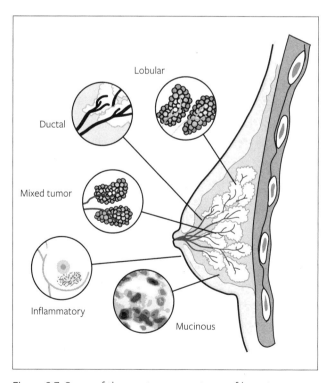

Figure 2.7. Some of the most common types of breast cancer

Invasive Breast Cancers

Invasive ductal carcinoma. About 80 percent of breast cancers are *invasive (infiltrating) ductal carcinomas* that have broken through the wall of the milk duct and entered the breast tissue (figure 2.8). Although invasive ductal carcinoma can affect women at any age, it's more common after age 55. Invasive ductal carcinoma also occurs in men.

Invasive lobular carcinoma. A small number of breast cancers begin when abnormal cells accumulate in the lobules. Instead of forming a lump like other breast cancers, *invasive (infiltrating) lobular carcinoma* (ILC) spreads through the breast tissue, making it more difficult to detect. Symptoms may include a swelling or thickness in an area of the breast, a change in texture or appearance, or a nipple that becomes inverted. While invasive lobular breast cancer exhibits different characteristics than invasive ductal cancer, it poses a similar risk for developing a new breast cancer and cancer that returns in the breast and elsewhere after treatment. ILC is more often diagnosed in women who are 60 or older.

Inflammatory breast cancer. *Inflammatory breast cancer* (IBC) occurs when cancer cells clog the lymphatic channels in the breast skin, preventing the normal flow of *lymph fluid* through the tissue. This is a fast-growing, aggressive disease, and symptoms may worsen in a single day. IBC has often spread to the lymph nodes and beyond by the time it's found, so recognizing the telltale signs and seeking prompt treatment is critical. Few women develop IBC, which behaves differently than other types of breast cancers. Instead of a lump, a large portion of the breast may itch, swell, feel warm, or turn dark; the breast skin may appear pitted (a condition called *peau d'orange*). IBC tends to occur at an earlier age than most other breast cancers; on average, at age 56 for white women and age 52 for African American women, who are more likely to develop IBC.

Paget's disease. A rare form of breast cancer called *Paget's disease* develops in the nipple ducts and then spreads to the nipple and the *areola* (the pigmented skin around the nipple). A red, scaly, crusty, or

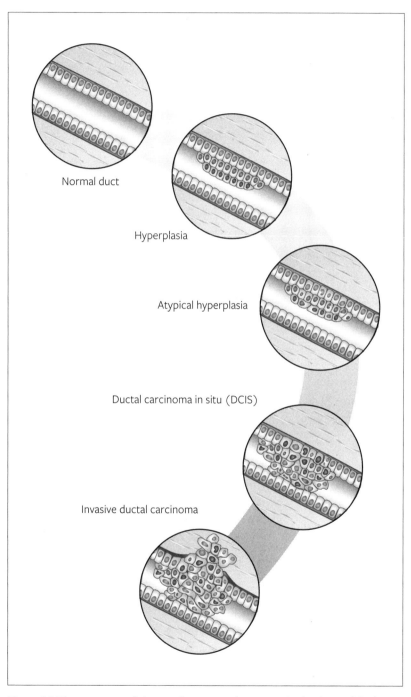

Normal duct

Hyperplasia

Atypical hyperplasia

Ductal carcinoma in situ (DCIS)

Invasive ductal carcinoma

Figure 2.8. The spectrum of changes from normal to cancer in the ducts of the breast

itchy nipple or areola can be a sign of this breast cancer—these same symptoms are sometimes misdiagnosed as eczema or dermatitis. Because most women with Paget's disease also have DCIS or invasive breast cancer, early diagnosis is very important.

Male breast cancer. Men have breast tissue and can also develop breast cancer, although their risk—just 1 in 1,000—is considerably lower than women's. The risk increases significantly for men who are obese or have gynecomastia, Klinefelter syndrome (a rare genetic disorder), or an inherited gene mutation that predisposes them to breast cancer.

Other types of invasive breast cancer. Three other less common types of breast cancer account for about 10 percent of all invasive breast cancers. Less than 2 percent of breast cancers are *mucinous carcinomas* that begin in the milk ducts and spread to surrounding tissue. Mucinous tumor cells are slow growing and contain unusually large quantities of mucous, or mucin. *Tubular carcinoma*, characterized by tubular-shaped cells and an area of the breast that may feel spongy, also accounts for less than 2 percent of breast cancers. Up to 5 percent of breast cancers are *medullary carcinomas*, which form in the ducts of the breast. Though these cancers divide aggressively, they often respond to treatment more successfully than other types of ductal breast cancers. Most medullary carcinomas occur in individuals who have a mutation in the BRCA1 (pronounced *brah-ca-one*) gene.

Ten Common Breast Cancer Myths

1. **Most women with breast cancer don't survive.**
   The majority of women who are diagnosed with breast cancer do
   survive. About 16 percent of women and 2 percent of men who are
   diagnosed die of breast cancer each year.

2. **Only women get breast cancer.**
   Although most breast cancers occur in women, men have breast
   tissue and can also develop malignant breast tumors.

3. **Breast cancer is an older woman's disease.**
   Women of any age can develop breast cancer, although 95 percent
   of diagnoses occur in women over age 40; half of all breast cancers
   are diagnosed after age 62.

4. **If you don't have a lump, you don't have breast cancer.**
   While a lump can indicate the presence of a tumor, most lumps
   cannot be felt, especially during early-stage cancer.

5. **Most breast lumps are cancerous.**
   Lumpy breast tissue is not uncommon, and most lumps are not
   cancerous.

6. **Most breast cancer is hereditary.**
   Most breast cancers are caused by genetic mutations acquired
   during one's lifetime; just 5 to 10 percent are inherited.

7. **Having an inherited mutation guarantees a diagnosis.**
   No one's risk for breast cancer is 100 percent. Even an inherited
   mutation, which greatly increases risk, doesn't ensure that breast
   cancer will develop.

8. **You can't develop breast cancer if none of your relatives has
   been diagnosed.**
   Most women diagnosed don't have a history of breast cancer in their
   family.

9. **Breast cancer doesn't occur during pregnancy.**
   Breast cancer is the most common cancer in pregnant women,
   primarily due to increased levels of estrogen.

10. **Most women know their risk for breast cancer.**
    Studies show that most women underestimate or overestimate their
    risk, sometimes greatly so.

CHAPTER 3

Demystifying Breast Cancer Risk

Although risk assessment isn't an exact science, it is becoming more precise as researchers continue to expand their knowledge of how cancers behave. The goal is to identify women who have a high risk of developing breast cancer and then to provide them with a personalized screening plan.

All men and women are at risk for breast cancer, but not everyone will be diagnosed. Some have a higher risk for breast cancer than others. What exactly does that mean? Risk is the probability of something occurring at a certain time. Climb a ladder, and you risk falling off. Drive in traffic, and you may be rear-ended.

Although risk describes the chance of something happening, it's not a guarantee that it will. The risk of being struck by lightning—about 1 in 1.2 million—for example, is an estimate based on how many people are struck in a given year compared to the entire population. Breast cancer risk is estimated in the same way. That one-in-eight breast cancer statistic we've all heard isn't quite as scary when it's put in its proper context. It's a statistical average calculated by the National Cancer Institute, based on the total number of breast cancer cases among all women in the United States. Currently, about 12.5 percent of women develop breast cancer at some point in their lives; divide that by 100 percent, and you get one in eight. (That same statistic also means that seven of eight women won't be diagnosed.) It's a broad statistic that applies only to the entire population of women.

It doesn't mean that between you and seven of your neighbors, one of you will definitely get breast cancer. One or more of you might, but you also might not. Until we know all the causes of cancer, we can't predict an individual's exact risk. In the meantime, scientists use population-based figures to describe the frequency of a disease, determine screening guidelines, and identify cancer trends.

ABSOLUTE AND RELATIVE RISK

Cancer risk is expressed in terms of absolute or relative risk. Knowing the difference between these two distinctly different views can help you put media reports of cancer studies in perspective and appreciate how your health care team refers to risk.

Absolute risk is the probability of developing cancer over a certain period: over the next 5, 10, or 20 years, for instance. It represents how often a disease occurs in a similar group of people over a certain

Doing the Math

Breast cancer risk estimates aren't always what they seem. When you hear that something inflates cancer risk by 10 percent, you need to know "higher than what?" as a baseline and over what period of time. Consider a woman who has a 10 percent risk of breast cancer over the next 10 years:

- Something that increases her risk by 20 percent leaves her with a 10-year risk of 12 percent (10 percent + 2 percent).
- A twofold increase leaves her with a risk of 20 percent (10 percent × 2).
- Having a single risk factor that decreases breast cancer by 10 percent and another factor that decreases it by 15 percent doesn't mean that her overall risk is 25 percent lower, because the interaction of all her risk factors is complex.
- Having a risk factor with a relative risk of 1.5 raises her risk to 15 percent compared to someone without that same risk factor. (A relative ratio of 1.0 means there's no difference between women who do or do not have the same risk factor. A ratio of 1.5 means that a woman with the risk factor has a 50 percent higher risk of breast cancer than someone without the factor.)

Table 3.1. Your Absolute Risk of Breast Cancer Increases as You Age

Current Age (years)	Absolute Risk of Breast Cancer in the Next 10 Years	Percentage Absolute Risk
20	1 in 1,429	0.07
30	1 in 217	0.5
40	1 in 67	1.5
50	1 in 43	2.3
60	1 in 29	3.5
70	1 in 25	4.0
80	1 in 34	2.9
Lifetime risk	1 in 8	12.5 (cumulative)

Source: N. Howlader, A. M. Noone, M. Krapcho et al., eds., "SEER Cancer Statistics Review (CSR), 1975–2017," National Cancer Institute Surveillance, Epidemiology, and End Results Program, April 15, 2020, https://seer.cancer.gov/csr/1975_2017/. Based on November 2019 SEER data submission posted to the SEER website.

period of time. The one-in-eight (12 percent) breast cancer statistic expresses an average woman's risk at some point in her life if she lives to age 85 (table 3.1). Your own risk isn't the same, because you're not average. Your risk of developing breast cancer is a moving target that changes throughout your lifetime, depending on your medical history, family history, lifestyle, and other personal *risk factors* that increase or decrease your odds of developing cancer compared to the "average" woman reflected in the one-in-eight statistic (table 3.1). It's a number that has limited value if you're considering ways to manage your current risk.

Relative risk compares how something reduces your risk compared to people who don't do the same thing: if you smoke, you're 15 to 30 times more likely to have lung cancer than nonsmokers. Expressed as a percentage (the number of people with the risk factor divided by the number of people without the risk factor), relative risk is based on observational studies. Reports that "eating berries every day reduces breast cancer by 30 percent" means that women who self-reported that they ate a daily serving of berries developed breast cancer 30 percent less frequently than women who didn't. Comparative risks like this example can be misleading, however, because they don't account for a person's age, weight, other behaviors, and all the other factors that influence risk or other factors that may have affected risk in the study participants. Nor does it mean that your risk of breast cancer will necessarily drop by 30 percent if you eat berries every day. Absolute risk more usefully conveys the true impact of something that influences risk.

The Problem with Headlines

Research on breast cancer is important, and becoming aware of new findings can add to your knowledge base. Unless you're a medical professional, you probably learn about research results through news and media reports. These stories often describe study data or share anecdotal information about breast cancer risk. But headlines and story content often exaggerate study findings or misrepresent the facts of a study. Some media stories neglect to mention that certain study results may be preliminary, uncorroborated, or based on limited or questionable research.

Frequently, research conclusions that seem promising but don't prove cause and effect are widely reported by the media. The problem occurs when journalists don't read or misunderstand the published paper, and too often, scientists don't have an opportunity to review these reports for accuracy before they're published. Social media then helps to spread this misinformation, causing additional confusion and perhaps negatively influencing patients' medical decisions. Headlines are often dramatic, and it can be easy to take them to heart. The best way to sort fact from fiction is to discuss research with your physician, the American Cancer Society, or some other reliable source that can set the record straight. You can also go directly to the source by searching www.pubmed.gov to find the published study.

RISK FACTORS

Breast cancer is one of the most studied diseases in the world, yet experts can't yet accurately predict which women will or will not develop breast cancer or when it might occur. Countless studies have tried to identify links between certain characteristics or behaviors and breast cancer. Despite urban myths and Internet rumors, breast cancer isn't caused by caffeine, hair dye, deodorants, cell phones, underwire bras, or exposure to power lines. Nor do breast reduction surgery or breast implants influence breast cancer risk. We know that women who have a strong family history of breast cancer or an inherited genetic predisposition are more likely to develop the disease, yet not all women in this high-risk group will have a diagnosis.

Breast cancer risk is personal. Your risk is not the same as your friend's, your neighbor's, or even other family members. That's because certain risk factors decrease or heighten your susceptibility for breast cancer, and collectively, your risk factors are different than someone else's. Risk factors don't cause breast cancer, but they do influence your risk. That's one reason why pinpointing someone's exact risk is so complex. Having several risk factors doesn't guarantee that you'll develop breast cancer, although it does mean that you're more likely to do so. Some risk factors, like getting older, raise the risk of many diseases, including breast cancer. Smoking, for example, increases the chance of developing lung cancer. Other risk factors help to reduce risk. Stop smoking, and you decrease the risk for lung cancer. In many cases, women who develop breast cancer have no known risk factors.

Risk Factors beyond Your Control

Gender. Although men develop breast cancer, it occurs about 100 times more often in women, who produce more estrogen and have more breast cells that are influenced by estrogen. About 2,000 men are diagnosed annually in the United States, compared to about 268,600 women.

Age. Your risk for breast cancer grows as you age. Although younger women can develop breast cancer, it most often occurs after age 50.

Race. White women develop breast cancer slightly more often than African American, Asian, and Hispanic women. But African American women are more often diagnosed before age 40, have more aggressive tumors, and are more likely to die of the disease.

Genetic factors. Up to 10 percent of all breast cancers are hereditary. People who inherit a mutation in a BRCA1, BRCA2, or other predisposing gene have a very high risk of breast and ovarian cancer. Family history can also influence risk: about one in four women with breast cancer have a family member who has also been diagnosed. The risk is greater depending on the number of relatives with breast or ovarian cancer and their ages at the time of diagnosis. Your risk is also higher if your family tree includes a first-degree male relative with prostate cancer (table 3.2).

A previous diagnosis of breast cancer or certain benign breast diseases. Having breast cancer in one breast raises your risk for a new cancer in the opposite breast by three to four times. This risk is greater if you're diagnosed before age 40 or you have a family history of breast cancer. The presence of atypical ductal hyperplasia or lobular neoplasia also raises breast cancer risk.

Previous radiation therapy. Having radiation therapy to the chest or breast, particularly before age 30, significantly heightens the risk of breast cancer, beginning 10 years after treatment. This applies to women who have had multiple chest x-rays as follow-up for tuberculosis or scoliosis. Women who were treated with radiation therapy for Hodgkin disease have a higher risk that begins about eight years after receiving radiation; their cumulative lifetime risk exceeds 30 percent. The risk is even greater if you have an inherited BRCA mutation and you were also exposed to radiation before age 20. Having one breast radiated to treat cancer doesn't increase the likelihood of cancer in the opposite breast.

Dense breast tissue. *Dense breasts* have more glandular tissue than fat, making them difficult to screen for cancer. Breast density can be inherited or develop from certain medications, including hormone replacement therapy. Women with dense breasts are five to six times

Table 3.2. Your Family History Affects Your Breast Cancer Risk

Family Member Diagnosed	Cancer Type	Your Relative Risk of Breast Cancer*
Maternal: first degree (mother, sister, daughter)	Breast or ovarian	Doubled
More than one first-degree relative diagnosed		2–4 times greater
Paternal: first degree (father, brother, son)	Prostate	14% greater
	Breast and prostate	66% greater
Second degree (grandmother, aunt, cousin)	Breast or ovarian	1.5 times greater

*Compared to women without the same family history.

more likely to develop breast cancer compared to women who don't have dense breasts.

Menstrual history. Estrogen levels are highest during menstruation. The more years you menstruate, the longer your breast tissue is exposed to the effects of estrogen. Beginning menstrual periods before age 12 and starting menopause after age 55 expose women to estrogen for a longer period during their lifetimes, increasing the likelihood of breast cancer. A lower relative risk is seen in women who:

- begin menstruating at age 15 or later
- begin menopause before age 45
- give birth to and breastfeed their first child before age 20

Diethylstilbestrol (DES). Women who took this synthetic estrogen between 1940 and 1971 to prevent miscarriage have a somewhat higher risk for breast cancer, as do their daughters.

Risk Factors within Your Control

Just about everything we do has the potential to increase our risk for harm, whether it's crossing a street, rock climbing, or just driving your car. Only you can decide how much and what kinds of risk you're happy to live with. That pertains to life generally and to breast cancer risk specifically. Although you can't change every risk factor that affects your odds of developing breast cancer, controlling others is a matter of choice.

Controlling your weight. If you're overweight or obese, especially after menopause, your risk for breast cancer is greater than the risk for women who are thinner. If you develop breast cancer, your risk of having a recurrence after treatment is also elevated if you're overweight.

Hormonal contraception. Using hormones to prevent pregnancy—pills, injections, a patch, a ring, or an intrauterine device (IUD)—may raise your risk of breast cancer. Most research on the relationship between birth control and breast cancer has involved oral contraceptives (OCPs), combinations of synthetic estrogen and progesterone that can fuel the growth of some breast cancers. A 2010 finding from the continuing Nurses' Health Study reported that OCPs slightly increase breast cancer risk. An analysis of more than 50 studies concurred, showing that breast cancer risk is somewhat higher in women who use OCPs and in women who have a strong family history of breast cancer. That risk decreases when OCPs are discontinued. Most of this research involved OCPs from the 1980s or earlier that contained higher doses of hormones than contraceptives in use today.

Danish researchers revisited the issue in 2017 with an observational study that followed 1.8 million women between ages 15 and 49 for an average of 10.9 years. Surprisingly, they concluded that women who were using newer, lose-dose formulations had a higher risk for breast cancer than women who had never taken them. The level of risk varied from 0 to 60 percent, depending on a woman's age, the type of OCP used, and how long it was used. Higher risk was observed in all types of hormonal birth control—pills, patches, vaginal rings, injections, progestin-only implants, and hormonal IUDs. This elevated risk quickly dropped back to the same levels as nonusers when stopped after short-term use. The small rise in risk remained in women who used hormonal contraception for more than 5 to 10 years. Experts generally agree that for most women, the risk of breast cancer associated with OCPs is quite small, even for those who used earlier versions with higher doses of estrogen. Women over age 40 or who have an elevated risk for breast cancer should talk with their doctors about birth control methods, such as an IUD that doesn't dispense hormones.

Pregnancy and breastfeeding. Pregnancy affects breast cancer risk in complex ways. By itself, becoming pregnant doesn't appear to affect this risk. Giving birth, however, is protective. Compared to women who complete their first pregnancy before age 20, having a first child after age 30 doubles the risk for breast cancer, even more than never being pregnant. Fertility treatments, miscarriage, and abortion haven't been shown to increase breast cancer risk.

Breastfeeding can be a special bonding experience that provides health benefits to mother and baby. These benefits are realized when you breastfeed exclusively for at least six months—meaning that your baby has only breast milk and no other liquids or solid food during this time. The longer you breastfeed, the greater the protective effect. Breast milk contains all the nutrients a baby needs, and its beneficial effects continue into adulthood. Nursing your baby for a year or more lowers your risk of both premenopausal and postmenopausal breast cancers, even if you have a family history of breast cancer. A study by the Collaborative Group on Hormonal Factors in Breast Cancer found that a woman's risk of breast cancer decreases by 4.3 percent for every 12 months she breastfeeds one or more children during that time. Lactation is protective in several ways. It delays menstrual periods, reducing lifetime exposure to estrogen and other hormones that can promote breast cancer. Nursing women also tend to eat more nutritiously, while avoiding alcohol and tobacco products.

Menopausal hormone therapy. Taking replacement hormones to alleviate the side effects of menopause increases breast cancer risk. Prior to 2002, hormone replacement therapy (HRT)—a combination of estrogen and the hormone progestin—was standard treatment to alleviate night sweats, hot flashes, and other symptoms of menopause in women who still had their uterus. It was also thought to have a protective effect on a woman's heart. Then the Women's Health Initiative discovered that postmenopausal women who took oral HRT had more blood clots, strokes, heart attacks, and were also more likely to develop breast cancer.

Now called *menopausal hormone therapy* (MHT), the estrogen-progestin combination is known to increase the risk of invasive breast cancer risk after five years of use (progestin is a synthetic hormone that is similar to progesterone). A meta-analysis of 58 studies that included more than 100,000 women of average risk found that the risks from MHT increased steadily the longer hormone replacement therapy was used, and lasted for up to 10 years after the women stopped using the medication. A greater risk was associated with estrogen-progestin therapies than for estrogen only. Every type of hormone replacement therapy, except for vaginal estrogens, was associated with excess breast cancer risks.

Estrogen alone appears to be safe for women who no longer have their uterus, but only for 10 years; after that, it increases the risk of breast cancer. It also increases the risk of ovarian cancer. The Sister

How Fertility Treatments Affect Breast Cancer Risk

Fertility drugs stimulate a woman's ovaries to produce more eggs than normal, considerably raising her estrogen levels. The Sister Study, funded by the National Institute of Environmental Health Sciences, collected data from women who were diagnosed before age 50, along with their sisters and biological parents. This study showed that women who conceived after using the fertility drug clomiphene citrate alone or with a follicle-stimulating hormone had a higher breast cancer risk (yet still below average) than women who used the same fertility drugs and didn't conceive. Researchers hypothesize that fertility drugs aren't protective against breast cancer; rather, women who cannot conceive on their own likely have below-average levels of estrogen and therefore have lower breast cancer risk.

Study observed that women who took estrogen-only hormone therapy were 42 percent less likely to develop young-onset breast cancer (before age 50), compared to their sisters who never had hormone therapy. MHT is not recommended for breast cancer survivors because some research shows that it may increase the risk for a recurrence and breast cancer in the opposite breast.

Smoking. Tobacco smoke contains more than 7,000 chemicals, at least 70 of which are carcinogenic to the human body. Because toxins in tobacco smoke can access almost all of the body's organs, smokers are more likely than nonsmokers to develop heart disease, stroke, and cancers of the lung, mouth, esophagus, and other organs. Smoking is also linked to a higher risk of breast cancer in younger, premenopausal women, and heavy exposure to secondhand smoke may increase risk in postmenopausal women. Smoking can also interfere with treatment by promoting infection, delaying healing, damaging the lungs after radiation therapy, and causing a higher risk of blood clots in women who are treated with hormonal therapies. It also reduces survival from breast cancer or any cause. Some evidence suggests that patients who formerly smoked more than 30 packs per year (about half a pack per week) had a 37 percent increased risk of recurrence and a 54 percent increased risk of breast cancer death compared to nonsmoking patients.

Environmental pollutants. Our modern world surrounds us with chemicals. What we put in and on our bodies and where we live, work, and play expose us to toxins that can affect our health. Scientists have long believed that exposure to pollution, pesticides, and industrial chemicals in plastics, cosmetics, and other common household goods may have something to do with the high rate of breast cancer in the industrialized world. This includes exposure to chemicals in the air we breathe, the food and beverages we consume, and the chemicals that come in contact with our skin. Many of these toxic substances, including bisphenol A (BPA), phthalates, and parabens can mimic estrogen or affect how estrogen and other hormones act in the body—research continues to study whether these and other environmental substances can influence breast cancer risk. Except for exposure to excessive radiation, however, no environmental toxins have consistently been linked to breast cancer.

More research is needed to better define the possible health effects of these substances and others like them. But isolating and observing the effects of these substances in humans is challenging, and few studies have done so. The National Toxicology Program lists more than 60 substances that cause mammary gland cancer in laboratory animals. Among them are food additives; pharmaceuticals; flame retardants, chemical solvents, and dyes in consumer products; vinyl and polyurethane foams; and pesticides.

The Environmental Working Group (www.ewg.org) provides safety information and a searchable product database of harmful chemicals. The Breast Cancer and the Environment Research Program (BCERP), a multidisciplinary network of scientists, clinicians, and community partners, is working to provide a clearer understanding of the effects of environmental exposures that may increase the risk of breast cancer.

Working night shifts. Women who work night shifts for several years develop obesity, diabetes, heart disease, and breast cancer at higher rates than women who work during the day. This might be because sleeping during the day and being awake in artificial light during the evening interferes with our circadian rhythm, the internal clock that tells us to sleep when it's dark and wake when it's light. A meta-analysis of 61 global studies found that nurses and other night shift workers in North America and Europe developed breast cancer 31 percent more often than women who didn't work at night. Women in Asia and Australia who worked nights didn't have the same increased risk. Although the World Health Organization classifies night shift work as "probably carcinogenic," the evidence is insufficient to be certain that night work causes breast cancer.

ESTIMATING PERSONAL RISK

Although risk assessment isn't an exact science, it's becoming more precise as researchers continue to expand their knowledge of how cancers behave. While it's not yet possible to accurately predict which women will or won't develop breast cancer, genetics experts can estimate an individual's risk based on personal and family medical histories and behavioral and lifestyle factors.

The Gail Model

Genetics experts use computerized risk assessment models to estimate an individual's probability of developing breast cancer within a certain time period—within 5 or 10 years or over a lifetime, for example—considering certain individual risk factors. These assessment tools aren't perfect, and each has its own strengths and limitations. They're most effective when a woman's personal and family history are similar to the study population on which the tool is based. The *Gail model* is the most common assessment tool used for women between ages 35 and 74. It scores the odds of developing invasive breast cancer over the next five years and to age 90, based on a woman's personal, reproductive, and familial risk factors, including:

- age
- age of first menstrual period
- age at first live birth
- number of first-degree relatives (mother, sister, or daughter) with breast cancer
- race and ethnicity
- number of previous breast biopsies
- number of biopsies showing atypical hyperplasia
- breast density

Updated versions of the Gail model also ask about alcohol use, breast density, and body mass index. Scores are based on the average five-year risk of women who have similar risk factors; a score below

1.6 percent indicates low risk, while a score above 1.66 percent indicates high risk and the need to consider more frequent screening and/or risk-reducing medications. This model doesn't consider an extended family history of breast cancer or environmental exposures, and it isn't recommended for women with a BRCA mutation or a strong personal or family history of breast cancer. In the following example, Jane's short-term and long-term risks are considerably greater than Denise's or the average woman's because of her personal risk factors (table 3.3).

Table 3.3. Gail Model Examples

Risk Factors	Denise	Jane
Age	61	61
Age at first menstrual period	12	9
Age at onset of menopause	55	60
Age at first childbirth	22	No pregnancies
Family history	No breast cancer	Several relatives with breast cancer
History of breast biopsies	None	One biopsy (atypical hyperplasia)
Gail risk five-year score	1.3% (average = 1.8%)	15.7%
Gail risk lifetime score	6.4% (average = 8.8%)	54.5%

Other Risk Models

The *Claus model* is more effective for women with a family history of breast or ovarian cancer. It calculates 10-year and lifetime estimates and is better suited to women who have one or more female relatives with breast cancer. Unlike the Gail model, the Claus model considers the number of first- and second-degree relatives with breast cancer and their age at diagnosis. It also distinguishes between maternal and paternal relatives; however, it doesn't consider a woman's nonhereditary risk factors, like a previous breast biopsy, smoking, or frequency of exercise. According to the American Cancer Society, a Claus model lifetime risk greater than 20 percent identifies patients who can benefit from heightened surveillance. A different model, the Breast Cancer Surveillance Consortium Risk Calculator, assesses risk in women between ages 35 and 74 who have never had breast augmentation, invasive breast cancer, DCIS, or a mastectomy. It also considers information about breast density and benign breast disease.

Other risk predictors estimate whether an individual is a likely candidate for genetic testing. The *Tyrer-Cuzick model* calculates the risk of having an inherited mutation in a gene other than BRCA1 or BRCA2. This model considers age; BMI; age at first menstrual period, at first live birth, and at menopause; hormone replacement therapy use; breast biopsies; atypical ductal hyperplasia or lobular carcinoma in situ (LCIS); and the history of breast and ovarian cancer in first- and second-degree relatives. It produces 10-year and lifetime risk estimates, which have been shown to be accurate for at least 19 years. BRCAPro considers a patient's age and ethnicity, the age of first- and second-degree relatives who had breast or ovarian cancer (including male breast cancer), and BRCA1 and BRCA2 mutations in the family. This model considers only risk factors that pertain to hereditary status; it doesn't include nonhereditary factors like smoking or obesity.

Risk Factors

Having any of the following risk factors indicates a higher-than-average chance for developing breast cancer:

- a previous breast cancer diagnosis
- atypical hyperplasia
- dense breasts confer a risk of five to six times greater than normal breasts
- an inherited breast cancer gene mutation
- a family history of breast cancer
- a Gail risk score of 1.66 or higher

Table 3.4. Assessing Your Breast Cancer Risk

	Lower Risk	Higher Risk
Age	30s (1 in 233 risk)	70s+ (1 in 8 risk)
Estrogen exposure	Menstrual period started at or after age 12	Menstrual period started before age 12
	Pregnancy before age 30	No pregnancies or pregnancy after age 30
	Breast-fed children	Never breast-fed
	Entered menopause before age 55	Entered menopause after age 55
	No birth control pills for 10+ years	Using birth control pills now
	No hormone replacement	Taking hormone replacement now
Previous breast biopsy	No	Yes—especially if atypical ductal hyperplasia was seen

CHAPTER 4

Strategies to Reduce Your Risk of Developing Breast Cancer

While no single behavior guarantees safety against disease, making positive changes in three areas—nutrition, physical activity, and body weight—significantly improves overall health. Managing these three lifestyle components is also the most balanced approach to reducing the risk of developing cancer.

You can't change how age, genetics, or other factors beyond your control influence your risk of breast cancer. But you can choose to change specific behaviors that lower your likelihood of ever hearing the words "You have breast cancer." Research shows that 40 percent of all breast cancers could be prevented with lifestyle changes. Although no single change can guarantee you won't get cancer, you can significantly improve your overall health and reduce your cancer risk by making positive changes in three areas: nutrition, physical activity, and body weight. Managing these three lifestyle components is the most balanced approach to minimizing cellular damage that leads to cancer. These same changes have been shown to improve outcomes and reduce the risk of recurrence in breast cancer patients. Failing to manage even one of the three—let alone all of them—jeopardizes your health and your cancer risk.

In 1940, a woman's lifetime risk of developing breast cancer was just 5 percent, compared to 12 percent today. What happened to more than double the rate of diagnosis? Our grandparents were more active and less sedentary. They had few fast food and processed food options, and they had less exposure to environmental toxins than we do now.

WHAT YOU EAT AND DRINK MATTERS

Increasingly, research shows that people who eat primarily nutritious, whole foods are less likely to develop cancer and other diseases. While no indisputable scientific evidence links specific foods and cancer, the indirect relationship is clear: nutritious dietary choices increase overall health and boost immune system response to DNA damage that often begins the cancer cycle. Unhealthy eating patterns promote inflammation, raise hormone levels, and contribute to excess weight; all three are known risk factors for breast cancer.

Unlike our ancestors, whose diets were limited to what they could find and catch, we can selectively decide what we eat. Yet most Americans choose boxed, prepackaged, and fast foods that are loaded with unhealthy fats, processed sweeteners, and chemical additives that extend shelf life and only mimic the texture and taste of the real foods they replace. These convenient yet unhealthy "empty calorie" foods now make up 61 percent of the average American's diet. Although they may satisfy our taste buds, they provide little in the way of nutrition. By eating too few whole foods and super-sized portions of the

---

**Risk Factors during Youth May
Increase Adult Breast Cancer**

Although children and teenagers rarely develop breast cancer, some influences during youth may raise their risk as adults. Data from the Nurses' Health Study found that teenage girls with poor diets—red meat, sodas, sugary foods, and white flour—were about 35 percent more likely to develop premenopausal breast cancer in their 20s, 30s, and 40s than girls who ate more salads and whole grains. In some girls, the onset of puberty now arrives at age 7 or 8. This "precocious puberty" is fueled by unnaturally high levels of estrogen that result from carrying extra weight and consuming hormones in food.

wrong foods, we're becoming obese while starving our bodies of the nutrients they need. A diet of mainly fresh or minimally processed foods instead of products with multisyllabic ingredients helps you to feel more energetic, fend off disease, and achieve and maintain a healthy weight.

The Relationship between Food and Cancer: Why So Mysterious?

It's difficult, if not impossible, to tie specific foods to cancer risk. Unlike medications that provoke specific, identifiable reactions in people, foods provide numerous beneficial compounds that are more difficult to identify. A group of women who eat a cup of blueberries each day may have lower breast cancer rates, for example, but we wouldn't know whether the improvement was due to a specific compound in the blueberries, other dietary factors, or other behaviors that may lower breast cancer risk.

Studies of food and cancer are observational, meaning that researchers arrive at their conclusions by analyzing participants' answers about their diets and observing how many people develop the cancer being studied. Short of limiting participants' diets to a single substance, while observational studies of a specific food can suggest a relationship, they don't prove cause and effect because so many other nondietary risk factors are involved. Nor is it practical or safe to require people to eat nothing but blueberries or fish for a few years while they're being studied. Self-reporting is also an imperfect study methodology, because too often, people don't remember exactly what they ate or drank or in what quantities. Even when researchers adjust study results for age, weight, family history, and other factors, they can't gauge the accuracy of self-reporting.

The Benefits of a Plant-Based Diet

The United States and other developed countries have higher rates of cancers, including breast cancer, than Africa, Asia, and other cultures where fruits, vegetables, and whole grains account for 50 to 90 percent of the average diet. Breast cancer rates in these low-risk cultures increase when their populations become Westernized or when native populations migrate to developed countries.

The American Institute for Cancer Research recommends meals that are two-thirds or more fruits, vegetables, beans, and whole grains, and one-third or less lean protein. The Mediterranean diet is one example of an eating plan that follows this recommendation. Rather than a diet in the traditional sense, it's recognized as one of the healthiest approaches to nutritionally balanced eating (figure 4.1).

The value and importance of plant-based foods are strongly supported by research. Plants manufacture an array of chemicals to stay healthy. As it turns out, many of those substances also benefit humans. *Phytonutrients* (also called phytochemicals) are naturally occurring substances that give fruits and vegetables their color, flavor, and fragrance. Plants make many types of phytonutrients, and each one helps our bodies in different ways (table 4.1). Nutritionists recommend eating a rainbow of colored fruits and vegetables, because phytonutrients are the source of those intense colors; eating a variety of produce across the color spectrum gives you a wide supply of nutrients. Even onions, garlic, pears, and other neutral-hued produce

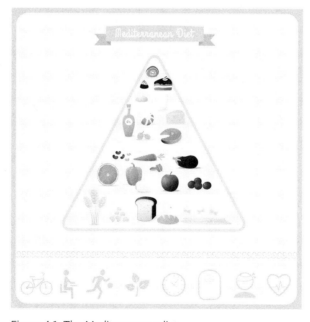

Figure 4.1. The Mediterranean diet

Table 4.1. Power Up with Phytonutrients

Category	Source	Benefits
Isoflavones	Soybeans, tofu, soy milk, other whole soy products	Inhibits tumor growth, slows production of cancer-related hormones, reduces heart disease
Flavonoids	Apples, onions, whole soy foods, soy milk, coffee, tea, citrus fruits, whole grains, onions, garlic, chives, shallots, leeks	Inhibits tumor growth, reduces inflammation, boosts immune system
Lignans	Flaxseed, sesame seeds, broccoli, apricots, strawberries	May reduce the risk of ovarian cancer; evidence is less clear for an association with breast cancer
Carotenoids: beta-carotene, lycopene, lutein	Tomatoes, broccoli, leafy greens, carrots, sweet potatoes, apricots, oranges, cantaloupe, watermelon; other red, orange, green fruits, and vegetables	Inhibits cancer growth, boosts immune system
Polyphenols: ellagic acid, resveratrol	Green tea, grapes, grape juice, red wine, blueberries, cranberries, citrus fruits, apples, whole grains, peanuts	May prevent damaged cells from becoming malignant, reduces inflammation

supply beneficial compounds. Fruits and vegetables are nutrient powerhouses with several cancer-protective mechanisms. They boost immune system response and reduce inflammation that provokes cancer growth, and they slow the growth of malignant cells. They also help to prevent DNA damage and help to repair it when it does develop. Phytonutrients in supplement form do not provide the same benefits as whole fruits and vegetables.

Fats

The link between fat and breast cancer is one of the most analyzed dietary relationships. The body needs fat, but all fats aren't the same.

The type of fat, rather than the amount consumed, is most important (figure 4.2). For decades, consumers were warned away from *saturated fats* found in red meat, dairy, palm oil, and coconut oil that raise cholesterol and increase the risk of heart disease and stroke. Newer information from researchers at the University of California and the Harvard School of Public Health shows that consuming saturated fat in moderation (less than 10 percent of total daily calories) minimally affects these conditions. (Chemically solidified trans fats in commercially prepared foods are the most harmful; they raise the bad type of cholesterol and lower the good type, and they have been banned in the United States since 2013.)

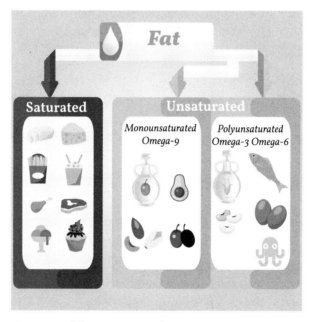

Figure 4.2. All fats are not equal

The European Prospective Investigation into Cancer (EPIC) study, which followed more than 300,000 women for more than 11 years, concluded that women who ate the most saturated fat and the most total fat had higher risks of estrogen receptor– and progesterone receptor–positive breast cancer than women who ate less of either

Yes or No to Soy?

Soy-based foods, including soy milk, tofu, edamame, soy nuts, and miso are rich with plant protein, fiber, vitamins, and all of the essential amino acids the body needs to function. While some studies show that a high-soy diet may lower the risk of breast cancer, others haven't. In past years, women were told that soy foods increased the risk of breast cancers that are fueled by estrogen. But experts now recognize that the isoflavone levels in whole soy foods are too weak to affect a woman's estrogen levels. In fact, soy isoflavones appear to balance hormone levels and reduce tumor cell proliferation. One to three half-cup servings per day of whole soy foods are a good protein replacement for meat and contribute to a well-balanced diet for women, including breast cancer survivors. Soy supplements, which contain higher levels of isoflavones, aren't recommended. If you're being treated for hormone receptor–positive breast cancer, talk to your doctor about how much soy you can include in your diet.

type of fat. Those who ate the most fat consumed about 47.5 grams of fat per day—in comparison, just one McDonald's Big Mac and one serving of French fries equals about 39 grams of fat. Women who consumed the least amount of fat per day ate 15.4 grams of fat or less. High-fat diets, like the ones assessed in the EPIC study, cause weight gain and obesity, which in turn increase hormone levels and breast cancer risk.

Monounsaturated fats from avocados, nuts, and nut oils and *polyunsaturated fats* from fish, plants, and nuts are more beneficial and less harmful than saturated fats (table 4.2). Olive, nut, and canola oils are healthier choices than margarine, butter, or tropical oils. Polyunsaturated fats also include omega-3 and omega-6 fatty acids, two essential fats that our bodies need yet can't make. Both types of omega fatty acids support immune system and heart function and lower blood pressure. Omega-3 fats are anti-inflammatory, while excess levels of omega-6 fats promote inflammation.

Some studies show that women who eat omega-3-rich foods have reduced breast cancer risk, possibly due to the anti-inflammatory properties of these omega fatty acids. Some research hints that the ratio of the two fats may be most important—a high omega-3-to-omega-6 ratio may lower premenopausal breast cancer risk. A diet that is high in omega-6s and low in omega-3s—like the typical Westernized diet—may increase inflammation, setting the stage for heart disease, arthritis, diabetes, Alzheimer disease, and cancer. Walnuts, soy, canola oil, pumpkin seeds, and flaxseed contain *alpha-linolenic acid*, a different type of omega-3. Foods are more reliable sources of omega fatty acids than fish oil supplements. Unless your doctor has prescribed fish oil supplements to lower your triglycerides, consider getting your omega fats from seafood or one or two daily servings of foods that supply alpha-linolenic acid.

Table 4.2. Sources of Healthy Fats

Monounsaturated Fat	Polyunsaturated Fat	Omega-3 Fatty Acids	Omega-6 Fatty Acids
Avocado and avocado oil	Soybeans, soy oil, tofu	Halibut, salmon,* trout, anchovies, oysters, sardines	Walnuts
Canola oil	Corn oil	Avocados, Brussels sprouts, kale, spinach	Flaxseeds
Olives and olive oil	Safflower oil		Pumpkin seeds
Nuts and nut oils	Walnuts		Sunflower seeds
Peanut butter and peanut oil	Sunflower seeds	Walnuts, soybeans	Soy
Sesame seeds, sesame oil, and tahini		Canola and flaxseed oils	Evening primrose oil
		Chia seeds	Acai

*Compared to wild salmon, farmed salmon tends to have more contaminants, more saturated fat, and less omega-3.

Vitamins and Supplements

Despite vigorous marketing claims, no vitamin, mineral, or herb has been proven to prevent breast cancer or to keep it from recurring. Because the US Food and Drug Administration doesn't regulate dietary supplements, vitamins, herbs, and other supplements, they

How Important Are Antioxidants?

Antioxidants are micronutrients that counteract the detrimental effects of oxidation on the body's cells and tissues. They're particularly effective fighting *free radicals*, which are toxic molecules that damage DNA and contribute to aging, disease, and cancer. Some free radicals develop naturally from the body's metabolic processes, while others are created from smoking, drinking, air pollution, and exposure to ultraviolet rays and other environmental substances.

Antioxidants are important because they can render free radicals harmless or destroy them before they do too much damage. Our bodies make small amounts of antioxidants, but we mostly get them from foods that are rich in vitamin A (liver, eggs, milk, butter), vitamin C (fruits and vegetables), and vitamin E (nuts, seeds, green leafy vegetables, canola oil). Foods that supply beta-carotene (carrots, peas, blueberries, peaches, and other brightly colored fruits and vegetables), lutein (green leafy vegetables, papayas, oranges), lycopene (tomatoes, watermelon, and other pink or red produce), and selenium (wheat, rice and corn products, poultry, fish, beef, eggs) also supply antioxidants. It's best to get antioxidants directly from whole foods. Taking antioxidant supplements is usually not advised during cancer treatment, because some studies show that they may interfere with treatment by protecting cancer cells as well as healthy cells.

are legally marketed and sold without proof of their effectiveness or safety. Unless your doctor has prescribed a particular supplement for a specific deficiency, whole foods are a better source of nutrients your body needs.

Vitamin D is critical for healthy muscles and nerves, and it also regulates cell growth. Along with calcium, it promotes bone strength and prevents osteoporosis. The recommended daily amount of vitamin D is 600 international units (IU) for ages 1 to 70. (Babies need 400 IU before age 1; adults over 70 need 800 IU.) Salmon, sardines, and oysters are good sources, as are fortified milk, yogurt, and cereals. The body converts sunlight into vitamin D—just 15 minutes of sunlight three days a week is enough. But concern about skin cancer from excessive sun exposure has resulted in vitamin D deficiencies in many populations.

Early studies suggested that vitamin D supplementation might increase breast cancer risk, although most research in several countries has disproved this theory. Along with sufficient calcium, vitamin D is especially important for breast cancer patients who are treated with tamoxifen or aromatase inhibitors, hormonal drugs that lower estrogen levels and promote bone loss. Some evidence suggests that vitamin D supplementation may lower the risk of recurrence for women with estrogen receptor–positive breast cancer, but it has no effect on estrogen receptor–negative tumors.

Folate is a B vitamin needed for cellular health. It occurs naturally in beans, green leafy vegetables, citrus fruit, and many other foods. Folic acid, the synthetic version of folate, is found in prenatal vitamins and in numerous fortified foods. Women in the Nurses' Health Study who had at least 300 milligrams of daily folate had fewer breast cancer diagnoses than women who had lower levels of folate. Most research doesn't support folate supplementation as a reliable way to reduce breast cancer risk, however. Folate supplements are sometimes recommended to reduce the increased risk of breast cancer associated with alcohol use.

Alcoholic Beverages

Consuming alcohol in moderation may be good for the heart and may protect against type 2 diabetes. But drinking alcoholic beverages is known to raise the risk of several cancers, and more than 100 studies have consistently linked increased drinking to a higher risk of breast cancer, possibly because it raises levels of estrogen, which can stimulate breast tumors. It may also impair the body's ability to detoxify cancer-causing substances. Drinking sabotages weight control by adding empty calories to your diet and priming your body to store fat and sugar, while modifying brain chemistry to increase appetite and create food cravings. All of these factors may translate into an increased level of risk for a first diagnosis or a recurrence. The more you drink, the greater your risk, and even a few drinks per week may somewhat increase the chance of developing breast cancer. (One standard drink is 12 ounces of regular beer, 5 ounces of wine, or 1.5 ounces—a shot—of hard liquor.)

Studies on alcohol and breast cancer have mostly blamed heavy drinking; many haven't found significantly higher risk among light drinkers. If you're of average risk for breast cancer, having one serving of liquor a day may raise your risk, although not significantly (table 4.3). If your breast cancer risk is high or you've already been diagnosed, it may be wise to forego alcohol or to have it only occasionally. Red wine is a better choice than white wine or cocktails because it contains resveratrol, which slows the formation and progression of malignant cells. If you drink at all, be sure that alcohol doesn't interfere with any medications you take.

**Table 4.3. How Daily Drinking Affects Women
with Average (12%) Breast Cancer Risk**

Number of Daily Drinks	Percentage Increase in Risk	New Risk
1	10.0	13.2
2	30.0	15.6
3	40.0	16.8
Each additional drink	Additional 10.0	Additional 1.2 for each drink

CONTROLLING YOUR WEIGHT

When considering the relationship of weight to breast cancer, size matters. Achieving and maintaining a healthy weight are the most important actions you can take to reduce your risk of breast and other cancers. Fueled by unhealthy diets and sedentary lifestyles, obesity is epidemic in much of the developed world, including almost 70 percent of American adults. Dangerously unhealthy, obesity dramatically raises the likelihood of hypertension, diabetes, stroke, heart disease, and other chronic diseases. Gaining weight after menopause is particularly risky, because although estrogen is no longer produced by the ovaries, it is made by fat cells. More fat means more inflammation, more insulin, and more estrogen—all three translate to a greater risk for a breast cancer. Obesity can also adversely affect treatment outcomes, raise the risk of recurrence, and shorten longevity.

You're considered to be overweight if your body mass index (BMI) is between 25.0 and 29.9, and obese if it's over 30. A higher score reflects obesity and a greater risk for several diseases, including breast cancer. You can calculate your own BMI: your weight in pounds ÷ (your height in inches²) × 703. A woman who is 5 foot 6 six inches and weighs 205 pounds has a BMI of 33 (205 ÷ 66² × 703). You can also find your BMI by using the online calculator at www.hopkins medicine.org/health/wellness-and-prevention/bmi. Waist circumference is another indicator for possible health risks related to being overweight or obese. Women with a waist measurement of more than 35 inches and men who have a waist measurement over 40 inches also have elevated risk of developing health issues, including serious and life-threatening diseases.

Weight Classification	BMI Score
Normal	18.5–24.9
Overweight	25.0–29.9
Obese	30.0 and above
Extremely obese	40.0 and above

Losing weight and keeping it off. Simply put, you gain weight when you eat more calories than you burn; excess calories are stored as body fat. More than any other factor, what you eat determines your weight. Although dieting may help you shed a few pounds quickly, the only successful way to achieve long-term balanced health and weight is to eat consistently in a way that satisfies your appetite, nourishes your body, and minimizes unhealthy foods. If increased weight raises the risk of breast cancer, does losing weight reduce that risk? In a follow-up study to the Women's Health Initiative, overweight women who lost 5 percent or more of their body weight lowered their breast

Tips for Long-Term Weight Control

If you've tried dieting, you know how difficult it can be to lose even a few pounds, especially if it requires changing your ingrained eating habits and curbing your cravings. These tips will help:

- Choose healthy, long-term eating habits over trendy diets.
- Prioritize nutrition; limit animal fats and "empty calorie" foods.
- Don't skip meals.
- Eat slowly, and be mindful of what you eat before you eat it.
- Keep portions moderate.
- Eat when you're hungry, and stop eating when you're full.
- Weight gained over months or years won't disappear overnight. Set realistic goals, such as losing 1 to 2 pounds per week.
- Don't buy what you know you shouldn't eat.
- Join a weight loss program if you need one.
- Be physically active every day.

cancer risk by 12 percent. Women who lost 15 percent or more of their body weight lowered their risk by 37 percent.

Counting fat grams isn't the best way to manage what you eat or reduce your breast cancer risk, and the low-fat, high-starch diets of the 1990s have been proven ineffective. Long-term follow-up studies, including the Nurses' Health Study, consistently show little relationship between the percentage of calories from fat and risks of breast cancer. Your body will know the difference if you consume 1,500 calories of soda, sugary foods, white bread, cookies, and chips compared to 1,500 calories of fresh fruits, vegetables, whole grains, and lean protein. Owing to the way insulin and other hormones determine how your body uses or stores fat, you're more likely to maintain a healthy weight with the latter diet, rather than the former, which provides primarily non-nutritious calories.

Your Sleep Habits Affect Your Weight and Your Cancer Risk

Most Americans don't get the recommended minimum nightly sleep the body needs to maintain and repair itself. The National Sleep Foundation recommends seven to nine hours of nightly sleep if you're age 18 to 65, and seven to eight hours if you're 65 or older. Sufficient sleep is critical for the health of your heart, body, and mind. Chronic sleep deprivation dulls reflexes, concentration, and decision-making in the same way as drinking alcohol. Poor sleeping habits are linked to heart disease, type 2 diabetes, and many other health problems. Unhealthy sleep patterns also affect weight gain by interfering with two hormones that regulate appetite: they can increase levels of ghrelin, a hormone that induces hunger, and reduce levels of leptin, which signals the brain that you're full. Insufficient or interrupted sleep can also cause mood swings that lead to cravings for high-fat and sugary foods, fueling weight gain and obesity. It can also raise levels of cortisol, a stress hormone that drops blood sugar and increases cravings for sugary, fatty foods.

Tips for better sleep
- Go to bed and wake at the same time every day, including weekends.
- Get plenty of light during the day.
- Don't nap or nap no longer than 30 minutes during the day if you have a difficult time sleeping at night.
- Avoid caffeine and alcohol late in the day.
- Wind down before bed by reading, meditating, or taking a warm bath.
- Turn off LED lights and electronic devices two to three hours before bedtime. The blue light that these devices emit activates the brain.
- Make your bedroom as dark and comfortable as possible.
- Replace your mattress and pillows if they're old or uncomfortable.
- Ask your doctor if you need a sleep study to determine if you have sleep apnea, a disorder where breathing stops for up to a minute while you're asleep.
- Exercise every day, but not just before bedtime.

MOVE MORE, SIT LESS

Physical activity is any action that moves your body and burns calories—a daily dose is the antidote for a sedentary lifestyle. More than 80 percent of American adults don't get enough exercise to meet the Department of Health and Human Services guidelines for optimum health. The good news is that even a small amount of daily activity provides short-term and long-term health benefits. And studies show that the more you exercise, the more likely you are to improve your diet.

Exercise influences your overall health, including the likelihood of a breast cancer diagnosis and recurrence. Women who are more active tend to have lower rates of mortality, heart disease, high blood pressure, stroke, type 2 diabetes, depression, and breast cancer. They're also more likely to maintain a healthy weight. The American Cancer Society recommends adults get at least 90 minutes of moderately intense activity or 75 minutes of vigorous activity each week, which works out to about 20 minutes of activity per day (table 4.4). For maximum benefit, strive for a combination of moderate- and vigorous-intensity activities, as well as stretching and resistance training of your major muscle groups at least twice weekly.

Getting some level of daily activity is more advantageous than getting a week's worth in a day or two. It's fine to break up your activity into several smaller increments so long as you sustain the activity for at least 10 minutes. Any amount of exercise is good, but more is

Table 4.4. Examples of Moderate and Vigorous Activities

Moderate-Intensity Activities	Vigorous-Intensity Activities
Modestly increases heart rate and breathing	Greater increase in heart rate and breathing; you need to take a breath after speaking a few words
Brisk walking	Jogging or running
Vacuuming, washing windows	Jumping rope
Dancing	Swimming laps
Leisurely bicycling	Fast bicycling (more than 10 mph)
Yoga or tai chi	Soccer, football, basketball
Doubles tennis	Singles tennis
Yard work	Hiking uphill

better and may further lower your breast cancer risk. If you're new to the idea of actively moving each day, begin slowly, gradually adding more time and effort as you become more fit.

Minimize the time you spend sitting. Standing and moving require more energy and burn more calories than sitting. In fact, excess sitting increases the likelihood of cancer and numerous other health conditions, especially for women. Extensive and uninterrupted periods of sitting, whether at a desk, in front of a screen, or in a car, can be harmful. An analysis of 13 studies involving more than one million people show that the risk of dying from sitting more than eight hours a day with no physical activity is similar to the risks of death from obesity and smoking. The same analysis found that 60 to 75 minutes of daily, moderately intense physical activity counters the effects of too much sitting. Experts recommend standing while speaking on the phone, using a standing desk, and standing or walking for a few minutes after 30 minutes of sitting.

A study by the American Cancer Society found that breast cancer risk increased by 10 percent in women who spent six hours or more sitting a day compared to women who sat less than three hours a day. The six-hour group had increased risk for other cancers as well, including a 65 percent increase in the chance of ovarian cancer.

What We've Learned from Sisters

The Sister Study identified links between lifestyle and breast cancer among 50,000 sisters of women with breast cancer in the United States and Puerto Rico. Observational findings included:

- A lower rate of breast cancer in obese premenopausal young women.
- A lower rate of breast cancer in postmenopausal women with higher levels of vitamin D or who reported taking vitamin D supplements at least four times a week.
- A lower rate of adult breast cancer in women who exercised or played sports more than seven hours a week when they were 5 to 19 years old.
- A higher rate of breast cancer in women who had sleep problems four or more nights per week.

(Increased odds of cancer were also observed in men who were obese and sat for long periods.)

MANAGEMENT STRATEGIES FOR HIGH-RISK INDIVIDUALS

Your likelihood of developing breast cancer is higher than average if you have any of the following risk factors:

- A positive test for a mutation in a gene that is known to increase breast cancer risk.
- A strong family history that elevates your lifetime risk to 20 percent or higher.
- A previous diagnosis of ductal carcinoma in situ (DCIS) or invasive breast cancer.
- A previous diagnosis of atypical hyperplasia or lobular carcinoma in situ (LCIS).
- Radiation therapy to the chest before age 30.

If you find yourself in this higher-risk category, experts recommend that you take extra precautions to avoid a diagnosis or to discover breast cancer early on, when it's more treatable. These decisions are complex, highly personal, and can be difficult. One alternative is to be screened for breast cancer more frequently than women in the general population. Heightened surveillance doesn't prevent or reduce the risk for breast cancer; it focuses on identifying early-stage cancer when it is more treatable. Screening recommendations for high-risk women are described in chapter 6.

Risk-Reducing Medications

If you're considering options to reduce your high risk of breast cancer, you have two choices: chemoprevention or preventive surgery.

For high-risk women who do not already have cancer, chemoprevention drugs proactively reduce their risk of a diagnosis. Taking these medications doesn't guarantee that you'll never develop cancer in your breasts, but it can significantly decrease your odds. Although it sounds like chemotherapy, it isn't. Tamoxifen and raloxifene treat estrogen-sensitive breast cancers by blocking the hormone's effect

Tamoxifen: From Pharmaceutical Failure to Superstar

Compound ICI 46474, as tamoxifen was first known, was discovered accidentally. It was synthesized in 1962 as part of a British research project to develop a morning-after contraceptive pill. The new drug wasn't a viable form of birth control because it stimulated ovulation and enhanced fertility rather than suppressing it. The lead researcher, however, believed that its anti-estrogen properties could be useful to treat breast cancer. And he was right. In 1977, following a series of successful clinical trials in humans, the US Food and Drug Administration (FDA) approved tamoxifen to treat advanced, estrogen-driven breast cancers. Several landmark studies in the 1980s then demonstrated that tamoxifen reduced the risk of breast cancer recurrence and death when given for one year after surgery; this benefit was even greater after three or five years. Additionally, tamoxifen lowered the risk of breast cancer in the opposite breast by 50 percent, inspiring the hypothesis that in addition to treatment, it might also be used to prevent breast cancer.

The research community now buzzed with excitement and hope: more and more, tamoxifen was looking like a breakthrough medication that could help so many people. In 1992, the National Cancer Institute sponsored the Breast Cancer Prevention Trial of approximately 13,300 high-risk participants. In this study, tamoxifen reduced the risk for invasive breast cancer by 49 percent. It did slightly increase the chance of deep vein thrombosis (blood clot in major veins), pulmonary embolism (blood clot in the lung), and uterine cancer in women over age 50. The reduction in breast cancer risk, though, was much higher than the risk of developing any of these complications.

The Study of Tamoxifen and Raloxifene (STAR) then compared tamoxifen with raloxifene, a related drug that was originally developed to treat osteoporosis. Both drugs similarly reduced the rate of noninvasive ductal carcinoma in situ (DCIS), while tamoxifen more effectively reduced the risk of invasive breast cancer. Raloxifene was less likely to cause uterine cancer, however. As a result of these invaluable studies, tamoxifen received FDA approval in 1999 as the first preventive medication for breast cancer in high-risk women. Today, it's widely recognized as the most important drug ever developed to prevent and manage breast cancer, and it's prescribed for many women to prevent or treat estrogen-sensitive breast cancers.

on breast tissue. Both drugs are also prescribed to reduce the risk of DCIS and invasive breast cancers in high-risk women: tamoxifen is prescribed for premenopausal or postmenopausal women over age 35; raloxifene has been used as a postmenopausal chemotherapy agent for breast cancer since 2007. When taken orally once a day for five years, both medications reduce the risk of estrogen-sensitive DCIS and invasive breast cancers by about 40 percent.

Aromatase inhibitors are used off-label for chemoprevention, meaning that they're approved by the FDA for treatment, although not specifically for prevention. But study results support the risk-reducing effectiveness of these drugs in high-risk, postmenopausal women. American Society of Clinical Oncology guidelines recommend that physicians discuss aromatase inhibitors as an alternative to raloxifene.

Risk-Reducing Surgeries

Surgical removal of both breasts, both ovaries, and the fallopian tubes is recommended for women who are predisposed to breast cancer due to a strong family history or a genetic mutation. You might feel that removing your healthy breasts and ovaries may be extreme, considering that they may never become cancerous. For now, though, these risk-reducing surgeries are the most effective method of ensuring that your genes don't dictate your future. Making decisions about these alternatives can be frustrating and difficult, and they shouldn't be made until you understand the benefits and limitations of each option. Taking drastic action to lower your risk as much as possible can calm the anxiety and angst you feel about a future diagnosis, especially if you've seen friends or family members wage war against breast cancer. Schedule a session with a genetics counselor to ensure that you don't underestimate or overestimate your risk and to learn how preventive surgeries will affect it.

Prophylactic bilateral mastectomy (PBM) is the most effective way of reducing the likelihood of breast cancer. Generally, PBM decreases breast cancer risk by 95 percent or more, lower than the risk of an average woman, and also reduces the odds of dying from breast cancer. Because it's not possible to remove every microscopic bit of breast tissue, a small risk remains. If you're at high risk and you have a mastectomy to treat breast cancer in one breast, preventive removal of the opposite healthy breast may be recommended to avoid a future diagnosis.

Choosing PBM is an important decision that deserves thoughtful evaluation of the advantages and disadvantages involved. Some women find that having the option for *breast reconstruction* after mastectomy softens the blow of losing their breasts (chapter 11). Consulting with plastic surgeons who perform breast reconstruction can help you understand your postmastectomy options and decide which, if any, is best for you. Consultations with a genetics counselor, breast cancer surgeon, and reconstructive surgeon will provide information that will inform your decision-making process.

Bilateral salpingo-oophorectomy (BSO) is a risk-reducing option for women who are predisposed to breast or ovarian cancer. Like risk-reducing mastectomy, it's an aggressive yet effective approach that improves the chance of diagnosis and survivability. For women with a BRCA1 mutation or a strong family history of breast or ovarian cancer, BSO is recommended between ages 35 and 40 or after childbearing is completed. Experts recommended BSO before age 45 for women with mutations in BRCA2, who tend to develop ovarian cancer 8 to 10 years later than BRCA1 mutation carriers. Guidelines for women with mutations in other predisposing genes vary, depending on the type of mutation. A genetics counselor can clarify how oophorectomy affects your risk and identify the best time to have the surgery.

In pre- and postmenopausal women, bilateral salpingo-oophorectomy lowers ovarian and fallopian tube cancer risk by about 90 percent. (A small risk of peritoneal cancer in the lining of the abdomen remains.) In premenopausal women, removing the ovaries stops production of estrogen and progesterone, reducing by half the odds of developing breast cancers that need these hormones to grow. Removing the ovaries eliminates the possibility of childbirth and causes premature menopause, with the same side effects that you would experience with natural menopause: hot flashes, changes in concentration or memory, sleep issues, and other symptoms can occur. Some of these symptoms can be treated effectively in the short term. Others, like increased risk for heart disease or a higher risk for osteoporosis, are long term and may require more serious intervention. Your health care team can discuss the advantages and disadvantages of taking menopausal hormone therapy to alleviate these issues.

CHAPTER 5

Hereditary Breast Cancer

For most women, we will never know why their breast cancer developed. It may be related to aging, hormones, environmental influences, or other factors. For a smaller group of women, *hereditary breast cancers* develop from genetic changes that are passed from parent to child from one generation to the next.

Women who develop breast cancer are often surprised that no one else in their family has been diagnosed, but most cancers aren't hereditary. The majority of breast cancers are *sporadic*; they develop from damage that our genes acquire as we age, rather than inherit. A small percentage of breast cancers are familial—they tend to run in families—with diagnoses of breast or ovarian cancers that occur across many generations and lead to the suspicion that hereditary factors may be the cause. Only 5 to 10 percent of breast cancers are caused by a known inherited gene mutation (figure 5.1). Inherited mutations have been identified in almost every country and culture, but they're more common in certain ethnic populations. For example, about 1 in 40 people who are of Ashkenazi (Eastern European) Jewish ancestry carry mutation in a BRCA1 or BRCA2 gene, compared to about 1 in 500–1,000 individuals in the general population (table 5.1). We still don't know why some *previvors*—people who are genetically predisposed to cancer but haven't been diagnosed—get breast cancer and others don't.

Hereditary breast cancers differ from sporadic breast cancers in important ways that may affect health care decisions.

- Tumors often develop at an earlier age.
- Cancers are often more aggressive and more difficult to treat, because they sometimes don't respond to treatments for sporadic breast cancer.
- Two tumors more often develop simultaneously in different areas of the same breast.
- Primary breast tumors are more likely to develop in both breasts.
- Recurrence is more likely.

Table 5.1. Incidence of BRCA Mutations by Ethnic Group

	BRCA1	BRCA2
African American	1%	3%
Ashkenazi Jewish	8%–10%	1%
Asian American	Less than 1%	Data not available
White (non–Ashkenazi Jewish)	2% to 3%	2%
Hispanic	4%	Data not available

Source: M. E. Malone, J. R. Daling, D. R. Doody et al., "Prevalence and Predictors of BRCA1 and BRCA2 Mutations in a Population-Based Study of Breast Cancer in White and Black American Women Ages 35 to 64 Years," *Cancer Research* 66, no. 16 (2006): 8297-308.

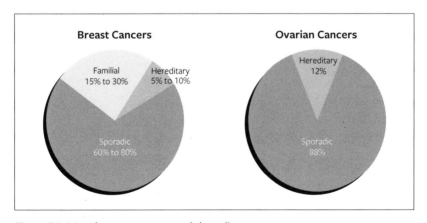

Figure 5.1. Most breast cancers aren't hereditary

MUTATIONS FROM MOM OR DAD

While sporadic cancers are caused by DNA damage from aging, hormones, environmental influences, or other factors, hereditary cancers develop from changes in genes called *genetic mutations* that are passed from parent to child. While you might thank your mother for your curly hair and your father for your height, if one or both of them have a cancer-causing gene defect, they could have passed that on to you as well. Although people often assume that breast cancer is a woman's disease and therefore genetic mutations are inherited only from one's mother, fathers can also pass genetic abnormalities to their sons and daughters. Children have a 50 percent chance of inheriting a parent's mutation and a high predisposition to cancer (figure 5.2). Children who don't inherit their parent's mutation have average risk for cancer.

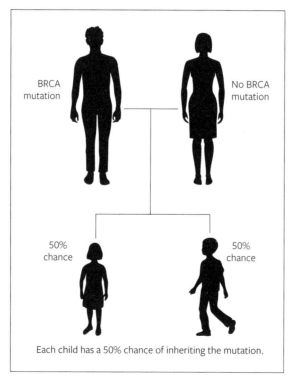

Figure 5.2. The probability of inheriting a BRCA mutation

Genetic mutations sometimes run in families, with multiple cases of breast, ovarian, and other cancers on the same side of the family. Even when a known genetic mutation can't be found in a family tree, breast cancer often occurs across many generations in a pattern that suggests hereditary factors are at work.

BRCA AND OTHER "BREAST CANCER GENES"

Most hereditary breast cancers are caused by an inherited mutation in the *BReast CAncer* (BRCA) genes. Mutations in the BRCA1 and BRCA2 genes predispose people to breast and ovarian cancer, and bestow a higher-than-average risk for some other cancers as well. While having a BRCA mutation doesn't guarantee a diagnosis, it does make it more likely.

We often hear that someone was diagnosed because of a "breast cancer gene," but that's a misnomer. Breast cancer doesn't occur because we have BRCA genes; everyone has them. In fact, we have two copies of every gene, including BRCA. Some mutations develop in *tumor promoter genes* that accelerate abnormal cellular activity. BRCA genes are *tumor suppressor genes*—when healthy, they repair DNA damage before cancer can develop. Breast cancer develops when a mutation in BRCA1 or BRCA2 prevents the gene from performing its job. When one BRCA gene is damaged and can't perform its repair job, the other one acts as a backup repair mechanism. That's why being born with a single BRCA mutation doesn't guarantee that you'll develop breast cancer, because your remaining BRCA gene can still repair cellular damage. If an error occurs in your remaining BRCA gene (called a somatic alteration), the entire protective function is lost, and nothing stops damaged cells from growing and reproducing. About half of hereditary breast cancers occur from mutations in the BRCA1 and BRCA2 genes. To a much lesser degree, mutations in ATM, CDH1, CHEK2, PALB2, PTEN, TP53, and other genes also play a role in breast cancer.

HBOC AND OTHER HEREDITARY
CANCER SYNDROMES

Mutations that are associated with multiple cancers cause *cancer syndromes*. *Hereditary breast and ovarian cancer* (HBOC) *syndrome* refers collectively to multiple cancers that are linked to BRCA mutations. Compared to their average-risk counterparts, men and women with HBOC syndrome have much higher lifetime odds of developing these cancers.

Other inherited syndromes also increase breast cancer risk. *Cowden syndrome* most often creates small, benign growths called hamartomas on the skin, mucus membranes, brain, or the intestinal tract. Caused by a mutation in the PTEN gene, affected patients develop characteristic skin lesions and have an increased risk of developing breast and thyroid cancers. Cowden syndrome also increases risk for benign and malignant tumors in the breast, uterus, and thyroid. *Li-Fraumeni syndrome* (LFS) increases the risk of developing breast cancer as well as leukemia, and cancers of the lung,

Discovering BRCA

Scientists have long known that genes pass from parent to child, along with any abnormalities in the genes that raise the risk for disease. Although a link between breast and ovarian cancer had been suspected for more than a century, most modern scientists believed that cancer was caused by a virus. Genetics scientist Dr. Mary-Claire King had a different hunch: she suspected that inherited genetic flaws that are passed from generation to generation cause the breast and ovarian cancers that run in some families. In 1990, she provided the world with a stunning discovery: proof that in some families, inherited mutations in a single gene significantly raise the risk of both cancers. She documented the general location of the first "breast cancer" gene. A frenzy of subsequent research followed, and in 1994, the precise location of that gene, BRCA1, was located on the 17th chromosome. Another predisposing gene, BRCA2, was pinpointed to the 13th chromosome the following year. With this new genetic road map, scientists knew where to look for BRCA mutations and soon developed a blood test to screen individuals for cancer-causing mutations in these two genes.

> ### Previvor or Survivor?
>
> Previvor is a term that is often used to describe someone who has an unusually high risk for cancer, inherited or otherwise, but hasn't been diagnosed. A cancer survivor is someone who has been diagnosed and treated successfully.

brain, adrenal glands, and soft tissue. LFS is less common than HBOC or Cowden syndrome; related cancers may appear anytime during a person's life, from childhood to adulthood. Most people with LFS have a mutation in the TP53 gene. *Lynch syndrome* (also called hereditary non-polyposis colorectal cancer syndrome) is one of the most common hereditary cancer syndromes. It develops from mutations in the EPCAM, MLH1, MSH2, MSH6, or PMS2 genes. It significantly increases the risk for colon, uterine, and ovarian cancers, and may also increase risk for pancreatic, prostate, and breast cancer.

RISK ASSESSMENT, GENETIC COUNSELING, AND GENETIC TESTING

The US Preventive Services Task Force, a panel of national experts that develops evidence-based guidelines for health care and prevention, recommends a three-step process to identify men and women who may be at high risk for cancers due to a BRCA mutation:

1. Primary risk assessment with a validated risk assessment tool by your primary care doctor.
2. Genetic counseling, if indicated by the risk assessment tool.
3. Genetic testing, if indicated by genetic counseling.

Primary Risk Assessment

Certain red flags can signal the possible presence of a harmful gene mutation in the family. If you have any of the following factors, your medical team will use the Tyrer-Cuzick, BRCAPRO, or other genetic risk assessment tool to determine whether you have a high likelihood of having a BRCA mutation and you should be referred to a genetic counselor. A *genetic counselor* can then further evaluate your personal and family history to determine whether you would benefit from *genetic testing*, a procedure that shows whether you've inherited a genetic change that predisposes you to disease or cancer. (A primary risk assessment isn't recommended if your personal history, family history, or ancestry doesn't suggest the possible presence of a harmful BRCA mutation.)

- A known genetic mutation in your family.
- A diagnosis of breast cancer before age 50.
- Ashkenazi Jewish heritage.
- A personal diagnosis of breast, ovarian, peritoneal, or fallopian tube cancer.
- A blood relative (grandmother, mother, sister, or aunt on either side) with breast cancer before age 50.
- A relative who had breast cancer in both breasts or had triple-negative breast cancer.

What If You Don't Know Your Family History?

If you were adopted at birth or you aren't aware of your family history, you may have a couple of options to find information about your biological family's health history. One option is to ask your adoptive parents or the adoption agency whether they have any information about your family medical history. Another option, if you have your birth parents' names, is to review public records such as birth or death certificates that may give you more insight into your family's background. If you were adopted through an open adoption, it may be possible to reach out to biological family members to inquire about their medical history. If this isn't possible, talk to your primary physician about whether following general medical practices for women at average risk is best for you. You may want to consider genetic counseling and testing if you develop breast or ovarian cancer before age 50. Genetic counseling is also warranted if you're a man with an unknown family history and you develop breast cancer at any age.

- Both breast and ovarian cancer in a single individual or on the same side of the family.
- Multiple relatives on the same side of the family with breast, ovarian, peritoneal, or fallopian tube cancer.
- A man in your family has had breast cancer.

Genetic Counseling

If you suspect that cancer runs in your family or your primary risk assessment indicates that you should have genetic counseling, a certified genetic counselor can interpret your family's *pedigree*, a chart of the cancers among multiple generations of family members, to determine whether a pattern of hereditary cancer exists (figure 5.3). It's important to obtain and document information about each relative's health condition, age of diagnosis, date of birth, and cause of death for relatives who are deceased.

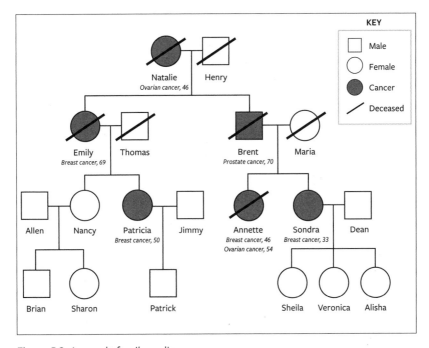

Figure 5.3. A sample family pedigree

The National Comprehensive Cancer Network (NCCN), a consortium of the nation's leading cancer experts who dictate standard-of-care guidelines in oncology, recommends genetic counseling before genetic testing. It's a critical first step, even if you decide not to be tested.

Trained and experienced in disease-related genetics and psychosocial counseling, genetic counselors don't try to persuade you to be tested or make decisions about testing for you. Rather, genetic counselors provide information and guidance before and after genetic testing, so that you and your family members can make informed medical decisions. They provide several services, including:

- Discussing the benefits and limitations of genetic testing.
- Identifying any hereditary cancer syndromes in your family.
- Determining which family members, if any, should consider genetic testing, and in what order.
- Deciding which genetic tests are most appropriate.
- Interpreting genetic test results and explaining what they mean.
- Estimating your cancer risk, whether or not you have an inherited mutation.
- Discussing ways to manage and reduce your cancer risk.
- Explaining how a mutation affects your risk of another cancer and clarifying treatment options if you've already been diagnosed.

Estimating Your Hereditary Risk

BRCA risk is calculated from studies of large multicancer families, so scientists can't be sure how much risk results from environmental exposures or lifestyle behaviors that are shared by family members. Lacking more definite estimates, genetics experts use a range of numbers to describe hereditary cancer risk, and even this range varies. Researchers at Johns Hopkins University developed composite

Questions for Your Genetic Counselor

- Does my family history show a pattern of inherited disease?
- Who in my family should be tested first for an inherited mutation?

If you're the best one to be tested
- For which mutations will I be tested?
- How reliable are the test results?
- What does the test mean for me and my family members?
- What are my options if I test positive?
- Will my test results change my treatment? (If you're currently being treated.)

estimates for decade-by-decade and lifetime BRCA risk based on the aggregate findings of nine studies (table 5.2). Knowing your 10-year risk is helpful when you're considering options to reduce it. As an example, if you're 34 years old and have a mutation in BRCA2, you might feel comfortable waiting to have preventive mastectomy until you near age 50, when your risk begins to escalate significantly. (Your personal risk factors for breast cancer also somewhat reduce or increase your chance of a diagnosis.)

Compared to the average male, men who carry a BRCA mutation have a higher lifetime risk for breast cancer: about 2 percent for men with a BRCA1 mutation, and about 7 percent for men with a BRCA2 mutation. Having a mutation in either gene also increases a man's risk for melanoma, prostate, and pancreatic cancer, so more frequent screening and careful surveillance are important. Some studies suggest that mutations in the PALB2 gene may also raise breast cancer risk in men, although to what extent is unclear.

Ask your doctor for a referral to a certified genetic counselor, or use the National Society of Genetic Counselors website (www.nsgc.org) or the National Cancer Institute's online directory (www.cancer.gov/cancertopics/genetics/directory). If there are no genetic counselors within a convenient distance, Informed Medical Decisions (www.informeddna.com) provides genetic counseling by telephone.

Table 5.2. Ten-Year Risks of Breast and Ovarian Cancer in Women with BRCA Mutations

	Percentage Breast Cancer Risk: BRCA1	Percentage Breast Cancer Risk: BRCA2	Percentage Ovarian Cancer Risk: BRCA1	Percentage Ovarian Cancer Risk: BRCA2
By age 30	<1	1	Almost none	Almost none
By age 40	2	10	4	2
By age 50	14	22	14	2
By age 60	32	36	28	10
By age 70	47	49	40	18
By age 80	57	49	40	18
Lifetime	64	56	55	31

Source: S. Chen and G. Parmigiani, "Meta-analysis of BRCA1 and BRCA2 Penetrance," Journal of Clinical Oncology 25, no. 11 (2007): 1329-33.

Genetic Testing

Genetic testing is a sort of medical crystal ball. The glimpse it gives of the future isn't a guarantee that you'll develop breast cancer, but it can tell you if your risk is steep. Testing gives you options to reshape your future, particularly if you have a risk-raising mutation: wait and see what happens, screen more often to detect cancer early, or preemptively act to reduce your odds of developing breast or other cancers.

Anyone with a family history of breast or ovarian cancer can benefit from genetic counseling, but not everyone will benefit from genetic testing, because most people don't have inherited mutations. Using a sample of your blood or saliva, genetic testing explores segments of BRCA or other genes where mutations are known to occur. Early genetic testing searched only for known mutations in BRCA1 and BRCA2. Newer *multigene panel testing* simultaneously checks for mutations in these genes as well as other genes that can be involved in hereditary breast cancer. Up to 50 percent of people who meet criteria for BRCA testing are found to have a mutation in a cancer-causing gene other than BRCA (figure 5.4).

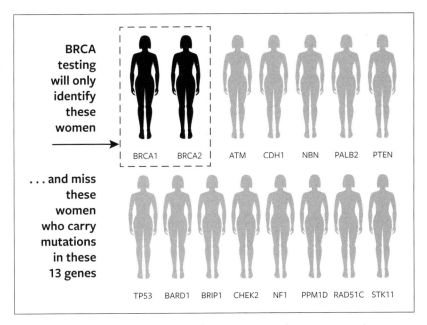

BRCA testing will only identify these women

BRCA1　BRCA2　　ATM　CDH1　NBN　PALB2　PTEN

...and miss these women who carry mutations in these 13 genes

TP53　BARD1　BRIP1　CHEK2　NF1　PPM1D　RAD51C　STK11

Figure 5.4. BRCA testing doesn't identify mutations in other cancer-causing genes

A genetic test result can be positive, negative, or unclear; any of these can have a significant psychological and emotional impact on you and your family. A positive result means that you have a known genetic mutation and an associated high risk for breast, ovarian, and other cancers. In this case, your genetic counselor will calculate your risk and explain how different risk management actions can reduce your chance of a diagnosis. Test results that are labeled *no mutation detected* mean that your test showed no evidence of known mutations in the genes that were scanned. This may mean that you don't have a mutation and that you have average risk for breast cancer. It may also be possible that you do have a mutation in a gene that wasn't tested or in a gene that is currently not known to be associated with increased risk. If you have a strong family history of cancer and test negative for a BRCA mutation, your risk is thought to be greater than that for a woman in the general population but less than the risk for someone who has a BRCA gene mutation.

If several people in your family have had cancer, a negative test result may mean that some unknown mutation is the culprit. A test result of *variant of uncertain significance* means that a change was recognized in one of your genes, but it's unclear whether that change increases cancer risk.

Identifying and confronting your risk for breast cancer can be frightening, but it's critical to do so. Knowing your risk, especially if it's high, provides the opportunity to be proactive about your health. Whether positive, negative, or unclear, test results can affect you and your entire family. Who else should be tested? Do relatives want to know your results? What, how, and when should you discuss test results with your children? Genetic counselors are trained to help you answer these questions as they support you and your family throughout the counseling and testing process (figure 5.5).

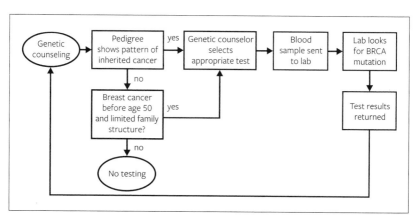

Figure 5.5. The genetic counseling and testing process

Health insurance usually covers the cost of genetic counseling and genetic testing if you have certain indicators that hereditary cancer might run in your family. Some insurance companies require that certain requirements are met, or they may cover the cost of certain tests but not others. Genetic testing can be costly, so it's a good idea to check with your health insurance company to verify coverage. A genetic counselor can also determine if your insurance will cover genetic testing and can help the process go smoothly. Your health insurer may pay for genetic testing only if you have first had genetic counseling. Medicare covers genetic counseling and testing only if you have already been diagnosed with breast cancer. Medicaid coverage varies by state; a genetic counselor or your state health commissioner can clarify your state's policy.

The Genetic Information Nondiscrimination Act (GINA) prohibits health insurers and employers from discriminating against you based on your genetic test results or simply because you have a BRCA mutation. Health insurers are prohibited from denying coverage, defining terms of coverage, or charging premiums based on your genetic information. Nor may employers make decisions about hiring, promoting, or terminating employment based on your genetic information. GINA is a federal law. Many states have legislation that provides additional protection. GINA does not apply to life, disability, or long-term care insurance, however.

PART TWO

Finding Breast Cancer and Dealing with a Diagnosis

CHAPTER 6

Screening Tools and Technologies

Mammography provides an early warning of precancerous changes, and since the 1970s it has been the gold standard for detecting early-stage breast cancer.

In the world of medicine, acting sooner is almost always preferable to acting later. The next best thing to preventing cancer is detection and early intervention before cancer cells can multiply and grow. Regular screening doesn't prevent breast cancer, but it can often identify the earliest stages of a malignancy, when it's most treatable and survival is more likely.

Women have long been schooled on the importance of checking their own breasts, having a doctor examine them, and getting routine *mammograms*, x-ray pictures of the breast. Although these three screening methods have been used for decades, the medical community disagrees about when, how, and even if women should continue using them.

BREAST SELF-EXAM

Screening methodologies for breast cancer are judged by how well they improve survival. Breast exams haven't been shown to do that. Even though 40 percent of women with breast cancer discover their own breast lumps, they tend to have the same rates of survival as women who don't, and twice as often, they undergo biopsies that don't find cancer. As a result, most medical organizations no longer recommend routine *breast self-exam* (BSE). The American Cancer Society's screening guidelines for women of average risk for developing breast cancer state:

> Research does not show a clear benefit of physical breast exams done by either a health professional or by yourself for breast cancer screening. Due to this lack of evidence, regular clinical breast exam and breast self-exam are not recommended. Still, all women should be familiar with how their breasts normally look and feel and report any changes to a healthcare provider right away.

You might argue that finding a tumor in your breast before it has a chance to advance is still quite important, and doing so might mean the difference between keeping and losing your breast. The benefit of BSE is that you may discover something unusual between mammograms—a dimpling of the skin or a nipple that has a discharge or becomes inverted. While the American Cancer Society (ACS) and some other organizations no longer recommend BSE, they agree that it should be optional, based on a woman's conversations with her doctor. Many physicians still believe in the value of breast self-exams, especially for finding fast-growing cancers that may be missed by other types of screening or that develop between screenings. National Comprehensive Cancer Network (NCCN) guidelines, which are generally recognized as standard clinical policy, recommend education about optional BSE at age 20 for women of average breast cancer risk.

How to Check Your Breasts

It's important to know how your breasts normally look and feel, so that you'll recognize any changes that occur. If you decide to examine your breasts, do so on the same day each month, three to five days after your menstrual period, when your breasts may be less tender, or any time of the month if you no longer have periods. Carefully examine both breasts in front of a mirror, in the shower, and while lying down (figures 6.1 and 6.2).

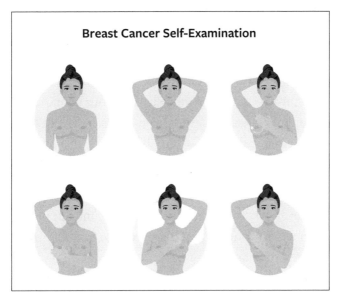

Figure 6.1. Look for changes in front of a mirror

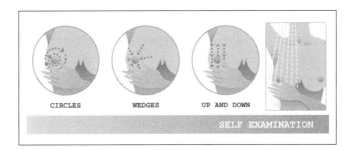

Figure 6.2. Feel for changes in the bath or shower

- Stand in front of a mirror as you visually inspect your exposed breasts. With your arms at your sides, face forward and then turn to one side and then the other, noting any skin irritation, swelling, or changes since your last exam.
- Check carefully underneath both breasts. Look for any discoloration or dimpling of the nipples. Gently pull on each nipple; notice any discharge (other than breast milk if you're nursing).
- Now put your palms on your hips and press firmly to flex your chest muscles. Look for any changes in your breasts as you

face forward and then repeat as you again turn from side to side. Note that your breasts are probably not exactly the same size or shape—most women don't have naturally symmetrical breasts.

- With your hands over your head, press your palms together, so that your chest muscles flex. Again, observe your breasts from the front and sides.

Press all around your breasts for lumps, bumps, and areas that feel unusual. (Soaping your wet hands will make this easier.) Using your fingers, feel everywhere you have breast tissue: in your breasts, up to your collarbone, in your underarms, across to your breastbone, and out to the sides of your ribs.

Move the pads of your fingers around your breast in a circular motion from outside to inside. Feel your underarms and just below your collarbone as well.

Feel for changes while lying down

- Lie down with a pillow under your left shoulder and your left arm behind your head.
- Move the pads of the fingers on your right hand up and down or in small circles around your left breast. Search your entire breast and underarm in this way, varying the pressure of your fingers as you lightly skim over the breast skin, then press deeper into the tissue.
- Gently squeeze your nipple to check for lumps or a discharge.
- Repeat the entire process on your right breast.

What Does a Breast Lump Feel Like?

Breast lumps may feel different depending on their location and whether they're benign or malignant. Lumps that are irregularly shaped, hard, painless, and don't move are more likely to be cancerous. Any lump that doesn't go away in a week or two deserves an appointment with your doctor. She may want you to have a mammogram or to watch the lump for any changes.

Having a breast lump doesn't necessarily mean that you have cancer. About 80 percent of the time, lumps turn out to be harmless. Many benign conditions can cause a lump to form, including the following:

- Cysts that are caused by blocked glands in the breast tend to be smooth or round, soft or hard, and may become sore just before your menstrual period.
- Fluid-filled cysts that develop just beneath the breast skin feel soft and a bit squishy. Cysts that are deeper in the breast tissue feel more like hard lumps.
- Fibroadenomas, benign tumors made up of glandular and connective breast tissue, usually feel smooth and rubbery.
- A mass of fat *necrosis* (dead tissue) that occurs from breast surgery, radiation therapy, or a blow to the breast usually forms a round and firm lump.
- *Mastitis*, a bacterial infection that can develop if your milk ducts become blocked while you're nursing, may create a warm, tender lump that you can easily feel.

Lauren's Story

Although Lauren found a lump in her right breast, her doctor didn't feel anything abnormal and suggested that she come back in three months. She decided to see him again in four weeks because she still felt the lump. Again, her doctor examined her breast, and again he found it to be normal. A subsequent mammogram also showed nothing suspicious. Lauren eventually consulted with another doctor who felt a subtle abnormality when he examined her breast. Soon after she had a biopsy, which revealed that the area was indeed cancer. The moral of this story is that it's important to follow your instincts, and even more so to biopsy any lump or thickening that persists even if the mammogram and other imaging studies are negative. It's possible and it's also important to be heard in the medical world, although it sometimes takes persistence.

CLINICAL BREAST EXAM

A *clinical breast examination* (CBE) gives your doctor an opportunity to find an early change that you might miss. Like breast self-exams, clinical breast exams haven't been shown to reduce breast cancer deaths, and they rarely find early cancers in women who have routine screening mammograms. The American Cancer Society no longer recommends CBE as part of a woman's overall screening regimen, while NCCN guidelines recommend a clinical exam every three years for women of average risk during their 20s and 30s, and annually starting at age 40 (table 6.1). If you feel more comfortable having your breasts examined by a professional, ask your doctor to include a CBE as part of your annual physical examination. During a clinical breast exam, your doctor will carefully inspect all around, over, and under your breasts and in your underarms to identify any lumps or changes that might warrant further investigation.

Table 6.1. Breast Exam Guidelines for Women of Average Risk

	Breast Self-Exam	Clinical Breast Exam
ACS	Learn about benefits and limitations	Every three years from ages 20 to 39; annually thereafter
NCCN	Breast self-awareness encouraged	Every one to three years from ages 20 to 39; annually thereafter
ACOG	Breast self-awareness encouraged	Every one to three years from ages 20 to 39; annually thereafter
USPSTF	Not recommended	Insufficient evidence to make a recommendation

Abbreviations are as follows: ACOG, American College of Obstetricians and Gynecologists; ACS, American Cancer Society; NCCN, National Comprehensive Cancer Network; USPSTF, US Preventive Services Task Force.

MAMMOGRAPHY

Mammography, x-ray technology that produces images of breast tissue, provides an early warning of precancerous changes, and since the 1970s it's been the gold standard for detecting early-stage breast cancer. While mammograms aren't foolproof, they identify about 87 percent of breast cancers, including those that are too small or too deep within the tissue to be felt by you or your doctor. This is important, because catching tumors when they're still quite small greatly increases survival. By one estimate, increased screening mammograms and treatment advances saved more than a half million lives between 1990 and 2018.

Screening mammograms look for cancer and abnormalities in breast tissue. They're noninvasive and are generally completed in about 15 minutes. You'll need to undress from the waist up, so it's a good idea to wear a shirt that you can remove easily. As you stand in front of the mammography equipment, a female technician places one of your exposed breasts between two plates of the machine; one plate holds the breast in place while the other takes the image (figure 6.3). Two views of each breast are taken, one from top to bottom and the other from side to side. Radiologists, medical doctors who

The Right Facility Makes a Difference

Studies show that you're less likely to have a false positive mammogram result if you choose an FDA-approved imaging facility that has up-to-date equipment and radiologists who are experienced in interpreting mammogram images. A safe bet is to choose a facility that holds an accreditation by the American College of Radiology, an organization that sets standards for training, equipment, safety, and quality assurance. Find the nearest location by using the search tool on the organization's website (www.acr.org). Ideally, look for a facility that is designated as a Breast Imaging Center of Excellence. Mammography callbacks are also less likely when your prior mammograms are available for comparison. If you're visiting a particular mammogram facility for the first time, bring an x-ray or a digital copy of your last mammogram with you.

specialize in interpreting medical images, review mammograms for unusual changes. They also look for irregularities in the breast, including *macrocalcifications*, calcium deposits that appear as large white dots that often develop from aging or benign breast conditions, and *microcalcifications,* small white flecks that are usually harmless, yet when clustered in certain patterns can signal breast cancer. If your natural breasts have been enlarged with breast implants, your mammograms should be performed in a facility with technicians who are specially trained to scan breast tissue with implants in place. Your doctor may want you to have an *ultrasound* as well to distinguish between the implant material and breast tissue.

Diagnostic mammograms can be used as a follow-up test if you or your doctor notice a change in your breast or if your screening mammogram shows something unusual. Diagnostic mammography takes more time because it provides more detailed images from multiple angles. A radiologist may also examine a woman and interpret her

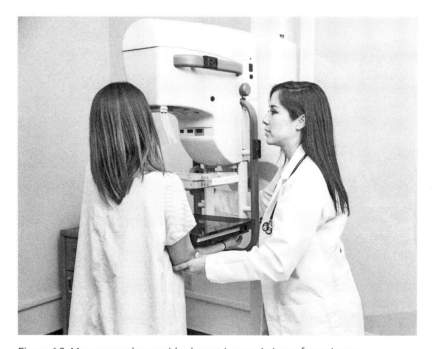

Figure 6.3. Mammography provides breast images in just a few minutes

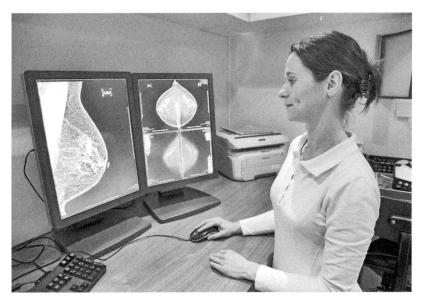

Figure 6.4. Evaluation of mammogram

x-ray findings. Results from a screening mammogram are usually available in about one week; diagnostic results may take less time if the radiologist is present or longer if old films need to be obtained and reviewed for comparison (figure 6.4).

Sometimes mammogram results are wrong. About 10 percent are *false positives*—questionable or suspicious results that require further testing or a biopsy, which then shows that the detected change is benign. After your first mammogram, the chance of having a false positive is about 7 to 12 percent, depending on your age. That rate is higher if you're younger and have dense breasts. After 10 annual mammograms, the chance of having a false positive result increases to about 50 to 60 percent. You're more likely to have a false positive if you have a family history of breast cancer, take estrogen replacement, or you've had previous breast biopsies. About 20 percent of mammograms, particularly in women with dense breasts, produce a *false negative*, meaning that they fail to detect existing breast cancer. False negatives are worrisome, because they fail to indicate active disease in the breast, thereby delaying diagnosis and treatment.

Tips for Minimizing Mammogram Discomfort

Compressing the breast to flatten it for several seconds gives a clearer image of the tissue. This isn't painful for most women, although some find the pressure to be uncomfortable. Here's how to minimize or avoid that discomfort.

- Schedule your mammogram just after your menstrual period when your breasts are least tender.
- Avoid caffeinated beverages, which can increase breast tenderness, for a couple of weeks before your mammogram appointment.
- Take an over-the-counter pain reliever about 30 minutes before your procedure.
- Let the technician know if you have fibrocystic breasts or if you typically have painful mammograms.
- Ask for a mammography pad, a thin rubber cushion that is placed between the breast and the mammography plate.
- Take a few deep breaths before the compression begins. Exhale and hold your breath for a few seconds while the image is taken.
- If you're breastfeeding, ask your doctor whether you should delay your mammogram until you're no longer nursing.

Types of Mammography

Mammograms can be taken with traditional, digital, and three-dimensional (3-D) technologies. All three modalities use low-energy x-rays to produce high-quality images of breast tissue. The experience is about the same regardless of which technology is used, although images and results can differ. Traditional mammography produces two-dimensional images on x-ray film, while newer *digital mammography* creates sharper computerized images that can be enlarged to more easily spot abnormalities—the difference is similar to taking photographs with film and then upgrading to a digital camera. A large clinical study, the Digital Mammographic Imaging Screening Trial, used traditional and digital mammography to screen the breasts of almost 50,000 women from ages 47 to 62. Both methods were equally effective, but digital mammography was superior in screening young women with dense breasts, so fewer of them needed to repeat the process. Digital technology is also somewhat safer: on average, a digital mammogram emits about 22 percent less radiation, although the amount of radiation in newer film mammography is also quite small.

Tomosynthesis (also called 3-D mammography) is a more advanced technology. It uses low-energy x-rays to capture several images of the breast from different angles. These images are then combined into a 3-D picture of the breast. Unlike the single images produced by standard and digital mammograms, three-dimensional mammography takes sharper views and multiple images of breast tissue segments than two-dimensional mammography. Viewing segmental images of the breast is more precise and more sensitive than traditional mammography, reducing the chance of false positives. Tomosynthesis identifies small cancers that standard mammography would miss and reduces callbacks for additional imaging. It's especially effective for women with dense breast tissue.

Screening Dense Breasts

Women who have dense breasts have more glandular tissue than fatty tissue. On a mammogram, dense tissue looks white, just as cancer does, making it more difficult to spot abnormalities. As women's health expert Dr. Susan Love says, "It's like looking for a polar bear in the snow." As women age, particularly after menopause, breast volume is mostly made up of fat, which allows malignant and other abnormal lesions to stand out in contrast.

Having dense breasts raises the risk for breast cancer. The risk is somewhat higher if you have mildly dense breasts. Your risk is four to six times greater if you have very dense breasts, and if you have dense breasts and you're diagnosed with breast cancer, you also have a greater likelihood of developing a tumor in the opposite breast. This elevated risk may be caused by cells in milk-producing lobules that actively divide and are more likely to mutate and become cancerous. Compared to fatty tissue, dense tissue surrounding the lobules may also produce more growth hormones that encourage cell division. Your doctor can advise whether your dense breasts should be screened with ultrasound or other imaging methods in addition to mammography. Some research shows that combined screening with digital or 3-D mammography, MRI, and ultrasound is most effective for dense breasts, but this is by no means standard.

Are Your Breasts Dense?

More than half of women in their 40s have some degree of density in their breasts, ranging from a mix of glandular and dense tissue to almost entirely dense. The level of density generally reduces as you get older and gain more fatty tissue—only 25 percent of women in their 70s still have the same breast density they had as younger women. Breast density needs to be confirmed by a mammogram; it can't be determined by the size of your breasts or how they feel.

Density can be inherited, so if your mother has dense breasts, you probably will too.

The Mammogram Controversy

Although the lifesaving benefits of mammography are well documented, some experts question whether improved treatments should get most of the credit. Mammography is unquestionably beneficial for women who are 50 or older, when most breast cancers occur, and generally, experts agree that women of this age should have regular mammograms. They disagree about mammography for younger women and the potentially harmful effects of cumulative lifetime radiation from mammograms.

For many years, the American Cancer Society recommended annual mammograms beginning at age 40. Then in October 2015, the guidelines were revised to recommend that women of average risk begin annual mammograms between ages 45 and 54, with continued screenings every other year until their life expectancy is less than

10 years. For young women of average risk, exposing the breasts to screening radiation before the age of 40 isn't recommended, especially since breast cancers are rare at this age.

In the absence of consistent, clear-cut screening directions, what should you do? Your doctor can help you understand the benefits and risks of having mammograms. Together, you can consider your personal circumstances and risk factors and decide when it's best for you to start and stop having mammograms (table 6.2).

Table 6.2. Mammography Screening Guidelines for Women of Average Risk

	Age at First Mammogram	Frequency	Age at Last Mammogram
ACS	40–44 (by choice)	Annually	When life expectancy is less than 10 years
	45–54	Annually	
	55+	Every two years, or annually by choice	
NCCN	40	Annually	When health conditions limit life expectancy
ACOG	40	Annually	After age 75, depending on health status and longevity
USPSTF	50	Every two years (ages 50–74)	Insufficient evidence to assess benefits/harms of screening after age 75

Abbreviations are as follows: ACOG, American College of Obstetricians and Gynecologists; ACS, American Cancer Society; NCCN, National Comprehensive Cancer Network; USPSTF, US Preventive Services Task Force.

MRI AND BREAST ULTRASOUND

While mammography adequately screens most women for breast cancer, *magnetic resonance imaging* (MRI) is also recommended for some women. Using magnetic fields and radio waves, MRI creates hundreds of detailed two-dimensional breast images from several angles that show the structures within the breast in great detail, even in dense breasts.

During a breast MRI, you're positioned face down with your breasts hanging through openings on a sliding table that has built-in electronics (figure 6.5). Once you're properly positioned, the table slides into the MRI machine and the imaging begins. It's very important to remain still during the exam. An MRI exam is noisy—you'll hear what sounds like loud hammering—and it can be an uncomfortable experience if you are claustrophobic. Keeping your eyes closed or having a cloth placed over them can help you remain relaxed and calm. Screening MRI exams are *outpatient procedures* that generally last between 30 and 60 minutes.

Mammography and MRI are complementary screening methods, with each capable of finding cancers missed by the other. MRI isn't an appropriate primary method of breast cancer screening, but it can provide additional information when mammography finds something unusual, and it can augment mammography in high-risk women. MRI is more sensitive than a mammogram. It can detect suspicious areas and very small tumors or groups of cancer that generally don't appear on a mammogram. It can also detect some areas that may represent ductal carcinoma in situ (DCIS) and may more precisely identify

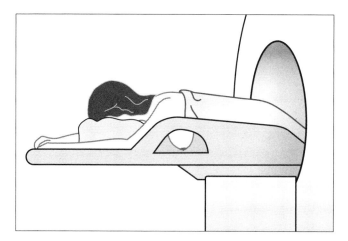

Figure 6.5. Screening with breast MRI

multiple masses in the same breast. Compared to mammography, breast MRI produces more false positives: it finds more abnormalities, both harmless and harmful. It's also more expensive and isn't as widely available.

Are Breast MRIs Safe?

Breast MRIs for women with high risk or dense breasts are performed with an intravenous contrast dye that includes the metal *gadolinium*. Injected into a vein before imaging, the dye "lights up" areas in breast tissue that have increased blood flow, as cancers do. Most gadolinium is excreted by the kidneys with 24 hours; however, there is some concern that small traces may linger and potentially accumulate in the brain, bones, and kidneys for several years and adversely affect a patient's health. While the FDA considers the dye to be safe for most patients, until its long-term safety can be studied, the agency doesn't recommend it for patients with kidney issues. Exposure to gadolinium may trigger nephrogenic systemic fibrosis, a rare kidney disorder, in some people with advanced kidney disease.

If your doctor recommends an MRI with contrast, let him know if you're pregnant, have kidney problems, are allergic to imaging dyes, or if you've had previous scans with gadolinium. Request a copy of the patient information for the dye, and read it carefully. If you're concerned about safety, ask which type of gadolinium will be used; the "macrocyclic" type doesn't appear to have the same risk as the "linear" type.

Breast Ultrasound

Breast ultrasound (also called sonogram) is safe, noninvasive, and painless. It uses high-frequency sound waves to create images of the breast interior. (It's the same technology that is used during pregnancy to assess the health of a fetus.) Ultrasound isn't routinely used on its own for breast cancer screening, but it is used to further investigate findings on mammography and to evaluate a palpable lump found during a breast exam. Ultrasound is a noninvasive way to determine whether a breast lump is a benign, fluid-filled cyst or a solid mass that could be malignant. Compared to mammography, ultrasound may provide clearer images of dense breast tissue, and it's the recommended method of evaluating young women with a palpable mass. During a breast ultrasound, you lie on your back while a technician applies a clear gel to your breast skin. Using a handheld device called a transducer, the technician sends sound waves through the gel and into the breast. The sound waves that echo back are collected by the transducer and converted into images by a computer.

Although ultrasound is most commonly utilized to investigate a specific area of concern, bilateral whole-breast screening ultrasound is sometimes used with mammography for screening high-risk women with dense breast tissue. The decision to undergo enhanced surveillance with either bilateral whole-breast screening ultrasound or MRI in addition to mammography should be based on your individual risk factors and estimated lifetime risk of developing breast cancer.

Mammograms, MRI, and Ultrasound: What's the Difference?

Breast imaging technologies have similarities and differences, and each plays a role in breast cancer screening.

- Mammography is a primary method of screening; MRI and ultrasound are most often used to follow-up on abnormalities found by breast exam or a mammogram.
- Mammograms capture images with x-rays, while MRI uses radio waves and ultrasound uses sound waves.
- Mammograms better detect microcalcifications than MRI or ultrasound. MRI and ultrasound can more clearly image dense breast tissue.
- MRI produces more false positives than mammograms.
- Mammograms and ultrasound are less expensive and more widely available than MRI.
- MRI usually takes 45 to 60 minutes compared to 15 minutes for a mammogram or an ultrasound.
- Digital or 3-D mammograms are recommended for high-risk women, but they are optional for women of average risk. MRI is recommended to routinely supplement mammography in high-risk women, but not for women of average risk.

OTHER IMAGING TECHNOLOGIES

Several other technologies are being studied, but they aren't considered to be sufficiently reliable for routine breast screening.

Ductal lavage, sometimes called a "Pap smear for the breast," may suggest an increased risk for breast cancer, but it doesn't usually confirm it. In this procedure, which isn't commonly used or standard, cells collected from the milk ducts are analyzed for precancerous and cancerous changes in high-risk women. If abnormal cells are found, additional imaging is needed before a biopsy, because ductal lavage doesn't identify the origin of the cells.

Molecular breast imaging (also known as an MBI, Miraluma test, or sestamibi scan) uses a radioactive tracer that is injected into the body. Breast cancer cells "light up" as they take up the tracers, and then a special medical scanner can see the highlighted cancer cells. This technology may be useful for women who have dense breasts or a higher-than-average risk for breast cancer, but more study is needed before it can be incorporated as standard of care.

Thermography (also called thermal imaging) measures the temperature of the breast skin. Breast cancer is thought to increase blood flow, which theoretically would increase skin temperature. This test doesn't reliably detect breast cancer, however, and is rarely used.

Paying for Screening Services

Most health insurance, including Medicare and Medicaid, covers the cost of recommended mammograms and other recommended breast cancer screenings. The Affordable Care Act requires health plans started after September 2010 to cover the cost of mammograms every one to two years for women who are 40 or older without co-payments or co-insurance, even if your annual deductible hasn't been met. If you don't have coverage for a mammogram or can't afford to pay the cost, contact the National Breast and Cervical Cancer Control Program (https://www.cdc.gov/cancer/nbccedp) or Susan G. Komen (www.komen.org) for information about low-cost or free screenings.

SPECIAL SCREENING FOR HIGH-RISK WOMEN

If you have a high risk for breast cancer, you need to be screened more aggressively and more often than women in the general population, because you're more likely to develop breast cancer (table 6.3). Some experts propose that beginning annual mammograms before age 30 may slightly increase breast cancer risk; little long-term research is available on the effect of radiation in BRCA mutation carriers. Additional screening with ultrasound or MRI is often recommended to identify "interval" cancers, particularly aggressive tumors that may grow between mammogram screenings. If you have a BRCA1 or BRCA2 mutation, you should also receive ovarian cancer screening, including pelvic examinations, transvaginal color-Doppler

Table 6.3. NCCN Screening Recommendations
for High-Risk Men and Women

Screening Method	Average Risk	High Risk*
Breast self-exam (BSE)	Education about breast changes and BSE at age 20	BSE training starting at age 18
Clinical breast exam	Every three years during 20s and 30s, and annually starting at age 40	Every 6–12 months, starting at age 25
Mammogram	See table 6.2	Annually with digital or 3-D technology, starting at age 25 if MRI is unavailable
MRI	Not recommended	Annually, starting at age 25
		Annually with mammogram, ages 30–75

Note: Screening recommendations for men with mutations in a BRCA gene include a baseline mammogram, and monthly breast self-exam training and annual clinical breast exam beginning at age 35.

*Includes women with a personal history of atypical hyperplasia, lobular carcinoma in situ (LCIS), ductal carcinoma in situ (DCIS), or invasive breast cancer; a family medical history that raises breast cancer risk to 20% or more; radiation to the chest before age 30; or an inherited mutation in BRCA gene. Discuss screening recommendations with your doctor if you have a predisposing mutation in a different gene.

ultrasound, and a CA-125 blood test every six months starting around age 35. Screening for ovarian cancer, however, may not detect ovarian cancer at an early stage. Therefore, as discussed in chapter 4, *oophorectomy* (removing the ovaries) is recommended as soon as you've finished having children or by age 40 if you have a BRCA1 mutation and by age 45 if you have a mutation in BRCA2.

CHAPTER 7

Making a Diagnosis

More than a million breast biopsies are performed in the United States each year, but fortunately 75 to 80 percent of them are benign. For a woman who is found to have breast cancer, the biopsy slides are reviewed and tested thoroughly by a trained pathologist to provide her and her oncology team with the information they need for a personalized and optimal plan of care.

A breast cancer diagnosis isn't made solely on the results of a physical exam or an x-ray, even though these may arouse suspicion. When a mammogram, MRI, or ultrasound show an abnormality in the breast, doctors then use a variety of diagnostic tests to further investigate and determine whether cancer is present. A breast biopsy identifies the type of cancer and how it behaves. Other tests determine whether it has spread beyond the breast. Together, these investigative steps paint a clearer picture of the cancer, determine your prognosis, and guide treatment decisions.

BREAST BIOPSIES

When the results of an initial screening are questionable or lead to a suspicion of cancer, a minimally invasive *biopsy* that provides a sample of cells or tissue is the only sure way to confirm or disprove that an abnormality is malignant. Many biopsies are performed with local anesthesia alone or with local anesthesia and "conscious sedation" that makes you sleepy but not unconscious.

Hearing that you need a biopsy can be frightening, especially if you're not sure what to expect from the procedure. But having a biopsy doesn't automatically mean that you have cancer. Out of the more than one million breast biopsies performed each year in the United States, 75 to 80 percent of them are benign. Whether you have a lump, a bump, or a thickened spot of breast tissue, anything that looks potentially worrisome on a mammogram, MRI, or ultrasound is normally followed up with a biopsy. Lumps that feel unusual, even if they can't be seen by mammography, are also biopsied. If the results of a biopsy are undetermined, the pathologist may ask for another opinion or request that a follow-up biopsy be performed. The type of biopsy depends on the size and location of the lesion and how many areas of the breast need to be investigated. If you need a biopsy, ask your doctor which type of biopsy you'll have and what you should expect.

Needle Biopsies

Needle biopsies are performed when a suspicious lump can be seen on a mammogram or felt. They provide only a small sample of cells or tissue for further analysis and aren't intended to remove the entire *lesion* (the area of abnormal change in the tissue).

A *fine needle aspiration* is the least invasive biopsy method. In this quick and typically painless procedure, a radiologist withdraws a few cells from the breast with a thin, hollow needle and a syringe (figure 7.1). This type of biopsy is rarely performed for breast lesions, since the few cells obtained provide the pathologist with limited information. Fine needle aspiration is still used to sample enlarged lymph nodes to determine whether cancer cells have spread from the breast to underarm lymph nodes.

A *core needle biopsy* is more often performed for breast irregularities because it provides a larger sample and more accurately predicts whether a mass is noninvasive or invasive. Compared to a fine needle aspiration, a core needle biopsy produces fewer false negative and false positive results. It's a bit more invasive because it requires a larger needle. After a local anesthetic is applied, a small incision is made to pass the needle through to the center of the lesion. The incision is small—up to one-quarter inch—and doesn't usually leave a noticeable scar. While a fine needle aspiration withdraws only cells, a core needle procedure provides four to eight small cylinder-shaped plugs of tissue. Recovery is minimal. The mild discomfort from bruising, bleeding, or swelling can be managed with an over-the-counter pain reliever (figure 7.1).

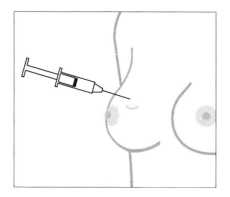 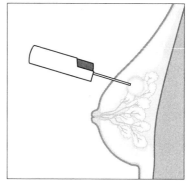

Figure 7.1. Fine needle and core needle biopsies

Image-Guided Biopsies

When a biopsy is needed on a lesion that can't be felt, radiologists or surgeons may perform an *image-guided biopsy*, which uses the same technology that identified the unusual area—mammography, MRI, or ultrasound—to guide the needle to the desired site in the breast (table 7.1).

A *stereotactic core biopsy* is accurate and minimally invasive. It uses mammography to pinpoint the biopsy site (figure 7.2). You lie on your stomach on a special table with your breast hanging through a hole beneath you. Your breast is compressed between two plates of a mammogram machine, and x-ray images are taken from different angles to guide placement of the needle. When the area to be biopsied is located, the breast is numbed with local anesthetic, and a small

Table 7.1. Image-Guided Biopsies

Breast Change Identified	Biopsy Imaging Used	Biopsy Performed By
Calcifications and other changes	Stereotactic core biopsy (mammogram guided)	Radiologist
A lesion seen only on MRI	MRI guided	Radiologist
A mass that is visible on ultrasound	Ultrasound guided	Radiologist or surgeon

incision is made. Then the machine rapidly pokes the needle into the incision several times to remove tissue samples from a few different areas throughout the lesion. Because the procedure compresses the breast, it isn't the best biopsy method for women with small breasts. Stereotactic biopsy may not be possible for lesions that are close to the underarm.

When an MRI finds a breast abnormality, an MRI-guided biopsy is used to position the needle. The breast skin is first numbed before the needle is inserted. Several passes with the needle may be needed to ensure an adequate sampling is provided before the incision is covered with surgical tape. The entire process takes about 30 to 60 minutes.

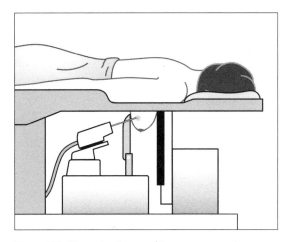

Figure 7.2. Stereotactic core biopsy

If a breast mass can be clearly seen with ultrasound, an ultrasound-guided biopsy is performed. The hour-long procedure is performed as you lie on your back. The physician makes a small incision in the breast and monitors needle placement with ultrasound. After the samples are removed, a biopsy clip is placed at the site, and the incision is closed with surgical tape.

Surgical Biopsies

When possible, it's preferable to have a core biopsy before surgically removing tissue. The needle procedure is less invasive, leaves a small cut, and if it turns out you don't have breast cancer, you're spared a needless operation. When a needle biopsy is inconclusive, a surgical biopsy is needed to confirm the diagnosis. Surgical biopsy may also be performed when a core biopsy shows atypical ductal hyperplasia or lobular carcinoma in situ—benign conditions that can be found alongside invasive cancer.

A surgical biopsy is a minor, outpatient procedure: either an *incisional biopsy* removes a small portion of the lesion or an *excisional biopsy* removes the entire lesion. Tissue is removed through an incision in the skin, which leaves a visible scar, and in some cases, it can cause a noticeable change in the shape of the breast. If you're scheduled to have a surgical biopsy, ask your surgeon beforehand about the placement and length of the incision. You'll be sedated with a local or general anesthesia in the operating room before the procedure begins. Bruising and slight swelling can occur at the biopsy site, but it's usually minimal and quick to heal.

When a breast lesion that needs to be surgically biopsied can't be felt, a *wire localization* is used to guide the surgeon to the questionable area in the breast. After locating the abnormal area with an ultrasound or mammogram, a radiologist then injects a local anesthetic into your breast to numb it before making the incision. Some women find this part of the procedure to be mildly uncomfortable. After your breast becomes numb, a small needle is positioned at the exact spot

Should You Get a Second Opinion Regarding Your Biopsy?

Based on a pathologist's examination of your tissue samples, your doctor can diagnose your disease, recommend treatment options, and form a long-term prognosis. But what if your biopsy result is wrong? While the majority of breast biopsies are considered to be accurate, several studies have found that mistakes can be made. Needle biopsies can fail to detect breast cancer if the tissue sample is taken from the wrong area. Surgical biopsies are less likely to miss a cancerous area, especially when wire localization is used, but even a surgical biopsy can remove tissue from the wrong area of the breast. Pathologists can also make mistakes if they misinterpret cancerous cells as benign, although they often seek another pathologist's input for tissue samples that are questionable or especially complex.

Getting a second opinion for a serious diagnosis like breast cancer can make a difference, especially if it changes your diagnosis and treatment plan. Consider this example: based on the results of your biopsy, you're diagnosed with a particularly aggressive type of breast cancer and your doctor recommends removal of both breasts followed by several rounds of chemotherapy. If another opinion confirms your biopsy result, you can at least be comforted knowing that your treatment is appropriately addressing your condition. If another opinion concludes that your diagnosis is actually a precancerous condition, such as DCIS, you would instead probably have lumpectomy and radiation and avoid losing your breasts and dealing with the toxicity of chemotherapy. Most health care policies cover a second opinion related to a biopsy. If a second opinion conflicts with your original diagnosis, you might even want to get a third opinion.

of the abnormality and threaded with a fine wire. A mammogram is performed to confirm and document the position of the wire in the breast. Now the surgeon knows exactly where to make the incision and remove the tissue sample. The wire is removed during the biopsy. Wire localization takes about 30 minutes.

Clear Margins

When an area of cancerous tissue that is removed during a biopsy is surrounded by a rim of healthy tissue, the biopsy is said to have negative or clear *margins*. This is good news, because it's an indication that all of the breast cancer was removed from the breast. Per published consensus guidelines, the margin required for invasive cancer is no tumor right at the edge. For ductal carcinoma in situ (DCIS), the margin required is 2 millimeters. Positive margins mean that cancer cells are close to or in the edge of the tissue sample, and that additional surgery will likely be needed to remove any remaining malignant cells left behind in the breast. A *close margin* isn't positive or negative. It means that cancer cells are near but not on the edge of the removed tissue.

Waiting for an Answer

After your biopsy, you'll be anxious to get your results, waiting and wondering whether you do or don't have breast cancer. You may have the results of a needle biopsy in two or three days; conclusions from an excisional biopsy can take 7 to 10 days. Not all hospitals have their own pathology labs, so if your biopsy sample needs to be sent to an outside lab for interpretation, the wait could be longer. If your biopsy result is indeterminate, your doctor may need to order additional imaging and testing before you have a definitive diagnosis.

INFORMATION AND ANSWERS FROM PATHOLOGY

Cancers are puzzles, and diagnosing a malignancy is the first step in putting the pieces together. Each bit of information about a lesion or a mass adds to the understanding of its unique nature. The right treatment can't be identified unless your doctor knows how the cancer behaves and understands its weaknesses. Providing such data is the role of the *pathologist*, a medical detective who carefully studies biopsy samples under a microscope in search of clues. Breast cancer *pathology* is a complex and multistep process. Pathologists analyze the biopsy sample for telltale shapes that identify benign, precancerous, or malignant cells. They can make a diagnosis by determining the origin of cancerous cells and whether they're noninvasive or invasive.

Even then, there is still much to discover about a cancer's behavior—what drives its growth and how it thrives—this critical information is ammunition for knowing how to destroy it. All of a pathologist's discoveries from your biopsy are recorded in a *pathology report*, a detailed document that tells your oncologist about the nature of your cancer. Federal law ensures your right to have a copy of your pathology report. If you're not given one after your biopsy, ask your doctor's office staff for a copy as a record of your diagnosis.

The Language of Pathology

Pathology reports differ, depending on the hospital and the procedure performed. A breast cancer pathology report is particularly detailed. It can be overwhelming and may seem to be written in a different language, and in a way, it is. Medical jargon can be confusing, but understanding the basics of the report will help you to better discuss your treatment options with your health care team. Here are a few of the most common pathology terms that you're likely to see on your report:

Origin: Where your breast cancer began—in the ducts, lobules, or, rarely, in the connective tissue.

Gross description: The size, weight, and color of the tissue sample.

Procedure: The type of biopsy—core needle biopsy, surgical biopsy, or other method.

Tumor size: The size of the tumor measured in centimeters.

Location: This describes where your tumor was found: in the upper inner quadrant, the upper outer quadrant, lower outer quadrant, lower inner quadrant, or the axillary tail (tissue that extends beyond the breast and into the underarm).

Position: Superior (top), inferior (bottom), lateral (toward the edge), medial (toward the middle), superficial/anterior (front), posterior/deep (back).

Multicentric: Cancer in different quadrants of the breast.

Multifocal: Multiple cancers that are isolated to one quadrant of the breast.

Microscopic description: How the cancer cells look under a microscope, including tumor stage, grade, and margins.

Histological grade: Describes the aggressiveness of tumor cells based on their appearance and how quickly they reproduce.

Surgical margins: How close cancer cells are to the edges of the tissue sample. Positive margins mean that cancer cells extend to the outer edge of the tissue sample. Clear margins mean that the outer edges of the sample are clear of cancer cells.

Lymph node status: Whether or not cancer cells were found in your lymph nodes (if they were sampled).

STAGING BREAST CANCER

When the type of breast cancer is identified, the next step is *staging* the tumor to describe its size, whether lymph nodes are involved, and to what extent malignant cells have spread within the breast or beyond. This is a complex but essential step for understanding your *prognosis*—your expected chance of recovery—and determining the best treatment. Information from seven categories is combined to assign an overall staging between 0 and IV. The formula includes the globally recognized tumor-node-metastasis (TNM) breast cancer staging system developed by the American Joint Committee on Cancer and four additional biological categories:

- size of the primary tumor (T)
- the degree of lymph node involvement (N)
- whether metastasis has occurred (M)
- tumor grade
- estrogen and progesterone receptor status
- HER2 status
- Oncotype DX Recurrence Score (for cancers that are estrogen receptor positive, HER2 negative, and are not found in the lymph nodes)

TNM Staging Categories

Tumor size. The size of the primary tumor is measured in centimeters at its widest point and is then classified as T1 through T4 (figure 7.3). If multiple tumors are found, the pathology report notes the size and location of each one.

Lymph node status. The "N" in the TNM staging system refers to the number of lymph nodes that contain cancer cells (figure 7.4).

Metastasis. If your biopsy shows that you have breast cancer, your doctor may use additional tests to gather information that will indicate whether it has migrated beyond the breast.

Tumor grade. Invasive breast cancers are assigned a *grade* based on how they appear and how abnormal they are compared to healthy cells. Noninvasive DCIS tumors are graded differently: a designation of low, medium, or high reflects the activity of the cell nuclei (the control center in each cell).

> Grade 1: The cancer cells are small and uniform like normal cells and are slow growing.
> Grade 2: The cancer cells are slightly larger than normal cells, vary in shape, and are growing faster than normal cells.
> Grade 3: The cancer cells appear different than normal cells and are growing faster.

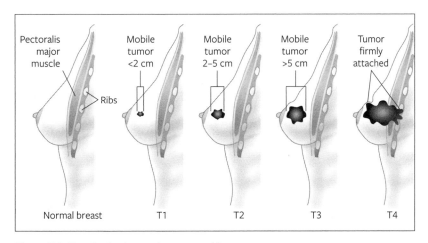

Figure 7.3. Tumor size in centimeters and breast cancer stage

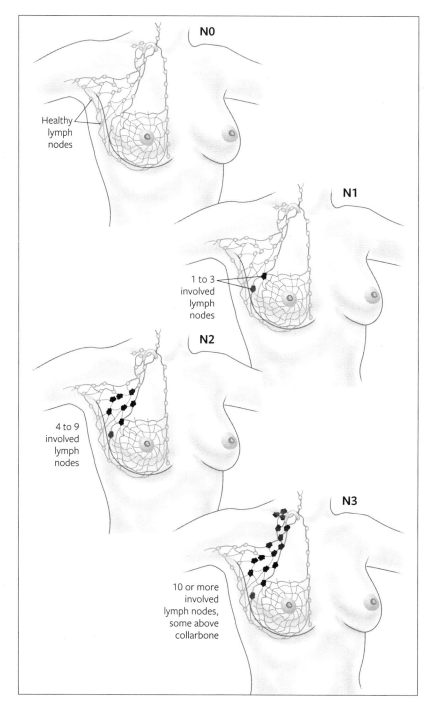

N0

Healthy
lymph
nodes

N1

1 to 3
involved
lymph
nodes

N2

4 to 9
involved
lymph
nodes

N3

10 or more
involved
lymph nodes,
some above
collarbone

Figure 7.4. Breast cancer spread to lymph nodes and breast cancer staging

Tumor-Node-Metastasis Staging Categories

Tumor-Node-Metastasis (TNM) status determines the diagnostic staging of a breast cancer. The National Cancer Institute defines the different stages as follows:

Primary tumor
T0: no evidence of cancer
Tis: ductal carcinoma in situ (DCIS)
T1: 2 centimeters (about three-quarters of an inch) or smaller
T2: greater than 2 centimeters but not more than 5 centimeters
T3: greater than 5 centimeters
T4: any size tumor that is growing into the breast skin or chest wall

Lymph nodes
N0: no node involvement
N1: cancer in one to three axillary (underarm) nodes and/or tiny amounts of cancer in the mammary nodes near the breastbone as identified by sentinel lymph node biopsy (removal of one to five lymph nodes, usually performed during breast cancer surgery, as discussed in chapter 10)
N2: cancer in four to nine axillary nodes
N3: cancer greater than 2 millimeters in 10 or more axillary nodes or in the nodes under the collarbone

Metastasis
M0: no metastatic disease
M1: metastatic disease in distant organs

Hormone receptor status. Most breast cancers are fueled by estrogen and/or progesterone, and the staging process reflects this status in a tumor. As these hormones circulate throughout the bloodstream, they bind to protein molecules called *receptors* on the surface of some cancer cells, triggering cellular growth. About 80 percent of all breast cancers are estrogen receptor positive. Some breast cancers are progesterone receptor positive; they grow in response to progesterone in the same way that estrogen fuels estrogen receptor–positive breast cancers. About 65 percent of breast cancers have receptors for both estrogen and progesterone. Some breast cancers lack receptors for either hormone.

HER2. HER2 is an *oncogene*, a gene that promotes cellular growth and division. Mutations in the HER2 gene overamplify the grow-and-divide message sent to cells. Compared to tumor suppressor genes that put the brakes on tumor growth, an amplified HER2 gene has the opposite effect. HER2-positive cancer cells develop faster and more aggressively because they're constantly bombarded with messages to divide and grow.

Adding It All Up

When all of the information for a tumor has been interpreted, pathologists assign a score between 0 and IV based on the cumulative results of all seven staging factors.

Stage 0 is the earliest stage of breast cancer, such as DCIS that remains within the boundaries of the ducts where it began. Paget's disease of the nipple is also considered to be Stage 0.

Stage I is the earliest stage of invasive cancer.

Stage IA cancer is 2 centimeters or smaller.

Stage IB cancer is less than 2 centimeters in the breast, but the axillary lymph nodes contain a small cluster of cancer cells between 0.2 millimeters and 2 millimeters. DCIS with small amounts of microinvasion—a small cluster of cancer cells that has spread into the surrounding breast tissue—is classified as Stage I.

Stage II is invasive breast cancer that is still confined to the breast but shows signs of growth. It often appears as a lump that can be felt during a breast self-exam or clinical exam. This stage has two possible scenarios.

Stage IIA may be a larger tumor in the breast measuring 2 to 5 centimeters with no lymph node involvement or a tumor in the breast that is up to 2 centimeters in size and involves one to three axillary lymph nodes. This stage also includes breast cancers in one to three lymph nodes in the underarm or near the breastbone where the primary tumor in the breast cannot be found.

A Stage IIB tumor is between 2 to 5 centimeters and involves one to three lymph nodes in the axilla or near the breastbone or is larger than 5 centimeters with no lymph node involvement.

Stage III has spread from the interior of the breast to other nearby tissues, including the breast skin or muscles and bones of the chest wall. It can be more than 2 inches in diameter and has already spread to several lymph nodes, but it hasn't metastasized elsewhere in the body. This stage has three subcategories: Stages IIIA, IIIB, and IIIC (table 7.2).

Stage IV is the most advanced form of breast cancer. At this point, malignant cells have grown beyond the breast and nearby lymph nodes and into the liver, brain, bone, or other parts of the body.

Table 7.2. Breast Cancer Staging Categories

Stage	Tumor Type	Tumor Size	In the Lymph Nodes/Beyond?
0	Noninvasive	0	No
IA (early stage)	Invasive	Up to 2 cm	No
IB (early stage)	Invasive	Up to 2 cm	Yes. Small clusters of breast cancer cells appear in the axillary lymph nodes
IIA	Invasive	Up to 2 cm or	Yes. One to three lymph nodes involved
		2–5 cm	No
IIB	Invasive	2–5 cm or	Yes. One to three nodes in axillary nodes, under the breastbone, or both
		>5 cm	No
IIIA	Invasive	>50 mm	Yes. Cancer has spread to one to three lymph nodes or has spread to four to nine nodes with or without a detectable tumor in the breast

(continued)

Table 7.2. (*continued*)

Stage	Tumor Type	Tumor Size	In the Lymph Nodes/Beyond?
IIIB	Invasive	Any size	Yes. Cancer has spread to the chest wall, to nodes near the breastbone, in nine or fewer axillary nodes, or broken through the breast skin
IIIC	Invasive	Any size or no tumor in the breast	Yes. Cancer has spread to the skin (inflammatory breast cancer), near the collarbone, breastbone, in some axillary nodes, or in 10 or more axillary nodes
IV (metastatic)	Invasive	Any size	Yes. Cancer has spread to bones, lungs, or other parts of the body

UNDERSTANDING YOUR PROGNOSIS

Your *prognosis*—the long-term prediction of your outcome after treatment—depends on the type of cancer, the stage of your disease, and how you respond to treatment. Doctors base a patient's prognosis on several factors, including population-based survival statistics from the National Cancer Institute's Surveillance, Epidemiology, and End Results (SEER) database. These numbers express survival as the percentage of women in the United States who live five years or more after a specific diagnosis, if they're in remission or are still undergoing treatment. These estimates, which include women who died of other causes, is updated only every five years, so they may not reflect the results of earlier diagnoses or newer, more effective treatments.

A different statistic, the disease-free five-year survival rate, is the percentage of women who are alive and free of cancer five years after their diagnosis. Five-year statistics are categorized as localized (no sign of cancer beyond the breast), regional (the cancer has spread beyond the breast into nearby tissues and lymph nodes), and distant (the cancer has spread to distant parts of the body). A number of organizations, including the American Cancer Society, provide information about the latest five-year survival rates for breast cancer and other statistics on their Cancer Facts and Figures website (https://www.cancer.org/research/cancer-facts-statistics/all-cancer-facts-figures/cancer-facts-figures-2020.html).

These five-year estimates don't mean that you won't live beyond five years; most women with breast cancer are treated successfully and live well beyond. Even when these general statistics appear discouraging, each individual is unique and may respond differently to therapy, and it's not unusual for patients to do better than expected.

These projections are only a general indication of how patients with a particular breast cancer respond to treatment; they aren't sufficiently personal to predict your outcome, because you're not average. No database is an exact match for you, because like your personality and your fingerprints, you're unique. Your personal strengths—level of fitness, healthy eating habits, your immune system response, and other factors—affect your prognosis. For these reasons, some women choose to ignore survival statistics. Your doctor can help you understand how effective your treatment is likely to be and the odds of your cancer recurring. Then you can decide whether survival statistics are too general or too impersonal to worry about.

CHAPTER 8

After a Diagnosis

CHARTING A COURSE AND ASSEMBLING YOUR TEAM

A patient who is diagnosed with acute appendicitis doesn't typically have multiple treatment options or discussion about her choice of treatment. After a diagnosis of breast cancer, however, women are asked to participate in complex, shared decision-making with their doctors. Women who are educated about their condition are more engaged in their own care, better equipped to participate in shared decision-making, and may have better outcomes.

Life changes when you hear, "It's cancer." What do you do now?

First, you need time to absorb the shock and disbelief you probably feel. You may ask yourself why you deserve cancer or what you did to cause it, especially if you exercise regularly and eat well. Even if you suspected that your biopsy might be positive for breast cancer, the reality can be more distressing than you may have expected. Talk with someone who is trusted and close, because you need the support they can provide. Give yourself time to grieve and to mourn what is happening in your body. Then lay out and execute a plan of attack to understand your emotions, learn everything you can about your diagnosis, choose your cancer care team, and decide on a treatment plan with your doctor (figure 8.1).

UNDERSTANDING HOW YOU FEEL

There's no right or wrong way to react to a cancer diagnosis. It's okay to be afraid, and it's all right to worry about the uncertainty,

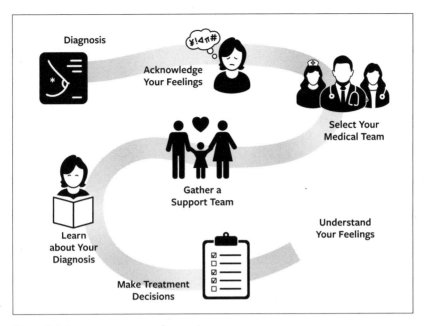

Figure 8.1. A strategy to move forward

numbness, or fear that you may feel—any way you react is normal. Dealing with the shock of a diagnosis can be difficult, and it's natural to feel afraid, angry, or any range of emotions as you absorb what you've heard. Chapter 20 describes these feelings: what to expect and how to manage them.

Right now, you may be unable to process any information or think about what to do next. At some point, though, it's important to accept and understand your diagnosis. Acknowledge your feelings, abandon negative self-talk, and focus on moving forward, rather than looking back to see what you might have done differently. Although this can be easier said than done, it's important to remember that breast cancer is treatable, and most often it's a curable disease.

You didn't cause your breast cancer. You may worry that your actions, such as coloring your hair, using certain cosmetics, getting too much or not enough sun, or injuring your breast may have caused breast cancer to develop. You're not to blame, and while many emotions are understandable, your diagnosis has no relationship to any single thing that you did or didn't do. Nothing you could have done would have prevented your breast cancer. At this time, we don't have a completely reliable medical or holistic strategy that can prevent breast cancer. The truth is that we don't know exactly what causes breast cancer. Some families are at higher risk, but for most people diagnosed with breast cancer, there is no identifiable cause.

Don't Panic

Whether you're a "glass half full" or a "glass half empty" type of person, coping with a breast cancer diagnosis is stressful. Your first reaction may be to panic, which can shut down your feelings, leaving you in a state of shock. While panic is a natural reaction to something so unsettling, it can make your situation seem worse than it actually is. When you're in this state, you're unable to think clearly, retain information, absorb what you hear, or make decisions. If you feel panic about your diagnosis, try these steps:

- If your heartbeat is racing, you feel confused, or you begin shouting or saying unreasonable things, recognize that you may be in a state of panic.
- Breathe deeply for a full minute or two to calm yourself and rid your body of adrenaline that's released during a panic.
- Understand your diagnosis, prognosis, and path forward. Having clear answers to these issues can restore your sense of control and replace fear with a sense of order and positive expectation.
- Talk to your doctor about what you fear. Or speak with someone you trust: your partner, spouse, friend, social worker, or a member of the clergy.

SELECTING YOUR MEDICAL TEAM

Cancer care is a team effort that involves multiple medical professionals who coordinate and provide your care. Although your primary physician or gynecologist may have delivered your diagnosis, you'll likely need a medical oncologist to coordinate your treatment. Over the course of your treatment, your medical team may change as you finish treatment with one specialist and begin with another. You may see a surgeon before and after a lumpectomy, for example; if you then require radiation or chemotherapy, you'll also begin seeing a radiation oncologist or a medical oncologist. Your treatment and outcome depend upon the knowledge, dedication, and ability of these experts.

- A *medical oncologist* specializes in cancer treatment. This is the doctor who will most likely coordinate your overall treatment plan.
- A *radiation oncologist* specializes in treating cancer with radiation, determines the appropriate type and amount of radiation you should receive, and supervises radiation therapy.
- A *breast surgeon* is usually who you see when you have a lump or an abnormal mammogram. Breast surgeons perform needle biopsies, and if cancer is diagnosed, they surgically remove part or all of the breast.
- An *oncoplastic surgeon* is a breast surgeon with *plastic surgery* training who can reshape the remaining breast tissue for better shape and symmetry after a lumpectomy.
- A *plastic surgeon* can reconstruct your entire breast if your treatment plan includes mastectomy.

Your cancer care may also involve other specialists. You might consult with a gynecologist if you're concerned about fertility issues related to treatment or have menopause-like symptoms from chemotherapy. Your doctor may recommend a physical therapist if treatment-related stiffness or pain develops, and a nutritionist can outline dietary choices that will give your body the balanced nutrition it needs during treatment. The support and guidance of a psychologist, social worker, or other counselor can help make difficult times easier.

Nurses and nurse practitioners can become friends and allies in the treatment process. They not only provide professional services—they're also understanding and compassionate sources of information and comfort. Oncology nurses do much more than take your vital signs. They may perform a physical exam, administer chemotherapy and other medications, answer questions, and generally strive to understand what you need and how to give it to you. You may find that they spend more time with you and get to know you better than your doctor.

Choosing Your Doctors

Where do you find the right doctor to lead your treatment? Your primary physician or the surgeon who performed your biopsy can recommend a trusted oncologist. The American Society of Clinical Oncology (ASCO) provides a free, searchable database of member oncologists available at www.cancer.net. Similarly, your oncologist will direct you to a radiation oncologist or other specialists that you need. Most community hospitals have staffs of excellent doctors with experience treating breast cancer, many of whom have been trained at larger academic centers before practicing in a community setting. Numerous major universities and community hospitals have breast cancer treatment centers with multidisciplinary teams of physicians in a single location. Representatives at your health insurance company can also provide the names of specialist physicians, although they can't vouch for their expertise. Family members and friends who have been previously treated can also be good sources of recommendations of who they do or don't recommend and why.

It's perfectly reasonable to ask your physicians about the extent of their experience treating the type of breast cancer that you have. They shouldn't be offended. The best physicians, those who are compassionate and excellent at their craft, will respond with honesty and humility, regardless of their age or experience. Not every doctor you meet will resonate with you. Some may be too impersonal, too impatient, or too abrupt for your taste. Choose doctors who have technical ability and empathy in equal measure, and who treat you with respect and solicit your opinion and concerns, because your relationships with them will last beyond your initial treatment consultation and into follow-up care.

AN EXPERT'S VIEW

Communication Is Key

A slide used in medical school depicts four types of patients. The first patient says, "Doctor, do whatever you want. I just want to live." The second patients says, "Doctor, I demand this of you." The third says, "I just can't make up my mind." And the fourth patient says, "Doctor, based on your clinical judgment and recommendation, and on my own personal understanding and desire, I think we'll go with . . ." It's a good slide because it demonstrates a range of starting points, a range of perspectives from which to seek a meeting of the minds between a woman and her doctor. The first patient relinquishes too much authority and power. As surgeons, we're here to offer guidance, not to make all the decisions. The fourth patient, at the opposite end of the spectrum, is empowered by her own care plan.

—*Theodore N. Tsangaris, MD*

The New Doctor-Patient Partnership

Physician-patient relationships have dramatically changed in the last decade. Doctors are more open, and patients tend to be more informed. Women who are educated about their condition are more engaged in their own care, are better equipped to participate in shared decision-making, and have better outcomes. Doctors frequently respond to communication cues from their patients. If you remain silent or ask few questions, your doctor may be less inclined to share information as liberally as you would like. Tell your doctor of your preferences: whether you prefer things described in lay terms rather than medical language, you do or don't want to know statistics, or you'd like to discuss treatment benefits and risks specifically or generally. Encourage your doctor to be open and clear about potentially distressing information, even when it's hard to hear (table 8.1).

Table 8.1. Optimal Doctor-Patient Communication

Your Doctor's Responsibilities	Your Responsibilities
• Encourage questions	• Be prepared; take lists of specific questions to your appointments
• Show empathy and give reassurance	
• Ask you how much you want to know	• Provide accurate and complete information
• Adjust the flow of information to your preference	• Be open and honest about your concerns
• Engage you to participate in developing your treatment plan	• Speak up if you need something explained, spelled, or repeated
• Pause frequently to make sure that you're taking in what's being said	• Actively participate in decision-making
	• Understand that not all treatment decisions need to be made immediately

What to Expect at Your First Appointment

A lot of things need to happen during the first appointment with an oncologist, including getting to know your history, performing a physical examination, reviewing laboratory studies, answering questions, and synthesizing all of this information into treatment recommendations. This first visit is also an opportunity to create a meaningful doctor-patient connection that calms your fears and worries, gives you a sense of hope, and builds a foundation of trust and a sense of forward motion toward getting and staying well. This appointment may also include a discussion of your treatment options, although your oncologist may first want to have the results of additional tests. Experts say that we forget 50 percent of what we hear in a doctor's office, because hearing so much new information at such

Questions to Ask Your Doctor about Treatment

It's easy to become so overwhelmed that you forget what you wanted to ask, so it's a good idea to be prepared before you meet with your doctor. Here are some questions to ask your doctor:

- Do I need additional tests before you can recommend a treatment plan?
- What are my treatment options and the associated benefits and risks of each?
- Which option do you recommend and why?
- What side effects should I expect?
- Will this treatment affect my daily activities and quality of life?
- Will this treatment cure me?
- If this treatment doesn't work, what other options do I have?
- What are the consequences of watchful waiting instead of treatment?
- When do I need to make decisions about my treatment?
- Is this treatment covered by my health insurance?

an emotional time can be overwhelming. If possible, bring someone with you who can provide emotional support and take notes while you focus on listening.

GETTING A SECOND OPINION

Having the right treatment the first time is important, although doctors sometimes disagree about what that should be. Pursuing a second opinion from another medical oncologist, radiation oncologist, or surgeon is a good idea to confirm your diagnosis and treatment plan. Getting another opinion isn't a rule or a requirement, though some insurance companies require one before providing coverage for certain treatments. Another opinion can be especially helpful if you're unsure, confused, or conflicted about how to proceed. In some cases, it's unwise to proceed without one, especially if you have a questionable diagnosis or if your doctor recommends an experimental or particularly toxic treatment. A second opinion can also inform you of newer treatment options that you may not know about.

To find an oncologist for a second opinion, ask your doctor for a referral to a breast cancer specialist who is in a different medical practice. Many local hospitals and academic medical centers have physician referral services that provide consultation for a second opinion. The National Cancer Institute's Cancer Information Service lists centers that provide state-of-the-art cancer treatment (www.cancer.gov /contact/contact-center). If you'd like an opinion from a well-known but distant cancer facility, ask about a telephone or video consultation. When you call for an appointment, explain that you're looking for a second opinion and ask what records or data you need to forward or bring with you—your mammogram films, pathology report, or other test results. Choose a physician who is experienced or an expert in treating your specific diagnosis. Most oncologists are adept at treating common breast cancers, for example, yet some may have less experience with advanced cancers or tumors that are hard to treat.

If a first and second opinion agree, you can be confident that you're on the right course and then decide which physician you prefer based on your interactions. If the second opinion favors a different treatment—one doctor may strongly feel you need radiation

Questions to Ask When Getting a Second Opinion

- What experience do you having treating my type of cancer?
- What is your success rate for the treatment you recommend?
- Have you treated breast cancer patients who have my underlying health issues (if you have any)?
- Will I need any other diagnostic tests before you make a recommendation?
- What treatment plan do you recommend and why?
- What clinical guidelines or evidence-based research supports your recommendation?
- What are the short- and long-term benefits and risks of the treatment you recommend?
- Have you recommended this treatment to other patients in my situation?
- Will my health insurance pay for this treatment?

after a lumpectomy while another may consider it unnecessary, for example—ask about its short- and long-term effects and why it would be beneficial for you. When two medical opinions are different, it's often helpful to discuss this openly with the physicians who provided them to understand whether the differences are minor or substantial. You can then evaluate the pros and cons of each one, follow up with your doctors, and discuss the matter with a friend or relative who is a reliable sounding board. Another option is getting a third opinion from another breast cancer expert. Ultimately, you may follow the original recommendation, but you have nothing to lose with getting an additional view.

FINDING THE RIGHT INFORMATION

Information empowers. It can answer your questions, give you confidence along each step of the breast cancer journey, and help to restore the control you felt that you lost when you heard your diagnosis. Understanding provides a clearer insight, resulting in more meaningful conversations with your doctor.

The Pros and Pitfalls of Internet Research

The modern world provides endless sources of information about breast cancer—books, articles, lectures, smartphone apps, and even podcasts. With millions of pages of breast cancer information, the Internet is often the first place patients turn to learn more. A few clicks of your mouse delivers mountains of free information to your desktop or mobile device. Much of it is helpful, but much of it isn't, and in many instances, information can be misleading or inaccurate. Consider these tips to make the most of your time online:

- Begin researching only after you know the type, staging, and prognosis of your cancer. Indiscriminate searches for information are bound to return unhelpful results like negative blogs and bad experiences on message boards, and many of them may not even apply to your circumstances. While you can spend countless hours looking for useful information, reading about patients who lost their hair and reacted badly to chemotherapy will unnecessarily worry you if your treatment plan doesn't include chemotherapy, for example. Be specific when you search. A Google search for "breast cancer" turns up more than 500 million individual items; a more specific search for "stage IIA HER2 breast cancer treatment options" returns far fewer results. It will still be an enormous amount of information; however, not all of the entries will be what you're looking for, and many will be duplicated.

- Stick to trustworthy sources. Anyone can publish medical information on the Internet, and it's not always easy to sort fact from fiction. As you sift through your search results, choose journal articles and physician-authored information for reliable, objective information. Pubmed.gov, a resource maintained by the US National Library of Medicine, is an excellent source for published, peer-reviewed studies. Check the publication date to ensure the information is timely. Other reputable sources of information include the National Cancer Institute (www.cancer.gov), the American Cancer Society (www.cancer.org), Susan G. Komen (www.komen.org), Breastcancer.org, and other trustworthy sources. Many large hospitals and cancer centers also provide credible information and videos.

- Know when to stop. Looking for information can quickly become obsessive. The more you learn, the more you want to know. Before you know it, you're stuck on the information merry-go-round, spending days in front of your computer, afraid to miss something important, yet not feeling any closer to the answers you need. At some point, endless searching becomes counterproductive. The goal is not to be your own physician, but to be an informed patient. Internet searches can provide accurate information and answers, but overdoing it can lead to a condition that psychologists call *cyberchondria*, which is when a person experiences heightened anxiety after consuming too much online information.

- Engage with the breast cancer community. Now, more than ever before, breast cancer patients and survivors willingly discuss their experiences. No matter where you are in the journey, a huge sisterhood of patients and survivors are happy to share the details of their treatment and recovery in chat rooms and on social media. (You'll also find online support groups for men with breast cancer.) Online message boards provide information and offer opportunities to interact and share experiences with a supportive network of fellow patients. These are safe places where you can give and receive support. Try the discussion forums at Breastcancer.org, Cancer Support Community (www.cancersupportcommunity.org), and the Johns Hopkins Breast Center (www.hopkinsbreastcenter.org /services/ask_expert). Some discussion groups focus on certain segments of the breast cancer population, such as newly diagnosed, going through chemotherapy, being high risk, and other facets of the breast cancer experience. Facing Our Risk of Cancer Empowered (www.facingourrisk.org) has a robust exchange of information and support for individuals with hereditary cancer. Consider joining a breast cancer support group that can help you as you move through diagnosis and treatment (chapter 21).

- Beware of the negative. It's easy to get caught up in personal blogs and social media. Patients who "have been there, done that" can give insight that a doctor cannot. Their tips and tricks can help you find a comfortable sleeping position after surgery, or sidestep undesirable side effects of chemotherapy and hormonal treatment. Realize, however, that women can be passionately positive or passionately negative about their personal experiences, which you may not share, and their choices may be not the best solution for you. For some people, the Internet is an anonymous outlet for bad experiences, so be wary of personal opinions that focus only on the negative.

- Be skeptical of information touting unique cures. Disregard or cautiously consider advertisements, blogs, or testimonials that claim to have discovered the cure for cancer.

CHARTING YOUR COURSE

One thing that hasn't changed in recent years is that women with breast cancer share the need to make a decision: "What's the best treatment option for me?" Now, more than ever before, women have choices about how their breast cancer is treated. The days of doctors making unquestioned medical decisions for their patients are history. Today's doctor-patient model is one of partnership and shared decision-making that provides a clear path forward and sidesteps the uncertainty that a diagnosis often creates. Women who are actively involved in making these choices, even if they rely heavily on their doctor's judgment, do better emotionally as long-term cancer survivors.

Many medical treatment decisions are straightforward and easily made, like taking antibiotics for strep throat or casting a broken arm. Other decisions are more pressing and need to be made quickly: a patient who is having a heart attack may have limited time to decide whether to give consent to undergo emergency surgery. Unlike these examples, decision-making related to breast cancer is often not straightforward. For most women, breast cancer treatment needs to be timely, but often not immediate. Your cancer developed over several years, and unless it's unusually aggressive, delaying treatment for one or two weeks to learn about your diagnosis, understand your treatment alternatives, and then let everything sink in so that you can make a good decision rather than a fast decision won't be harmful. Some breast cancers, including triple-negative, HER2-positive, and inflammatory breast cancer may be more aggressive, so initiating treatment and getting a second opinion should be done quickly.

Organize Your Information

Dealing with breast cancer means accumulating lots of notes and information. A medical binder can help you keep everything neatly organized in one place. You'll then have everything you need, when you need it, in a single place. Create your own binder or order a sectioned, three-ring medical binder from Cancer101 (cancer101.org). Your binder might have several sections, including:

- a copy of your health insurance card
- your personal and family medical history
- your medicines and doses
- your pathology report
- your medical team contact list
- your support team contact list
- test and scan results
- a calendar of your doctor appointments and treatments
- questions for your doctor appointments
- notes from your doctor appointments
- log of side effects
- list of helpful websites
- insurance information, medical bills, and payments
- blank paper

You may fear that your cancer is getting worse and "spreading" minute by minute and feel a sense of urgency to get rid of it as quickly as possible. Most experts believe, however, that the natural history of breast cancer is measured in months and years rather than days or weeks. At some point, moving forward becomes a leap of faith. You've done your research, have your doctor's input, and know what to expect from each of your treatment options. Now it's time to make informed decisions about your path forward and have confidence in the treatment plan that you and your team decide on.

🔵 AN EXPERT'S VIEW

How Newly Diagnosed Women Address Decision-Making

For most people, a diagnosis of breast cancer is initially terrifying, and clear thinking seems impossible. First there is the diagnosis. Then there are all these medical terms coming at you, all these statistics. And there are so many options— almost as soon as you learn about your choices, you're asked to make decisions. All you want is a guarantee of good health, but you are asked to navigate a path through a strange landscape. Last week, you gave no thought to this path. Today, you must decide which direction to take and who will be your guide. When asked to choose the best surgical option, many women say they feel ill equipped, uninformed, and emotionally strained. "Wait," you think. "I know how to manage real estate, sew my own clothes, practice law, or homeschool my children, but how in the world can I be expected to make crucial medical decisions about breast cancer? I'm no doctor."

—Laura Siminoff, PhD

SHARING YOUR DIAGNOSIS

There are no rules or etiquette about whom to tell or how much to say about your diagnosis. The nature of your relationships will guide you about what to divulge. At first, it may be difficult to talk about your situation. Talking is often therapeutic, however, and most women find that the more they talk about having breast cancer, the easier it gets.

The culture of communication in your family will dictate what you say to relatives. You may not feel comfortable openly discussing the details of your diagnosis if your family isn't close or doesn't talk about health issues. Go with your instincts and do what feels right. Start by talking with a parent, sibling, or the relative with whom you're closest.

Decide when you want to tell your friends, who'll learn about your diagnosis sooner or later—and what you want them to know. The extent you share will be different depending on your relationships. Likewise, you'll decide who will be told in person with a hug or who to inform with a phone call. For friends who are outside your innermost circle, you might even decide to do a group e-mail or video chat. Another option is to create a group website, such as at CaringBridge (www.caringbridge.org), a free source where you can post updates about your condition for friends and family to access.

You'll also need to inform your workplace. You may consider your coworkers to be extended family, as many women do, or prefer not to draw attention to yourself or be treated differently because of your diagnosis. At a minimum, you might explain to your supervisor that you'll be treated for cancer. Decide how much more you want your boss and coworkers to know, or whether you prefer to keep much of the details confidential. As your treatment plan is clarified, you'll need to be more candid with your supervisor about how treatment might affect your workload and schedule and if you'll need an extended leave.

Strange and Wonderful Reactions

Most people react with care and compassion when they learn someone has cancer. It can be surprising, then, when some people seem insensitive or speak disrespectfully when they hear your news. You may feel guilty or pressured by the things people say, even from wellmeaning friends who may need time to get over the shock of your diagnosis, just as you probably did.

Cancer is a universally frightening concept, and hearing that you're coping with it may trigger someone else's fears or memories of coping with their own past experiences with cancer. Although they may feel badly about your circumstances, they may also feel embarrassed, uncomfortable, or unsure of how to act around you. Sometimes people are so shocked when they hear of a diagnosis, they don't understand that what they're saying isn't in your best interest. While most people tend to offer encouragement and support, others may let something unfortunate slip out before they've had time to filter their response. Don't take it personally if people react in an off-putting way.

Your approach to the conversation will set the tone for others; if you deal with it openly, they probably will too. Friends and family often react to the information in response to how you frame the information and present it to them. If you're feeling positive and confident, they probably will too. If you're feeling worried and anxious, they may reflect this back to you as well. This doesn't mean that you need to always present a positive face or attitude. You do, however, have the opportunity to share different information and feelings with different people in your life. Realize that most people know someone who has had cancer, and they may want to share that with you, even the gruesome details. It's okay to speak up if you're offended or upset.

CREATING A SUPPORT SYSTEM

Some patients say that being diagnosed with breast cancer feels like being forced into a club that no one wants to join. It can be confusing, highly emotional, and at times it can be lonely. But no one should cope with breast cancer alone. That's why it's so important to have a support system in place for times when you need it. A healthy support system of people who want to stay connected and committed to you and help you is critical, because it can relieve the stress of living day-to-day with breast cancer. Studies show that having a good social support system during cancer can even improve your outcome.

Help takes many forms, whether it's to accompany you to medical appointments, bring you meals when you're tired or feel ill, or just offering a heartfelt smile or a nonjudgmental ear when you feel overwhelmed, frustrated, or sad. Emotional support, including input from others who have experienced cancer, is also important. Yet even the most caring friends and family won't always know what to say or do. If they don't offer, reach out and ask for help when you need it. If you're independent by nature and you're not used to asking for help, you might need to practice a few times before it gets easier.

Your support system may include:

- family
- friends
- coworkers
- neighbors
- caregivers
- your health care team
- a counselor or social worker
- spiritual or faith-based groups
- breast cancer support groups

PART THREE

Understanding Treatment Choices and Making Decisions

CHAPTER 9

Local Therapy

BREAST CANCER SURGERY

As you make decisions with your medical team, it is important to learn about your breast cancer diagnosis, understand your treatment choices, and carefully consider how breast-conserving therapy or mastectomy will affect your quality of life. For many or most women with breast cancer, both surgical options offer an equal chance of becoming a long-term breast cancer survivor.

Treatment for breast cancer needs to address two separate problems. *Local therapy*—surgery with or without radiation—removes malignant cells in the breast and lymph nodes and prevents cancer from returning there. *Systemic therapy* uses *chemotherapy* and other medications to eliminate breast cancer that has spread beyond these areas. This chapter focuses on surgery, which is the primary local treatment for almost everyone who has breast cancer.

You have a right to choose treatments that you feel are right for you. It is important that you understand and carefully consider the benefits, risks, and side effects of the two major types of treatment: breast-conserving therapy and *mastectomy*. Understand your future risk and talk to your surgeon about the advantages and disadvantages of breast-conserving surgery, mastectomy, or contralateral mastectomy before making your decision.

LUMPECTOMY

Lumpectomy is the most common local treatment for small, early-stage breast cancers. It's also called *breast-conserving surgery* or *partial mastectomy* because it removes the tumor while preserving most of the breast (figure 9.1). Lumpectomy is almost always followed by radiation therapy to destroy any lingering cancer cells in the breast. When a larger tumor is involved, a *quadrantectomy*, which removes about a quarter of the breast, may be performed, although it's an uncommon procedure in the United States.

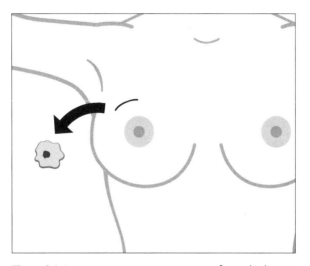

Figure 9.1. Lumpectomy removes a tumor from the breast

Lumpectomy is an outpatient procedure that takes about an hour. Working through a small incision in the breast, your surgeon carefully removes the tumor, along with a border of surrounding tissue. It's important that this rim of tissue has a *clear margin*, free of cancer cells. A *positive margin*, meaning that cancer cells extend to the edge of the tissue removed, indicates a higher risk of recurrence. In that case, a *re-excision*, a second surgery to remove an additional margin of tissue, is performed. Subsequent attempts can be made to remove additional tissue to get clear margins, depending on breast size and the volume of tissue that has already been removed, and whether you're strongly motivated to preserve your breast. When these additional surgeries also fail to obtain clear margins, a mastectomy to remove the entire breast is the next step.

Oncoplastic Surgery

Although lumpectomy preserves most of your breast tissue, it can change how your breast looks. Removing a small area of tissue may not cause more than a dent or dimple along the incision line. When a larger mass is removed, it can cause a noticeable loss of volume or distortion of breast shape, particularly if the area is large in proportion to your breast. *Oncoplastic surgery,* a combination of lumpectomy and plastic surgery, remedies this situation. An experienced *surgical oncologist* can give you the best cosmetic appearance by rearranging your remaining breast tissue to fill in the space left when the lump is removed. If needed, your opposite breast can be lifted or reduced for better symmetry while you're still sedated. If you don't have access to an oncoplastic surgeon, a plastic surgeon can step in to rearrange your remaining tissue after your breast surgeon removes your lump.

If your breast tumor isn't palpable, a radiologist may perform a *seed localization* procedure a week or two before your lumpectomy to mark the location of the tumor. Using a mammogram or ultrasound for guidance (similar to a guided biopsy), a tiny radioactive seed is fed through a thin needle to the lumpectomy site. You'll be awake during the 30-minute procedure, but your skin will be numbed to prevent pain. During your lumpectomy, your surgeon will locate the seed with a handheld radiation detection device and then remove it along with the tumor. No radioactivity remains in your body when the seed is removed. Alternatively, a wire may also be placed to localize a nonpalpable tumor on the same day as the lumpectomy. The wire can be placed using ultrasound or mammographic guidance while you are awake with local anesthesia to numb the skin; sometimes it may be placed using ultrasound guidance in the operating room after you are asleep. The wire helps guide the surgeon to the tumor during surgery; it's removed along with the tumor.

After a lumpectomy, you may feel tired and the area around your incision will be tender for two or three days, but pain is usually minimal and well managed with either prescription or over-the-counter medication. You'll need to wear a support bra around the clock (except when you shower) for at least one week. Bruising may last for a week or two. If some of your lymph nodes were also removed, you'll need a bit longer to recover; you may feel numbness or tingling in your armpit for a few additional weeks or even longer. It may take three or four months before the swelling in your breast completely subsides.

Breast-Conserving Therapy

Most women who have a lumpectomy also need radiation to eliminate any remaining cancer cells that aren't visible but may linger in the breast. *Breast-conserving therapy* (BCT)—lumpectomy with radiation—is standard treatment for early-stage breast cancer to reduce the risk of cancer returning in the breast. Occasionally, radiation is omitted in women who are elderly, in poor health, or who have a particularly small tumor or low-grade ductal carcinoma in situ (DCIS). You're unlikely to have a recurrence in the same breast after BCT. If your cancer does return, however, the entire breast then needs to be removed. You're a good candidate for BCT if you meet all of the following conditions:

- You have DCIS or early-stage invasive breast cancer.
- Your tumor is small relative to your breast size.
- You have only a single area of cancer or close multiple areas that can be removed without distorting your breast.
- You've had no previous lumpectomy or radiation in the affected breast.
- You're willing to have radiation therapy and can meet the radiation schedule.
- You aren't pregnant (this should be considered on a case-by-case basis).
- You don't have scleroderma, lupus, or another connective tissue disease.

The Evolution of Breast Cancer Surgery

Removing more breast tissue was traditionally believed to be the key to a good outcome—a principle that was perhaps true in the treatment of colon, thyroid, and other cancers, but didn't apply to breast cancer. Beginning in the late 1890s, a *radical mastectomy* was the only treatment for breast cancer. This invasive procedure removed a woman's entire breast, her underlying chest wall muscle, and all of her lymph nodes. Although this aggressive approach saved some lives, it also disfigured women for the rest of their lives. Then in the 1970s, the less invasive modified radical mastectomy proved to be equally effective to eradicate breast cancer, while leaving the chest muscle in place.

Recognizing that the primary threat from breast cancer is its ability to advance in the breast and spread to other parts of the body—which can't be resolved with surgery alone—surgeons pursued the possibility of preserving even more breast tissue if surgery was followed by radiation. The NSABP B-06 trial in 1976 further advanced breast cancer surgery when it compared modified radical mastectomy, lumpectomy alone, and lumpectomy with radiation for stage I or stage II invasive breast cancers that were 4 centimeters or smaller. Follow-up at 5, 12, and 20 years showed that long-term survival was similar among the three groups, but rates of local recurrence were quite different. Overall, 14.3 percent of women had a recurrence after lumpectomy and radiation compared to 39.2 percent of women who had lumpectomy alone. Of the mastectomy group, 10 percent had a local recurrence in the chest wall. This important research showed that while more extensive surgery is associated with fewer local recurrences, long-term survival is affected most by the risk of cancer recurring elsewhere in the body, independent of the type of surgery.

In 1990, lumpectomy and radiation became standard of care for early-stage breast cancer when the National Cancer Institute declared it to be "preferable" to mastectomy. Today, with advances in systemic therapy and radiation, the five-year risks of local recurrence are much lower:

- 10 to 15 percent after lumpectomy alone
- 3 to 7 percent after lumpectomy and radiation therapy, depending on the hormone receptor status of the tumor
- about 2 to 4 percent after mastectomy when lymph nodes are clear; the risk is significantly higher when lymph nodes are positive for cancer cells, and radiation therapy reduces this risk to about 6 percent
- the risk of developing a distant recurrence is the same whether you have lumpectomy and radiation or mastectomy

MASTECTOMY

Unlike lumpectomy, which removes a portion of the breast, the goal of mastectomy is always to remove as much breast tissue as possible. Mastectomy is recommended if you have any of the following circumstances:

- Multiple areas of cancer in different parts of the same breast.
- A cancerous area that is too large to remove with lumpectomy.
- A tumor that is large relative to the size of your breast; removing it would eliminate a large portion of your breast.
- Clear margins can't be obtained after lumpectomy and one or two attempts at re-excision.
- Previous radiation to the breast or chest.
- Scleroderma, lupus, or other connective tissue disorder.
- You're in the first trimester of pregnancy (lumpectomy could potentially be performed if chemotherapy were to be given following surgery, and then radiation after delivery).

Types of Mastectomies

A *total mastectomy* removes the entire breast, including the nipple and areola (figure 9.2). Total mastectomy is appropriate for women who have unclear margins or DCIS in multiple areas of the breast. It's also used prophylactically to reduce inherited breast cancer risk. A *modified radical mastectomy* is similar, but it also removes most of the underarm lymph nodes (figure 9.2). Radical mastectomy, which includes removal of the chest wall muscle, is performed rarely and only when cancer has advanced to the chest wall.

A *unilateral mastectomy* (removal of one breast) takes about two hours under general anesthesia; a *bilateral mastectomy* (removal of both breasts) lasts about four hours (figure 9.3). Your mastectomy will take longer if you have breast reconstruction at the same time. If you're having mastectomy alone, your breast tissue and most of your breast skin, including your nipple and areola, are removed through a broad elliptical incision across your chest. All visible breast tissue

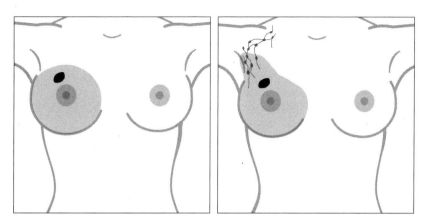

Figure 9.2. Total and modified radical mastectomy

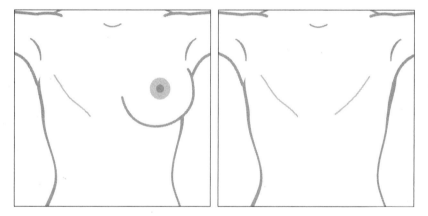

Figure 9.3. Unilateral and bilateral mastectomy

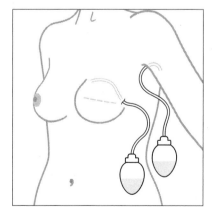

Figure 9.4. Placement of surgical drain after mastectomy

from the collarbone to the ribs and from the breastbone to the side of the ribs is separated from the chest wall and removed. The edges of the incision are then pulled together and closed around a surgical drain, which remains in place for a few days to siphon fluids away from the chest and encourage healing (figure 9.4).

Skin-Sparing and Nipple-Sparing Mastectomies

If you have breast reconstruction at the same time as your mastectomy, a *skin-sparing mastectomy* will remove your breast tissue, nipple, and areola while preserving most of your breast skin. You might also be interested in a *nipple-sparing mastectomy*, which preserves almost all of the visible breast, including most of the skin, nipple, and areola. It requires a breast surgeon with the skill and experience to carefully remove tissue without damaging the delicate blood vessels that support the nipple. If this vital blood supply is compromised, some or all of the nipple may die. To reduce the chance of that happening, nipple-sparing mastectomy incisions are made under the breast, beneath the areola, or along the outside of the areola (figure 9.5).

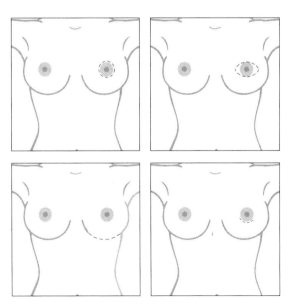

Figure 9.5. Skin-sparing and nipple-sparing mastectomy incisions

Questions for Your Breast Surgeon

- What are my options?
- Why do you recommend this procedure?
- What are the benefits and risks of this surgery?
- What is your experience with this procedure?
- What can I do to prepare for surgery?
- What should I expect in the hospital?
- How long will I be hospitalized?
- What should I expect from recovery?
- What complications can occur?
- When can I resume my normal activities?
- Can you recommend a plastic surgeon for breast reconstruction?

During a nipple-sparing mastectomy, a sample of the tissue at the base of the nipple is removed and sent to pathology. If it's clear of cancer cells, the nipple and areola can be preserved. If the tissue sample contains cancer cells, the nipple and areola are removed.

If you have nipple-sparing mastectomy, your nipple may not look, feel, or react exactly as it did before your surgery. The extent of sensation in the nipple varies between women. Nipple-sparing mastectomy is safe for most women who have small, non-aggressive tumors that aren't located close to the nipple, and for women who have mastectomy to reduce their high risk of breast cancer. You're not a candidate for this procedure if you have tumors or DCIS close to the nipple, you smoke, or you have diabetes or other reasons for poor blood flow. Women with larger breasts may also be poor candidates for nipple-sparing mastectomy, since blood flow to the nipple may be inadequate.

After a mastectomy, you'll spend at least one night and maybe two in the hospital. You may need to stay longer if you have breast reconstruction at the same time. The muscles in your arm, shoulder, and chest will feel tight and sore; you'll need to avoid stretching, pulling, or lifting until your surgeon says it is okay to do so. Your nurse will show you how to care for your surgical drain and how to slowly and gently stretch your shoulder and arm to regain full range of motion and strength. Although you'll be up for short walks the day after your surgery, you'll need extra rest for several days. You'll do better each day, but you may need three to four weeks before you're able to resume all of your normal activities.

CHOOSING LUMPECTOMY OR MASTECTOMY

Because mastectomy removes more tissue than lumpectomy, it seems only logical that it's therefore more effective, but that isn't always the case. Breast cancer is most often diagnosed at an early stage, when the prognosis is generally excellent, so having more extensive surgery isn't necessarily beneficial. Although the risk of a local recurrence is slightly higher after BCT, the chance of metastasis and long-term survival is the same whether you remove or keep your breast.

Breast-conserving therapy is a good choice if your priority is to preserve your breast. (Mastectomy would be necessary if your cancer returns after BCT, because it isn't safe to radiate the same breast more than once.)

For some women, mastectomy is clearly a better treatment choice. It's the best option for the following situations:

- the tumor is large in proportion to the breast
- cancer is in the breast skin
- you've already had radiation to that breast
- you're unable or unwilling to have radiation treatments
- you have separate areas of cancer in two or more different quadrants of the breast; BCT may be possible when the areas are close together

Personal reasons may compel you to opt for mastectomy, especially if keeping your breasts or having them reconstructed isn't critical to your body image. If you're uncomfortable with your risk for recurrence, you may feel that removing your breast will give you greater peace of mind. Choosing mastectomy also adds more complexity to decision-making and lengthens recovery. Should you have breast reconstruction? And if so, are you prepared to have it at the same time as your mastectomy, or sometime in the future? This is another layer of decision-making that requires additional research and careful assessment of advantages and disadvantages of either decision.

Women's decisions about breast conservation vary in different regions of the United States: lumpectomy is more common in the Northeast and Pacific West, while mastectomy occurs more often in the South and parts of the Midwest. Physicians in metropolitan areas and locations where radiation facilities are plentiful are more likely to recommend BCT. Your surgeon's age and medical training may also influence his or her treatment recommendation.

If you have stage I or stage II breast cancer that can be treated with breast-conserving therapy or mastectomy, your doctor will likely leave the choice up to you. If you're struggling to decide which surgery is better for you, consider the comparisons in table 9.1. Weigh the pros and cons of BCT compared to mastectomy, and then make the informed decision that is best for you.

Table 9.1. Comparing Breast-Conserving Therapy and Mastectomy

Lumpectomy and Radiation	Mastectomy
Preserves most of breast	Removes the breast
May need additional surgery	Less likely to need additional surgery
Outpatient procedure	Requires overnight hospital stay
Requires follow-up radiation	Radiation not required if lymph nodes are clear
Shorter recovery	Longer recovery
Risk of local recurrence: 1% per year	Risk of local recurrence: <1% per year
Low risk of metastasis	Low risk of metastasis
Continued mammograms advised	Mammograms no longer needed*

*After unilateral mastectomy, routine mammograms of the remaining breast are still recommended.

AN EXPERT'S VIEW

Personal Feelings Can Affect Decisions

Some women base their decisions about surgery on medical fears that may be unwarranted. Some may choose mastectomies simply because they feel that getting rid of the entire breast is safer. Although they would most likely have the same positive outcome with lumpectomy followed by radiation, the decision to undergo more drastic surgery gives them the peace of mind they need. One breast cancer survivor explained that even though she knew an analysis of the facts showed that she would be a good candidate for lumpectomy with radiation, she had to go with what felt best: "Knowing myself, I knew I would be checking my breast and worrying, so I knew I better go for mastectomy. I discussed it with my husband who stated that he married me because of who I am and not because of my breasts. Mastectomy it was." A woman's "personal relationship" with her breasts is also a major part of the decision-making process. Some women consider their breasts to be their best feature and don't want to part with them, even if it means losing their life. The importance of a woman's breasts in regard to her intimacy with her partner is another personal factor in decision-making. We should never underestimate the impact of a spouse or partner's opinion on a woman's choice. Conversely, for some women, physical appearance is a comparatively trivial factor in the decision-making process, and they don't let anything interfere with their focus on health.

—*Lillie Shockney, former administrative director,*
Johns Hopkins Breast Center

Kathleen's Story

My tumor was found during a mammogram, and I saw the surgeon the same week. After my biopsy, he informed me that the tumor was definitely malignant and said that either lumpectomy or mastectomy was appropriate for me. The "plus" of going with mastectomy was that it would require no radiation treatments. My surgeon said that many women felt that removing their breast gave them the greatest peace of mind that the cancer was gone and "couldn't come back." He wanted to go back in and make wider margins and take out some lymph nodes to determine if the cancer had spread. The tumor turned out to be bigger than he had first thought. That was worrisome, and he was noncommittal about which surgery I should have, saying that it was totally my decision. I made appointments with a radiation oncologist to see if I was a candidate for lumpectomy and radiation. I also saw a plastic surgeon to see what reconstructive surgery would involve if I chose mastectomy instead.

Meanwhile, several well-intentioned breast cancer survivors called to tell me their stories. Several had chosen mastectomy and encouraged me to just "get it off." It was too much information, and I went back and forth about lumpectomy or mastectomy. My husband's roommate, who was a general surgeon, strongly recommended lumpectomy. He talked to me as a good friend, not as a patient. He said he had removed too many healthy breasts where the pathology showed that no other cancer remained in the breast after the lump was removed during biopsy. I wanted to keep my breast, but I wanted a guarantee that all would be well. He looked right at me and said, "Kathy, you could leave here and be killed going home on the highway. There are no guarantees in life." Boy, did I need to hear and think about that! In my panic and fear, I forgot that I needed to make a decision based on knowledge and then trust in my doctors' and my own ability to meet this challenge.

I decided to go with lumpectomy and radiation for several reasons. I had clean margins, and my surgeon felt he had gotten it all. I trusted his judgment, and I didn't want to lose my breast unless it was absolutely necessary. I had such a positive experience with the radiation oncologist, who was so knowledgeable but also so warm and compassionate. My surgeon put me in touch with one of his patients who had a lumpectomy several years before. She was supportive, and it was calming to talk to her during this decision-making period.

Contralateral Mastectomy

Facing the loss of one of your breasts, what should you decide about the other? Increasingly, women, especially younger women, choose *contralateral prophylactic mastectomy* (CPM), removal of their healthy breast to reduce their risk of a future diagnosis. Rates of contralateral mastectomy rose significantly in the past decade, even though it doesn't improve survival or the risk of recurrence any more than lumpectomy and radiation. Health experts are concerned that most women who choose CPM don't really need it—the growing CPM trend is greatest among women of average risk who are prime candidates for breast-conservation therapy. If the risk of contralateral breast cancer is remote for most women, why do so many decide to sacrifice their healthy breasts, even when their doctors advise against it? Here are some reasons for the rising CPM rate:

- Overestimation of risk. Less than 10 percent of women who have lumpectomy or unilateral mastectomy develop breast cancer in the opposite breast. Studies show, however, that women commonly believe their risk is much higher.
- Increasing use of MRI scans before mastectomy. Women who have preoperative MRIs are more likely to request CPM when the scan shows early-stage abnormalities in the healthy breast.
- Fear of repeating diagnosis and treatment. Many breast cancer patients prefer the most aggressive action to avoid another diagnosis, treatment, and potentially another mastectomy.
- Better reconstructive results. Women often view CPM as an opportunity to have both breasts reconstructed at the same time, which may result in better symmetry.

National Comprehensive Cancer Network guidelines recommend CPM only on a case-by-case basis for women who have a high risk of breast cancer in the opposite breast due to a BRCA mutation or Li-Fraumeni syndrome. The American Society of Breast Surgeons agrees and cautions against contralateral prophylactic mastectomy for women of average risk. The organization recommends that patients be engaged in decision-making and have all the information they need to make their decision based on a clear understanding of their risk. The guidelines suggest that contralateral prophylactic mastectomy:

- should be considered for women who have a significant risk for contralateral breast cancer, including women with a predisposing genetic mutation, a strong family history of breast cancer, or a history of chest radiation before age 30
- may be considered for women with other genetic risk or no identified genetic risk but a strong family history of breast cancer
- may be appropriate for other women to limit contralateral breast surveillance, improve symmetry from breast reconstruction, and to manage risk aversion or extreme anxiety
- should be discouraged for women of average risk with unilateral or advanced breast cancer, a high risk for surgical complications, and women who test negative for a known genetic mutation in their family, including a mutation in a BRCA gene

Some women who are at high risk of developing a second breast cancer choose to have ongoing surveillance of the other breast, while others choose to undergo a prophylactic mastectomy. Mastectomy is a choice that cannot be reversed, even with breast reconstruction. Understand your future risk, and talk to your surgeon about the advantages and disadvantages of contralateral mastectomy before making your decision about keeping or removing your healthy breast.

LYMPH NODE SURGERIES

The *lymph system* is the body's filtering and drainage network. Colorless lymph fluid circulates through the body, collecting and transporting cellular debris, bacteria, harmful microorganisms, and cancer cells to small, bean-shaped *lymph nodes*, where they're mostly destroyed by the immune system. Lymph nodes also filter impurities from lymph fluid and then recycle the cleansed lymph fluid back through the system. Our bodies have hundreds of these nodes clustered together like knots on a string.

Lymph nodes are the gateway to the bloodstream and the rest of the body, so when invasive breast cancer is diagnosed, it's important to know if cancer cells have reached any of your nodes. Cancer cells can drain with fluids from the breast through the bloodstream to nearby lymph nodes in the axilla (underarm), above or below the collarbone, or to the internal mammary nodes in the chest and near the breastbone. Removing lymph nodes helps to determine whether breast cancer has spread beyond the breast. It also provides important information that can be used to stage the cancer and help plan your treatment.

Sentinel Lymph Node Biopsy

Removing most or all of the axillary nodes was once thought to be the best way to reduce the risk of metastasis. As we learned with breast cancer surgery, however, removing more isn't always better. We now recognize that removing lymph nodes in the axilla is important to determine the stage of the cancer, but it doesn't improve the chance for a cure as chemotherapy and other systemic treatments do. Removing them can impair the lymph system's ability to adequately filter body fluids, which may then collect in the arm, causing mild to severe *lymphedema*. It's a lifelong condition that is characterized by chronic swelling and numbness that can occur months or years after lymph nodes are removed. Leaving healthy nodes undisturbed or removing as few nodes as possible is preferred.

When early-stage cancer is diagnosed and the lymph nodes appear normal, a minimally invasive *sentinel lymph node biopsy* (SLNB) is performed. If cancer cells spread beyond the breast, they'll first reach the one or two *sentinel lymph nodes* that are closest to the tumor. A sentinel lymph node biopsy begins by injecting a small amount of a harmless radioactive tracer or blue dye into the breast near the

Breast Cancer Surgeries

- Breast-conserving surgery is another name for lumpectomy. Breast-conserving therapy refers to lumpectomy and radiation.
- Lumpectomy removes the cancerous area of the breast along with a margin of healthy tissue.
- Unilateral mastectomy removes one breast.
- Bilateral (double) mastectomy removes both breasts.
- Total mastectomy removes the breast tissue and may also remove the nipple and areola.
- Modified radical mastectomy removes breast tissue and underarm lymph nodes.
- Sentinel lymph node biopsy removes one to four underarm lymph nodes.
- Axillary lymph node dissection removes multiple underarm lymph nodes.

tumor. Lymph nodes then take up these substances as they travel from the breast through the lymph system (figure 9.6). Any cancer cells that spread to the lymph nodes will take this same route. The sentinel lymph nodes closest to the breast that take up the tracer or turn blue show your surgeon which ones to remove. When the radioactive tracer is used, the surgeon uses a handheld Geiger counter to identify nodes that contain the tracer. The sentinel lymph nodes are removed, along with any others that look or feel abnormal, and sent to pathology. If the sentinel lymph nodes are found to contain cancer cells, additional lymph nodes may need to be removed.

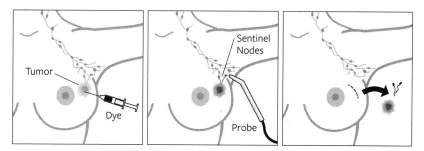

Figure 9.6. Sentinel lymph node biopsy

If the sentinel lymph node (or nodes) is free of cancer, the remaining axillary lymph nodes are also assumed to be clear, and no additional nodes are removed. This approach precludes having more extensive node surgery. Removing fewer lymph nodes means a shorter and less painful recovery, and reduces the risk of developing lymphedema. The ACOSOG Z0011 trial and other studies demonstrated that women who have lumpectomy with radiation with no suspected lymph node involvement gain no benefit by having additional lymph nodes removed, even if pathology finds evidence of cancer in one or two sentinel nodes. Overall survival and the risk of recurrence in the breast or in the axilla is similar whether or not additional lymph nodes are removed, likely due to the effects of radiation and systemic therapy that most women with invasive breast cancer receive.

Axillary Lymph Node Dissection

Compared to sentinel node biopsy, *axillary lymph node dissection* (ALND) is a more extensive procedure that removes more lymph nodes. It's usually performed during a lumpectomy or mastectomy, but it can also be done in a separate operation. An incision about 2 inches long is made under the arm. The pad of fat in the hollow of the underarm, which usually contains most or all of the *axillary lymph nodes*, is then removed and sent to pathology to test for the presence of cancer cells. The number of cancerous nodes you have influences your prognosis more than the extent of cancer found in a single node. Women tend to have different amounts of lymph nodes, so it's difficult to know how many are contained in the fatty tissue until it's examined by a pathologist. Usually, fewer than 20 lymph nodes are removed, but in some women, ALND involves up to 30 or 40 lymph nodes.

The axilla contains three levels of lymph nodes (figure 9.7): level I, below the lower edge of the pectoralis minor muscle; level II, underneath the pectoralis minor muscle; and level III, above the pectoralis minor muscle. A standard ALND removes the lymph nodes from levels I and II. This more invasive procedure carries a higher risk of lymphedema—up to 30 percent compared to just 5 percent after a

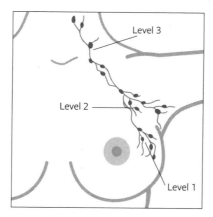

Figure 9.7. Levels of axillary lymph node dissection

sentinel lymph node biopsy. Removing level III nodes doesn't justify the risk of damaging the nerves and blood vessels. Nor does it provide significant benefit, because women with level III lymph node involvement are usually treated with chemotherapy and radiation.

While removing axillary nodes helps to determine the extent or stage of the cancer, it doesn't improve long-term survival, and newer research suggests that removing or radiating nodes is equally effective at keeping recurrence at bay. Radiating nodes is less invasive than removing them, although radiation therapy directed at the lymph nodes increases the risk of lymphedema; the risk with nodal radiation is about half of that with axillary dissection. The combination of axillary dissection and nodal radiation increases the risk of lymphedema compared to either treatment alone, but it's sometimes necessary for patients with many positive nodes to receive both.

Before sentinel node biopsy became the procedure of choice for women with early-stage breast cancer, ALND was the typical way to determine whether breast cancer cells had reached the lymph nodes. It's still recommended in certain situations:

- When the sentinel node can't be identified.
- When enlarged or suspicious lymph nodes are felt on a physical exam or seen on mammogram, ultrasound, MRI, or a *positron emission tomography* (PET) *scan*, an imaging procedure that

uses a radioactive tracer to produce detailed computerized images of the tissues and organs.

- When a needle biopsy confirms cancer in the lymph nodes.
- When three or more positive sentinel lymph nodes are found.
- When the diagnosis is inflammatory breast cancer.

Based on findings of the ACOSOG Z0011 trial, ALND isn't recommended when only one or two sentinel nodes are positive. For women undergoing mastectomy with one or two positive sentinel lymph nodes, management of the remainder of the axillary lymph nodes typically involves a multidisciplinary discussion with surgery and radiation oncology. The multidisciplinary team will weigh the pros and cons of performing an axillary dissection or proceeding with postmastectomy radiation to the chest wall and the area around the lymph nodes.

Guidelines for Lymph Node Biopsies

American Society of Clinical Oncology (ASCO) guidelines for sentinel lymph node (SLN) dissection and biopsy in patients with early-stage breast cancer include:

- SLN biopsy may be offered to women with operable breast cancer and tumors in different parts of the breast, women with DCIS who will have mastectomy, women who had previous breast and/or axillary surgery, and women who were treated with systemic therapy after surgery.
- SLN biopsy shouldn't be performed on women with large or locally advanced invasive breast cancer, inflammatory breast cancer, or DCIS when breast-conserving surgery is planned.
- ALND may be offered to women with SLN metastases who are planning to have a mastectomy; this should be based on a discussion of the pros and cons of ALND versus postmastectomy/nodal radiation.
- ALND shouldn't be performed for women who don't have SLN metastases.

- ALND shouldn't be performed for women with one to two positive sentinel nodes who plan to have breast-conserving surgery with whole-breast radiation.

Recovery Time from Breast Cancer Surgery

- After lumpectomy *without* a sentinel node biopsy, you're likely to feel well enough to resume normal activities and return to work after two or three days to a week or two, depending on the type of work you do.
- After mastectomy *without* breast reconstruction, recovery takes three to four weeks. Fatigue can last several weeks as your body heals.
- After mastectomy *with* breast reconstruction, recovery time can range from four to eight weeks depending on the reconstructive procedure.

FOLLOW-UP SCREENING AND CARE

Unless both of your breasts are removed, regular screening mammograms are still important after surgery.

- After radiation or chemotherapy, which can cause changes in the breast tissue and skin, mammogram images can be more difficult to interpret. A new baseline mammogram is recommended six months after your last radiation treatment, and then generally each year after that.
- When one is breast removed, your remaining breast should still be screened annually with mammography.
- It isn't necessary to image breasts that have been surgically reconstructed after mastectomy, because the breast tissue has been removed. A clinical breast exam every six months is recommended, followed by ultrasound if any concerning findings are detected.

CHAPTER 10

Radiation Therapy

Radiation is a powerful and effective part of breast cancer treatment. Healthy cells can often repair radiation damage and continue to function properly, but cancer cells can't usually make such repairs. Radiation helps to eliminate them.

Radiation therapy (also known as "irradiation" therapy) has been used to treat cancers for more than a century. Initially it was used only as *primary treatment* for individuals whose breast cancer recurred after mastectomy. As the effectiveness of radiation therapy was better understood, it became an important adjunct to lumpectomy for newly diagnosed patients with early-stage breast cancer. Radiation therapy almost always follows lumpectomy, and it is sometimes given after mastectomy. It can also be used to treat recurrent and advanced cancers and occasionally to shrink large tumors so that lumpectomy or mastectomy can be performed.

Radiation is a local therapy: it destroys cancer cells that may have been missed by surgery. Not all men or women with breast cancer need radiation, but it's often recommended as an added measure to reduce the risk of recurrence, and for some individuals, it also decreases the risk of death from breast cancer. The risk of a local recurrence is slightly higher after lumpectomy and radiation than mastectomy, but long-term survival is equivalent for both treatments. Although radiation lowers the chance of a recurrence in the breast, it doesn't treat metastatic disease that is already outside the area receiving radiation. For patients who have breast cancer in their lymph nodes, radiation therapy to the axilla (under the arm) may reduce the risk of developing metastatic disease.

The goal of radiation therapy is to destroy malignant cells while minimizing damage to healthy tissue. With advances in radiology, newer radiation options are now accelerated, more precise, and more convenient. Depending on the diagnosis and pathology of a breast cancer, radiation may be given to the breast, the chest wall, and/or to the lymph nodes. It can be delivered from outside or inside the body and to the entire breast or only to the area that is most susceptible to recurrence. Radiation therapy can be given in a single large dose or in doses that are delivered over multiple treatments.

RADIATION THERAPY BASICS

Invisible and without immediate side effects, radiation therapy produces *free radicals*, unstable atoms that damage the DNA of cancer cells so that they can't continue to grow and reproduce. Although radiation is carefully planned to minimize damage to healthy tissue surrounding the tumor, it's a *cytotoxic* treatment, meaning that it's harmful to both cancer cells and normal cells. Healthy cells can often repair radiation damage and continue to function properly. Cancer cells can't usually make such repairs. They progressively weaken in the days, weeks, and months after treatment until they die; the body then breaks them down and rids itself of them. Traditional *whole-breast radiation* treats the entire affected breast. More recently, *partial-breast radiation* in appropriately selected patients with early-stage breast cancer has been studied as a means to shorten radiation therapy treatment time by delivering doses only to the areas at highest risk around the site of initial disease.

Starting with a Plan

Before any radiation is given, you'll meet with a *radiation oncologist*, a doctor who specializes in radiation treatment. This is the time to ask what type of radiation therapy is recommended for you and why, how many sessions you'll need, how your treatment will affect the chance of your cancer returning, and what side effects may occur. Your radiation oncologist will consider how much radiation you need based on the size, type, and location of your tumor; the surgery you had; and how many of your lymph nodes, if any, are to be radiated. The shape and size of your breast and your chest anatomy are also considered. Based on this information, your radiation oncologist then calculates the total amount of radiation and dose per treatment needed to reduce your risk of recurrence while minimizing harmful effects to nearby tissue. The radiation oncologist designs your treatment plan with the help of a dosimetrist, who helps to create the plan using a specialized computer system, and a radiation physicist, who helps to ensure the safety and accuracy of radiation delivery. A single dose of radiation absorbed by breast tissue is measured in units of "Gray." For example, if your radiation oncology team determines that you need a total of 40.5 Gray over 15 treatments delivered to the whole breast, you'll receive 2.7 Gray during each session. Your radiation oncologist will monitor you throughout your treatment, and adjust the amount of radiation you receive, if necessary. After those 15 treatments, you may then receive an additional dose of 10 to 14 Gray to just the tissue around the surgical site.

TRADITIONAL EXTERNAL BEAM RADIATION THERAPY

Traditional *external beam radiation therapy* for breast cancer is usually an outpatient procedure that begins three to six weeks after surgery. If chemotherapy is recommended after surgery, external beam radiation often starts about three weeks after the last chemo treatment. Patients who are treated with chemotherapy before surgery often begin radiation treatments three to four weeks after their surgery. External beam radiation therapy targets the treatment area with high-energy x-ray beams, in sessions of two to three minutes. Before your first session, you'll have a one-hour planning appointment called a "simulation," to mark the boundaries of your breast area that will be radiated. This

Myths about Radiation

- It's painful. Most patients feel nothing unusual while radiation treatment is being delivered.
- It makes you radioactive. External radiation therapy leaves the body immediately after the machine is turned off. Afterward, neither you nor the people around you are exposed to harmful rays. Internal radiation therapy is active while a radioactive implant is in your body; you're not radioactive after it's removed.
- It makes you nauseous. Although radiation to the brain, liver, or digestive tract to treat metastasized breast cancer may cause nausea, radiation directed to the breast or lymph nodes doesn't. Your radiation oncologist will warn you of this risk if it's expected to happen, and will discuss whether an antinausea medication can be used to manage this side effect.
- It makes you lose your hair. Hair on the head and on other areas of the body is unaffected by radiation; however, any hair on your breast or under your arm may temporarily disappear.

is usually plotted with a *computed tomography* (CT) scan. A *radiation therapist* marks the perimeter of your treatment area with a few tiny dots, which are usually permanent and look like pinpoint tattoos. If your oncologist uses a semipermanent marker, try to avoid washing them off until all of your treatments have been completed so that they don't need to be remarked. Once the marks are made, the CT images are uploaded into the radiation computer. These images help the radiation oncologist develop a plan that ensures that the radiation beams will be accurately lined up for each of your sessions.

During each of your radiation treatments, you'll change into a hospital gown, and a radiation therapist will position you on the treatment table. Positioning is critical to ensure that the radiation is delivered only within the boundaries outlined by the dots. (Positioning sometimes takes longer than the treatment.) You'll need to lie very still in exactly the same position during each treatment. The radiation therapist will then leave the room and turn on the radiation machine, which delivers a precisely calculated dose of radiation to your breast area. You should notice no immediate effects after your treatment and be able to continue with your day.

External beam radiation is delivered to the breast by a *linear accelerator*, a machine that has several built-in safety measures to ensure that it delivers the prescribed dose. The machine generally sends out two beams that pass through the breast from opposite sides of the body; this reduces the amount of lung and heart that is directly exposed to radiation. One beam stretches from the side of the breast to the breastbone; the other begins at the breastbone and moves toward

Protecting Your Heart and Lungs

Because the heart and lungs lie just beneath the chest, care is given to minimize their exposure to harmful radiation. When breast cancer occurs in the left breast, extra care must be taken to protect the heart, which can be damaged and develop issues years after treatment unless it is shielded from radiation. Improved radiation procedures have greatly reduced the risk for heart issues, but it can still be problematic, particularly for people who already have heart problems. Fortunately, contemporary radiation therapy can minimize these risks with a few safety measures:

- Radiation fields can be angled to skim across the chest, rather than passing deeply into the area of the heart.
- Special shields can be positioned in the path of the radiation beam to block its passage into the heart.
- Radiation can be delivered as you lie face down with your breast suspended beneath you. This pulls the breast away from the chest wall, creating greater distance between the radiation field and the heart.
- *Deep inspiration breath hold* moves the heart toward the back and away from the chest. You take a deep breath to fill your lungs with air and hold it while radiation is delivered to your breast. Air in the lung often pushes the chest wall farther from the heart, thereby reducing the radiation exposure to this organ. "Respiratory gating" and "respiratory motion management" techniques may be used to monitor your breathing.
- Three-dimensional conformational therapy and intensity-modulated radiation therapy use advanced software to accurately and evenly deliver radiation to the treatment area while limiting incidental radiation to nearby healthy tissue.

the side. The area or "field" of radiation depends on your surgery and the pathology of your tumor (figure 10.1).

- After a lumpectomy, the entire breast is generally radiated. The radiation field usually extends from the collarbone (or a few inches below) to an inch or two beneath the bottom of the breast. For some patients, treatment may be restricted to the tumor area.
- After a total mastectomy (without lymph node removal), radiation targets the chest wall. In many cases, the radiation field may include the mastectomy scar and any spot on the body where surgical drains were placed.
- If lymph nodes are found to be positive for cancer, the underarm area may also be radiated. Depending on your pathology, the lymph nodes above your collarbone and under your breastbone may also receive radiation therapy.

Can You Have Radiation More Than Once?

Although healthy tissue can tolerate radiation and recover from its effects, radiating the same area more than once can cause more serious complications than the first time around. While a future cancer that may develop in a different area of your breast, in your opposite breast, or elsewhere in your body may be treated with radiation therapy, a recurrence in the same breast is usually—but not always—treated with mastectomy. If you have a recurrence after a mastectomy, surgically removing the tumor followed by radiation therapy may be possible.

Until 2018, daily low-dose external beam radiation treatment was given five days a week—usually Monday through Friday—for five to seven weeks. To ease the burden of such prolonged courses of treatment, shorter courses of radiation are now common in many cases. *Hypofractionated whole-breast radiation* delivers slightly higher doses per day during fewer sessions with the same effective amount of radiation. Clinical trials show that for many individuals with early-stage breast cancer, these shorter regimens are as effective as longer courses of treatment and may have fewer side effects.

American Society for Radiation Oncology guidelines recognize this shortened regimen, preferably 40 to 42.5 Gray given in 15 to 16 doses over three to four weeks, as standard of care for most patients after

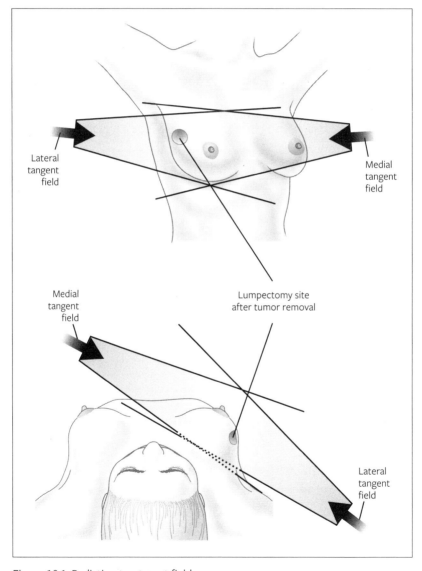

Figure 10.1. Radiation treatment fields

lumpectomy. The five-to-seven-week regimen is still recommended to treat inflammatory breast cancer; breast cancers in the skin, chest wall, or lymph nodes; and/or after mastectomy. An extra "boost" of radiation is often given at the end of the treatment for patients who are younger than age 50, have ductal carcinoma in situ (DCIS), close surgical margins, or high-grade tumors. While the bulk of radiation focuses on the whole breast, the boost targets the most likely area of recurrence, where the primary tumor was located prior to surgery.

ACCELERATED PARTIAL-BREAST IRRADIATION THERAPY

Treatment that is directed only to the lumpectomy site and surrounding tissues rather than the entire breast is called partial-breast radiation. When this type of radiation is delivered over a short period of time (usually one week or less) using relatively high doses of radiation per treatment, it is called *accelerated partial-breast irradiation* (APBI). APBI can be delivered using external beam and internal radiation techniques. This approach is appealing because the area immediately surrounding surgical site is precisely where 85 percent of local recurrence develops. Generally, because a smaller area of the breast is treated, radiation exposure to nearby tissues, including the heart and lungs, may be reduced. Because the course of treatment is much shorter, APBI is often more convenient than standard whole-breast radiation therapy.

The ability to use APBI may be limited by the size and location of the surgical area. Recent research suggests that patients treated with APBI may have a slightly higher chance of developing recurrent breast cancer than those who are treated with radiation therapy to the whole breast. But the chance of recurrence remains so low with either treatment that for many patients, the benefits of APBI may outweigh this small risk.

American Society for Radiation Oncology guidelines identify candidates for APBI as those who meet the following criteria:

- Women who are age 50 or older. Women between ages 40 and 49 with breast cancers that meet all other conditions are considered cautionary for APBI. It isn't recommended for individuals who are under age 40.
- Women who have small areas of low-risk DCIS or small, low-risk invasive breast cancer.
- Women who have negative surgical margins of 2 millimeters or more. Patients with close margins or clear margins less than 2 millimeters may be eligible.
- Women who have no evidence of cancer cells in the lymph nodes.

External Beam APBI

APBI can be treated with external radiation beams that are directed at the breast area, but unlike whole-breast radiation therapy, it targets only the surgical site and the immediately adjacent breast tissue. External beam APBI is given as an outpatient procedure twice a day for five days.

Three-dimensional conformal radiation therapy uses external radiation beams that are delivered from a linear accelerator. A CT, MRI, PET, or PET/CT scan provides 3-D images of the tumor, which are then analyzed by a computer that designs radiation beams that conform to the precise shape of the tumor. This more effectively targets tumor cells with higher doses of radiation than traditional external beam radiation therapy, while exposure to healthy nearby tissue is reduced.

Sometimes the extent of disease or specific patient anatomy requires a special type of radiation planning called *intensity-modulated radiation therapy* (IMRT). IMRT uses special software to bring numerous beams of radiation from many different angles to achieve adequate doses to the breast and/or lymph nodes. This strategy is sometimes needed when cancer is visible on postoperative imaging, the lymph nodes under the breastbone need to be treated, and/or when tissue expanders (used to aid in breast reconstruction with implants) have been placed in the chest. Although IMRT may be useful in reducing high doses of radiation to the heart, lungs, or other organs, it generally exposes a larger area of the body to low doses of radiation compared to 3-D conformal therapy. This is why 3-D conformal planning is used in most cases.

Internal Radiation APBI

APBI can also be delivered with *internal radiation therapy* or *brachytherapy*, as it's commonly known. Brachytherapy can be given as a single treatment during surgery or as a postoperative outpatient procedure over several days. It's delivered with a small amount of radioactive material that is placed in the tumor bed after the malignancy has been removed. In some cases, brachytherapy can also be used to shrink a tumor before surgery or to provide a boost at the end of a traditional external radiation therapy regimen.

Although the overall benefit is the same, brachytherapy procedures may differ depending on the dose of radiation given. High-dose radiation usually involves several 15- to 20-minute outpatient sessions. You're free to leave once the material is removed. Low-dose brachytherapy continuously releases radiation over several days and requires that you be hospitalized during your treatment. Because the radioactive material remains inside your breast during this time, visitors are restricted as a precaution until the radiation source is removed and you're no longer radioactive.

Brachytherapy can be delivered with a single catheter (a hollow tube) or multiple catheters. The most common delivery method uses a special catheter with a balloon at one end. This is sometimes referred to as "Mammosite radiation." Mammosite is the brand name of the first internal delivery system approved by the US Food and Drug Administration (FDA).

The balloon end of the catheter is placed into the space where the tumor was removed, while the opposite end sticks out of your skin (figure 10.2, *left*). Correct placement is then verified with a CT scan. You'll need to visit your medical center twice a day for five days, when the catheter will be plugged into a special device for 10 minutes while radioactive seeds are fed into the balloon. When the machine is unplugged and the seeds are removed, your body is free of radiation. You'll leave each session with the catheter and balloon in place; they'll be removed after your final treatment.

A different method of brachytherapy called *interstitial radiation* uses multiple catheters to treat a larger area of the breast. Between 10 and 20 of the tubes are inserted through small punctures in the skin, implanted around the perimeter of the tumor cavity, and then sutured in place. Guided by a CT image or ultrasound, radioactive seeds are placed into the tubes for a few hours each day. The seeds are then removed, and the catheters are closed but left in place for the next treatment. This multi-catheter procedure is more precise than the balloon method, but each catheter leaves a small scar on the surface of the breast. It's also more difficult to perform and it isn't used frequently, but some radiation oncologists who are highly skilled with this technique recommend it (figure 10.2, *right*).

Brachytherapy is less commonly used than external beam radiation. It's a somewhat newer and promising therapy, although it doesn't have the benefit of long-term studies, as traditional external radiation does. A study involving 16 European cancer centers that randomized 1,300 women with stage 0 to stage II breast cancer to have either whole-breast radiation or brachytherapy found that after five years

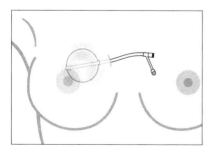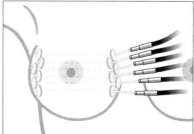

Figure 10.2. Single catheter (*left*) and multi-catheter brachytherapy (*right*)

of treatment, brachytherapy appeared to be as effective as traditional radiation and caused fewer long-term undesirable cosmetic effects.

Physician expertise and candidate selection are both important; at least one study has shown that many patients who have brachytherapy aren't good candidates for the procedure. More studies and long-term follow-up are needed to confirm the safety and effectiveness of this procedure.

Table 10.1. Comparing Radiation Therapies

Whole-Breast External Radiation	APBI External Radiation	APBI Internal Radiation
Targets entire breast; may include an extra "boost" of radiation to the surgical site	Targets the surgical site and minimal surrounding tissue	Targets the surgical site and minimal surrounding tissue
Takes three to six weeks	Takes about one week	Takes about one week
Painless	Painless	Can be painful at the catheter site
Delivered by linear accelerator	Delivered by linear accelerator	Delivered with small radioactive seeds
Multiple low doses	Fewer high doses	Fewer high doses
Outpatient procedure	Outpatient procedure	Outpatient or inpatient procedure
Can cause side effects in the whole breast and the surrounding area	Minimizes side effects outside the surgical site	Minimizes side effects outside the surgical site
Reduces risk of recurrence throughout the whole breast	Reduces risk of recurrence at the surgical site	Reduces risk of recurrence at the surgical site

OTHER RADIATION THERAPIES UNDER RESEARCH

Scientists continue to search for ways to make radiation even more precise, more effective, and more convenient for patients. Although the following examples of new radiation therapies are offered in some treatment centers, they require specialized equipment, are not standard of care, and may not be covered by your health insurance.

GammaPod, another type of radiation system, delivers higher doses in one to five treatments, reducing treatment time. The continuously rotating system combines thousands of beam angles that target the tumor but spare surrounding tissue. Approved by the FDA in 2017, GammaPod has not been widely studied and so far, it has limited availability.

Proton therapy uses positively charged energy particles that deliver radiation to treat breast cancer in a precisely defined area. It begins four to eight weeks after surgery or chemotherapy and lasts five to seven weeks. In some cases, proton therapy results in lower doses of radiation to the heart and lungs than x-ray therapy. While this may be a particularly important advantage when treating tumors in the left breast, early evidence suggests other side effects like skin irritation may be high with proton therapy as compared to x-ray therapy, and use of protons requires special training and expertise among the radiation oncology team. This is a relatively new type of radiation delivery that requires further long-term study.

Intraoperative radiation therapy (IORT) is a method of partial breast radiation that delivers radiation through the lumpectomy incision at the time of surgery. Once the tumor is removed, the applicator of an IORT machine is inserted into the lumpectomy incision to deliver a single, high dose of radiation directly into the tumor site for 25 to 30 minutes. The applicator is then removed and the incision is closed—lumpectomy and radiation are completed in a single visit to the operating room. Radiation is limited to the lumpectomy site, with minimal dose delivered to neighboring tissue and organs. IORT provides direct line-of-sight accuracy—the physician can see the area that needs to be treated. It's more convenient for the patient, generally results in fewer side effects, and is less expensive than conventional radiation treatment. Two large trials that compared whole-breast external beam radiation to IORT, however, found that although

Lumpectomy without Radiation

Patients often ask if they can be successfully treated by lumpectomy without radiation, but unfortunately, lumpectomy alone doesn't eliminate all microscopic cancer cells. For most women with early-stage cancer, destroying cancer requires a one-two treatment punch, and postoperative radiation is that second punch. The risk of recurrence in the breast after lumpectomy alone can be up to 30 percent over 20 years. Radiation therapy decreases that risk to about 14 percent or less, which is close to the average woman's odds (12 percent) of having a diagnosis. But a small, select group of patients who have lumpectomy can forego radiation, including those over age 70 who have small estrogen-positive tumors that will be treated with hormone therapy. Women who have a serious or life-threatening illness or who are too elderly or too frail to tolerate radiation can instead be followed carefully after lumpectomy. Radiation therapy would probably be recommended for a 40-year-old woman who has a lumpectomy to remove a 2-centimeter infiltrating ductal cancer, but not for an 88-year-old woman with multiple serious medical illnesses who has a lumpectomy for a 1-centimeter, low-grade area of DCIS and who will start hormone treatment after her surgery.

survival rates were similar, IORT had a higher rate of breast cancer recurrence in the treated breast. Another disadvantage of IORT is that the final pathology isn't available until after the procedure. If the surgical margins or the sentinel node contain cancer cells, additional whole-breast radiation is then necessary.

Candidates for IORT are individuals over age 50 who have small areas of DCIS or small early-stage invasive cancers that have clear surgical margins and no lymph node involvement. For well-selected patients, the gamble that no additional radiation will be needed may be worth the effort. If you're treated with IORT, you'll need routine long-term follow-up for at least 10 years to screen for any recurrence.

RADIATION AFTER MASTECTOMY

Many women who have a mastectomy don't require adjuvant radiation treatment, but it's an important part of treatment if you have a higher-than-average risk of recurrence in the chest wall or in the axilla. After mastectomy, the risk of local recurrence in the chest wall is 2 to 4 percent; cancer found in the lymph nodes may significantly raise the risk of a future recurrence in the chest wall or the lymph nodes. Radiation after mastectomy would be recommended for a 65-year-old woman with a 5-centimeter breast cancer that extends into her chest wall and multiple axillary lymph nodes with cancer. It probably wouldn't be recommended for a 60-year-old woman who had a 1-centimeter invasive breast cancer who had a mastectomy with a negative sentinel lymph node biopsy.

If you plan to have breast reconstruction after your mastectomy, radiation treatment can affect the timing of your reconstruction and the plastic surgery procedure you choose. Read more about this in chapter 11.

Do's and Don'ts of Radiation Therapy

- Do keep the treated area out of sunlight.
- Do wear loose-fitting, cotton clothes to avoid further irritating the treated area.
- Do let your radiation oncology team know about any side effects or problems.
- Do eat nutritionally balanced meals and stay hydrated.
- Do pursue mild exercise and get plenty of rest.
- Do use a reliable method of birth control to prevent pregnancy (radiation can harm a developing fetus).
- Do tell your radiation oncologist if you have a history of collagen vascular disease or autoimmune disease, which may increase the risk of side effects from radiation therapy.
- Don't wash away the ink dots or remove markers that are placed on your breast skin (if you're having external radiation).
- Don't apply ice packs or heating pads to the treated area.
- Don't rub or scratch the treated area.
- Don't apply any lotions, deodorants, soaps, or creams to the treated area before checking with your doctor.
- Don't use razors or hair removal products under your arms if your lymph nodes are being treated.
- Don't wear an underwire bra unless your doctor says it's okay.

Your doctor may recommend radiation after mastectomy if you have any of the following:

- an area of cancer that is 5 centimeters or larger
- positive surgical margins that can't be improved with additional surgery
- cancer in four or more lymph nodes (radiation for one to three positive lymph nodes is determined on a case-by-case basis)
- cancer in the chest muscle or the skin

SIDE EFFECTS

Improved radiation technologies decrease adverse side effects. Most people do well during treatment, and many have no troublesome side effects at all. Some effects accumulate during treatment, but most resolve on their own in the weeks and months after treatment ends. Other longer-term effects can develop months or years after radiation treatment ends and can be permanent.

Short-Term Effects

- *Skin changes.* Radiated skin may redden, darken, or otherwise become irritated as if it's sunburned. It may also feel warm or slightly swollen. In some people, the skin underneath the breast or in the underarm peels towards the end of treatment, causing sensitivity that's known as a *moist reaction.* Taking special care of your skin is important during radiation therapy and can help to minimize unwanted skin changes. Protect your skin from the sun while you're being treated, and when you wash or shower, carefully pat rather than rub your breast dry. Your radiation oncologist will recommend skin lotions that are moisturizing and advise the best way to manage these conditions.
- *Fatigue.* Mild to moderate fatigue can develop from the cumulative effects of radiation, especially when it follows chemotherapy. Getting plenty of rest and eating well will help.

- *Soreness.* Some women report mild discomfort or aching in the breast as radiation progresses. An over-the-counter pain reliever usually provides relief for this type of tenderness.
- *Costochondritis.* Radiation to the breast can cause a temporary type of arthritis that creates inflammation in the cartilage that connects a rib to the breastbone. Costochondritis pain is sharp and feels like a pressure; when experienced on the left side of your chest, it can be similar to symptoms of a heart attack. Once diagnosed, it often resolves on its own in several weeks, or it can be easily treated with anti-inflammatory medications.

Long-Term Effects

Fortunately, serious long-term side effects of radiation for breast cancer are rare, but some can require treatment. Complications that may develop include:

- *Lymphedema.* Chronic swelling of the arm or chest wall can develop after surgery and radiation to the axilla or regional lymph nodes, especially if you're obese or smoke. The risk increases when more lymph nodes are removed during surgery, although removing even a few nodes can be problematic.
- *Breast changes.* Radiation treatment can cause changes in the breast, including discoloration of the skin, an unusual firmness, or reduced size. While significant changes can occur, most are minor and are difficult to see once you're dressed. Radiation therapy after lumpectomy can distort the shape and size of the remaining tissue. It may also adversely affect the appearance of a reconstructed breast after mastectomy (see chapter 11). If needed, your radiation oncologist or breast surgeon may recommend a specialty bra to minimize the appearance of these changes.
- *Fibrosis.* Painful scarring of the breast tissue, which often begins with inflammation during radiation therapy, may develop after radiation. Fibrosis hardens the tissue, and sometimes a firm

area of fibrosis can feel like a cancerous mass. It most often appears in the first two years after radiation, but it can show up 10 years after your treatment. Although fibrotic changes are irreversible and affected tissues never recover, over-the-counter pain medication, physical therapy, and applying heat to the affected area can reduce discomfort. If you develop fibrosis, it's important to have it treated as soon as possible, because it can worsen over time. Your doctor may recommend medications that will slow the progression of your fibrosis if it's severe.

- *Radiation pneumonitis.* Inflammation of the lung typically develops within two or three months after completing radiation therapy. Symptoms often include a dry cough or a low-grade fever, shortness of breath, and mild to severe chest pain. Taking steroids for several weeks is typically recommended to reduce inflammation, and most patients recover without any lasting effects. Left untreated, radiation pneumonitis can cause scarring of the lungs.

- *Decreased milk production.* Nursing women can experience reduced milk production because radiation therapy damages tissues in the milk ducts and lobules. If you're nursing, your radiated breast may still make milk, although it may be darker and thicker than normal, and the supply may be diminished. Depending on the amount of radiation you have, your treated breast might be unable to produce any milk. Milk production from your unaffected breast will be normal.

- *Heart damage.* While it is possible for radiation to potentially harm the heart muscle, modern therapy techniques considerably reduce this risk. The chance of heart attack or heart failure after radiation is extremely rare; it's highest for individuals who already have diabetes, high blood pressure, high cholesterol, a past history of heart attack, or other risk factors for heart disease. It's important to discuss any of these preexisting risk factors with your radiation oncologist.

Does Radiation Therapy Cause Other Cancers?

Patients with breast cancer who subsequently develop another cancer often blame radiation, but recurrence is unlikely because radiation to treat breast cancer doesn't spill over into other organs in the body. Nevertheless, lung cancer, esophageal cancer, and cancers of the bone, muscle, and soft tissues in the radiated areas have been found following radiation treatment. Although these cancers may be secondary to radiation, they can also develop due to aging, hereditary influences, environmental exposures, and lifestyle behaviors. Some experts believe that if your immune system is vulnerable enough to develop one cancer, it may be more susceptible to another one. Although developing a secondary cancer from radiation is relatively rare, the likelihood of certain cancers can be somewhat increased after breast radiation. The chance of having a breast cancer recurrence without radiation, however, is far greater.

- Radiation doesn't usually increase the odds for a new cancer in the opposite breast, particularly with newer methods that deliver radiation to a focused area in the affected breast and minimize exposure to healthy tissues.
- Radiation-related sarcomas, cancers in the blood and lymphatic vessels, are slightly more common, especially 10 to 15 years after treatment, but they occur only rarely.
- Certain blood cancers, including leukemia, are more likely to develop after breast radiation, but the risk is very low.
- Radiation may increase the risk for lung cancer; this risk is highest in people who are current smokers. Tell your doctor if you smoke, and ask about resources that can help you to quit.

AN EXPERT'S VIEW

Knowing What to Expect

Radiation is probably the most mysterious of the treatment options. Almost everyone knows something about what happens in surgery—the surgeon goes in and cuts out the tumor. Similarly, almost everyone also knows something about chemotherapy: it can make you throw up, and you may lose your hair. Radiation treatment suffers a bad reputation, but like any other treatment, it has possible side effects. It is helpful for patients to have realistic expectations about side effects so that they aren't shocked when they occur. I go over these in detail with patients. I let them know what their risk of having these side effects is depending on their cancer and their anatomy. I try to emphasize which effects they're likely to get, the ones they may or may not get, and the effects that happen only rarely. Some patients want to believe that they are going to have no side effects, and then when they do, they don't handle it well emotionally and have a difficult time getting through their treatment, even when side effects are minimal.

—*Luther Ampey, MD*

MAKING TREATMENT DECISIONS

Depending on the facility where you're treated, you may have only one choice or multiple options for radiation therapy (figure 10.3). Like all treatment-related decisions, the choice you make is a balance between risk and benefit. Discuss each alternative for external and internal radiation with your treatment team. Ask about the benefits and risks of whole-breast and partial-breast alternatives and standard accelerated procedures. Consider not only the time and scheduling required, but also the overall short- and long-term effects of each type of radiation technique.

If you have a choice between lumpectomy and radiation or mastectomy, carefully consider the benefits and limitations of each treatment before you choose one or the other. The course of treatment you decide is something that you should discuss with your radiation oncologist to ensure that it's as effective as possible. If you're worried about the effects of radiation, talk to your radiology team about your specific concerns. Be clear about how these choices affect your risk of recurrence, and then make the decision that feels best for you.

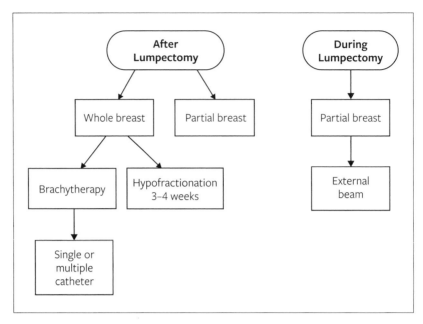

Figure 10.3. Comparing radiation treatment options

CHAPTER 11

Rebuilding Your Breasts
after Mastectomy

Years after their breast reconstruction, the overwhelming majority of women report that they're happy with the
choice that they made.

Facing the loss of their breasts, women often fear that they'll never
again look and feel the same. Breast reconstruction helps to soften
the effects of mastectomy by restoring breast volume and shape. It
isn't perfect; reconstruction can't reestablish sensation or restore the
ability to breastfeed, which are lost when tissue and nerves are removed during mastectomy. But it can give you soft, rounded breasts, so
that you can wear the same clothes you wore before mastectomy and
look natural without them. Breast reconstruction isn't right for every
woman who has a mastectomy, but many say that knowing reconstruction is a possibility makes the loss of one or both breasts a bit easier.
Years after their breast reconstruction, the overwhelming majority of
women report that they're happy with the choice that they made.

No reconstructive procedure is one-size-fits-all. Your breast tissue
can be replaced with synthetic implants or your own living tissue,
and each method has its own advantages and disadvantages. Implant
reconstruction is quicker and less invasive with a shorter recovery.
Reconstruction with your own tissue is more invasive and requires a
longer surgery and recovery. Although many surgeons still prefer tried-
and-true traditional methods, surgical innovations and improvements
in recent years have streamlined both implant and natural tissue procedures, improved results, and reduced recovery time.

Most reconstruction involves three steps: restoring breast volume; a secondary operation to revise and improve symmetry, fullness, or problems and to create a new nipple; and finally, tattooing the new nipple and areola for a more natural appearance (figure 11.1).

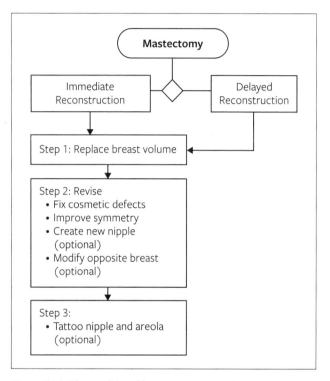

Figure 11.1. The traditional breast reconstruction process

TIMING YOUR RECONSTRUCTION

Having *immediate breast reconstruction*—at the same time as your mastectomy—isn't a must, but it has definite advantages. It's a two-in-one procedure; mastectomy and reconstruction are performed in one visit to the operating room with a single recovery. If you have immediate reconstruction, your breast surgeon will perform a skin-sparing mastectomy, removing as much breast tissue as possible while leaving an envelope of breast skin intact. Usually, this involves removal of the nipple and areola as well, but if you have a

Going Flat

Not all women want to have their breasts replaced. You may feel strongly against having new breasts that aren't the ones you were born with, or you might want to avoid any additional surgery and recovery after your treatment has ended. Perhaps you'd like to try going flat before committing to a reconstructive procedure. If you decide to remain flat and you want to fill out your clothes, you can use a *breast prosthesis*, a temporary breast form that fits into your bras, swimwear, lingerie, or adheres to your chest. Available in different shapes, materials, weights, and skin tones, you can put them on and take them off as needed. Wearing a prosthesis after a unilateral mastectomy will balance your posture and symmetry when trying to fit into clothes. A qualified fitter in a mastectomy boutique or department store can help to fit you correctly. If you change your mind about reconstruction, you can still have it any time in the future.

nipple-sparing mastectomy, your nipple and areola will be preserved. Your mastectomy incision will be minimized and positioned to be less obvious and may be completely hidden on your reconstructed breast. Once this is completed and while you're still under anesthesia, your plastic surgeon will then replace your breast tissue with a temporary expandable implant, a full-sized breast implant, or a segment of your own tissue, depending on the reconstructive technique you've chosen. You'll wake up with partial or complete new breasts, so you'll never have a completely flat chest. If you don't have immediate reconstruction, your surgeon will remove your breast tissue and most of your breast skin as described in chapter 10. *Delayed reconstruction* can be performed any time after your incision has healed, even years later, but it requires additional surgery and recovery, and your mastectomy scar will remain on your new breast.

SALINE AND SILICONE BREAST IMPLANTS

The least invasive breast reconstruction uses *breast implants* that are filled with either sterile *saline* (salt water) or thick *silicone* gel. Saline implants are firm, while silicone more closely mimics the softness of breast tissue. Breast implants are either round or teardrop shaped, with a smooth or textured surface, and have different widths and levels of projection. Before your reconstructive surgery, talk with your plastic surgeon about how large or how small you want your new breast to be; your surgeon will select an implant that best fits the dimensions of your chest.

Implants can be placed under or over the chest muscle, in a single procedure or as a two-stage procedure over the course of several months. *Tissue expansion* is required for women who don't have enough breast skin to cover an implant after mastectomy or for those who want to be slightly larger than their original breast size. This involves placing a temporary *tissue expander* above or behind the muscle and gradually inflating it with saline every 7 to 10 days in the surgeon's office (figure 11.2). Over the course of several weeks, the skin—and the muscle if it's above the expander—stretches to make room for a more permanent breast implant.

Tissue expansion can feel like one long recovery, as discomfort can occur as muscle and skin stretch. Your chest will be numb and may ache or feel heavy for several days, and you may feel tired for two weeks or more after your surgery. Any discomfort you feel should be adequately controlled with pain medication. Although you'll feel better each day, the chest tissues need four to six weeks to fully heal.

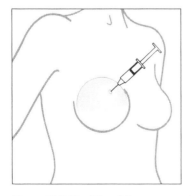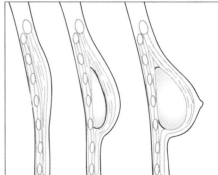

Figure 11.2. Traditional tissue expansion

A quicker, do-it-yourself expansion lets you control when, where, and how much you expand—you use a remote-control unit to inflate the expander with small bursts of carbon dioxide. When the skin has stretched enough, it's replaced with an implant during a second, shorter operation. The entire expansion-to-implant process can take six months or longer.

Direct-to-implant reconstruction is the quickest method of breast reconstruction. It places a full-sized implant above or below the muscle without expanding the skin or muscle. Using an *acellular dermal matrix* (ADM) makes this possible. ADM is an FDA-approved, sterilized biologic mesh of donor skin that retains collagen but has been stripped of DNA. When an expander is placed behind the muscle, stitching a patch of ADM onto the bottom of the muscle forms a supportive sling at the base of the implant (figure 11.3). When an expander is placed over the muscle, ADM adds a cushioning layer between the implant and breast skin. Compared to traditional expansion, recovery is shorter and easier after direct-to-implant reconstruction.

This "one-step" procedure requires a skin- or nipple-sparing mastectomy. Mastectomy and reconstruction are completed in a single trip to the operating room, and you enter and leave with full-sized breasts. Unless a problem occurs, no *revision surgery* is necessary. The downside of direct-to-implant reconstruction is that there is

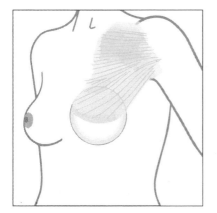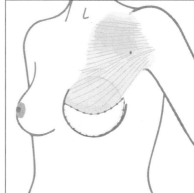

Figure 11.3. Direct-to-implant breast reconstruction

less control over the size (you can only place what fits at the time, whereas with tissue expanders you will have some control over the size prior to the final reconstruction). Also, placing a full-size implant at the time of mastectomy puts more tension on the breast skin; this can affect the blood supply in your breast skin, which is diminished when tissue is removed. Although the intent of this procedure is to complete reconstruction in a single step, some women do need revision surgery to address asymmetries or to improve the cosmetic appearance of their breast.

Like most manufactured devices, complications can develop with breast implants. They don't last a lifetime; experts estimate that implants last between 10 and 20 years, although other problems can develop that require sooner medical intervention. While newer-generation implants are thought to be more reliable, follow-up operations to fix asymmetry, position, or infection aren't unusual. Still, not everyone with implants develops these problems, and many women are perfectly happy with their implant reconstruction.

The most common problem, *capsular contracture*, occurs when scar tissue that naturally forms hardens and squeezes the implant. Mild capsular contracture may go unnoticed; severe cases can be painful, distort breast shape, and require removal of the implant, which can then be replaced with a newer model.

Implants that leak or rupture must be removed and/or replaced. If you have reconstruction with silicone implants, an MRI is recommended three years after your initial implant reconstruction and every two years after that to evaluate for any leak or rupture. This surveillance isn't required for saline implants because they deflate in an obvious way if they develop a leak or rupture.

Most implants are smooth, but some teardrop-shaped models are textured—they have a roughened exterior to help keep them in place. *Textured breast implants* are associated with a rare, treatable type of cancer called *anaplastic large-cell lymphoma* (ALCL). In the general population, only three women in 100 million develop this type of lymphoma. If ALCL is diagnosed, the breast implant is removed, along

---

Will Insurance Pay for Your Reconstruction?

The *Women's Health and Cancer Rights Act* of 1998 (WHCRA) requires group health plans and health insurance companies that cover mastectomy to also pay for all stages of breast reconstruction, including surgery to the opposite breast to achieve a symmetrical appearance and treatment for any related complications. The WHCRA also requires coverage for mastectomy bras and prostheses. Insurers must provide coverage with the same deductibles and co-payments that are consistent with your existing plan benefits. (Some plans provided by the government and religious organizations are exempt.) Medicare pays for breast reconstruction, and Medicaid coverage varies by state. Most states have laws that also mandate coverage for reconstruction.

---

with any suspicious masses or lymph nodes. Radiation and chemotherapy may also be recommended. Allergan's Biocell textured implants are specifically linked to ALCL and were voluntarily recalled worldwide in 2019.

OPTIONS FOR USING YOUR OWN TISSUE

Autologous tissue flaps are more complex and require more advanced surgical skills than implant reconstruction. Breasts made with your own living tissue feel more natural.

Flap procedures form full-size breasts during the initial operation. Skin and fat can be transferred from your abdomen, back, buttocks, hips, or thighs to your chest and sculpted into a breast (table 11.1). Abdominal flaps are the most common, because that's where women most often carry excess weight—removing abdominal fat is essentially a tummy tuck. If you're thin and don't have enough fat in one area to remake your breast, more than one flap of tissue can be "stacked" to add more volume.

A *pedicled tissue flap* is a segment of fat, skin, and the underlying muscle that is moved under the skin from the donor site to the chest while it remains connected to its original blood supply (figure 11.4).

The muscle is included in pedicled tissue flaps because it contains essential blood vessels that the flap needs to survive. Removing muscle increases the length of recovery and can reduce some functionality at the donor site. A *perforator flap* (also called a "muscle-sparing" flap) removes the same amount of fat from the same area but spares the muscle—the flap is disconnected from its existing blood supply and reconnected to blood vessels in the chest. Perforator flaps are less invasive at the donor site since the muscle is left in place, but they require a specially trained *microsurgeon* to reconnect the tiny blood vessels. The new breast looks the same with either type of flap, but the difference on the inside is significant (figure 11.4). Although reconstruction with pedicled flaps is still widely available, perforator flap reconstruction is increasingly available as more surgeons are trained and become experienced with this advanced technique.

Table 11.1. Autologous Tissue Flaps

Source	Flap	Type
Abdomen	Deep inferior epigastric perforator (DIEP)	Preserves muscle
	Transverse myocutaneous (TRAM)	Uses muscle
Back	Lumbar artery perforator (LAP)	Preserves muscle
	Latissimus dorsi (LAT)	Uses muscle
Buttocks	Gluteal artery perforator (GAP)	Preserves muscle
Inner thigh	Transverse upper gracilis (TUG)	Uses muscle
Upper posterior thigh	Profunda artery perforator (PAP)	Preserves muscle

Recovery varies depending on the type of reconstruction you have. Muscle-sparing procedures generally heal faster with significantly less discomfort than procedures that remove muscle. Swelling in the new breast will last for a month or two, and the breast and donor area may remain numb for 6 to 12 months. Most women don't have significant problems during or after reconstruction, but like all surgeries,

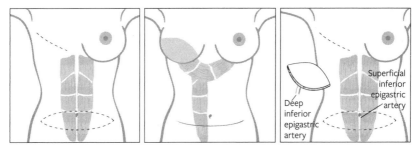

Figure 11.4. TRAM (*left and center*) and DIEP (*right*) flaps

How Radiation Affects Breast Reconstruction

Radiation is an important and necessary part of treatment for many women, but it makes for a more challenging breast reconstruction. Some women have satisfactory reconstructive outcomes after radiation, but radiated tissue can be unpredictable. The chance of developing multiple complications is especially high when breast implants are used for breast reconstruction after radiation. Tissue expander and implant reconstruction after radiation greatly increase the risk of infection, slow wound healing, skin that breaks down from the pressure of the implant, capsular contraction, and other complications, often requiring one or more corrective operations. Even then, however, the new breast may feel hard or shrink as radiated tissue contracts. Padding the radiated mastectomy site with an acellular dermal matrix or injections of fat can help. Autologous tissue reconstruction, which brings healthy tissue and blood vessels to the chest 6 to 12 months after radiation is completed, is more likely to provide a better long-term outcome.

If you're unsure at the time of your mastectomy whether you'll need radiation, a *delayed-immediate reconstruction* can preserve your breast shape and breast skin. A *tissue expander* is placed under your chest muscle and fully inflated after your breast tissue is removed. If you don't need postmastectomy radiation, you can proceed with implant or tissue flap reconstruction. If you do need radiation, your breast reconstruction can be started in 6 to 12 months, when your skin has had a chance to heal. The expander can then be removed and replaced with a tissue flap. It could also be replaced with an implant, but the risk of capsular contraction and skin fibrosis is high after radiation and may make the cosmetic outcome less desirable in some patients.

infection, *delayed wound healing*, and other issues can develop. A *hematoma* (excess blood under the skin) or a *seroma* (excess fluid under the skin) may occur and need to be drained, or a portion of the flap may die if the blood supply is insufficient. Rarely, the entire flap may die and must be removed. Women who smoke or are obese are especially susceptible to these complications. Tissue flaps require a longer and more intense recovery than reconstruction with implants (table 11.2). Generally, pedicled flaps take longer to heal and make for a more uncomfortable recovery than muscle-sparing flaps. Routine screening isn't required after flap reconstruction; however, some surgeons recommend having a baseline mammogram that can be compared to any future changes in the breast.

Table 11.2. Comparing Breast Implants and Tissue Flaps

Breast Implants	Tissue Flaps
Incision/scar at mastectomy site	Incision/scar at mastectomy and donor sites
Creates breast contour	Creates breast contour; improves shape at donor site
Shorter surgery	Longer surgery
Hospital stay: one to two days*	Hospital stay: three to five days*
Recovery: two to six weeks*	Recovery: four to eight weeks*
May not require revision#	Almost always requires revision
Eventual replacement	Lifelong
Prone to long-term problems that require corrective surgery	May have complications related to surgery, but rarely develop complications after recovery
Widely available	Fewer experienced surgeons, especially for muscle-sparing flaps
Very rare link to ALCL	No link to disease

*May vary depending on the procedure and individual recovery.

#Direct-to-implant reconstruction after nipple-sparing mastectomy.

FAT GRAFTING

Fat grafting is a versatile tool for improving and fine tuning almost any reconstruction. It involves three distinct steps. Fat is liposuctioned from the belly, thighs, buttocks, or "love handles" and processed to remove impurities and fluids. It's then loaded into syringes and injected precisely where it's needed to improve contour defects in the breast. Injecting multiple, minute amounts of fat increases the likelihood that they'll connect with healthy blood vessels in the breast and survive. Fat that doesn't form these connections is resorbed back into the body. It's difficult to predict how much fat will stay put, and results vary between surgeons. Generally, about 50 to 70 percent of injected fat remains in the breast.

Fat grafting can:

- add up to a cup size to your reconstructed breast
- smooth contour irregularities and fill in dents
- further define or improve your cleavage
- fill in a sunken area above your breast
- hide rippling and wrinkling on the surface of the implant
- soften and improve the texture of previously radiated tissue
- refine the appearance of scars

Fat grafting can be performed during a revision surgery under general anesthesia or as a separate outpatient procedure. Two or three rounds of fat grafting at least three months apart are usually needed for the best results; improvement is obvious after each session. Unlike cosmetic liposuction, where removed fat is discarded, a surgeon's expertise, skill, technique, and method of introducing the fat into the reconstructed breast affect results, so careful handling of fat is an absolute requirement. If your surgeon suggests fat grafting, be sure to ask about his or her experience with this procedure, and ask to see before-and-after photos of patients who have had fat grafting to improve their breast reconstruction.

Breast Reconstruction for Men

Men who develop breast cancer are often treated with lumpectomy and radiation or modified radical mastectomy that removes their breast tissue, nipple, and areola. Some men are candidates for nipple-sparing mastectomy, though in most cases of male breast cancer, the tumor is too close to the nipple and areola to preserve either area. Because men have far less breast tissue than women, removing a tumor can leave a noticeable cosmetic deformity in the chest wall.

Breast cancer is uncommon in men, and few plastic surgeons are experienced with male breast reconstruction, but chest contour can be restored in three ways.

1. With a small, low-profile breast implant placed under the muscle. Although expensive, a custom-made silicone breast implant offers the best chance of restoring a man's unique chest structure.
2. When mastectomy removes a man's chest muscle, a small portion of the latissimus dorsi muscle from the back can be transferred to the chest as a replacement.
3. Fat grafting, which is the most common method of male breast reconstruction, can replace volume that is lost when breast tissue is removed.

Male nipples can also be reconstructed and tattooed, either with or without breast reconstruction. Men are entitled to the same health insurance coverage for breast reconstruction that is mandated for women by the Women's Health and Cancer Rights Act, even if the name of the law implies that it's just for women.

RE-CREATING NIPPLES AND AREOLAS

The final step in reconstruction is re-creating the nipple and areola. (This step isn't necessary if you've had a nipple-sparing mastectomy.) This optional surgery marks a physical and psychological milestone for many women. It's the final touch in the sometimes long process of replacing a lost breast. The simple and straightforward minor procedure is most often done during revision surgery.

Nipples are formed from mini-flaps of breast skin. A pattern is first marked on the breast. Shallow incisions are then made along three sides of the pattern to free a small flap of skin and fat. In a bit of surgical origami, the sides of the flap are folded around to meet in the center, the top part is folded down over them, and the edges are stitched together (figure 11.5). The entire process takes less than an hour. It's easy and painless, with no downtime or surgical drains. The new nipple will be protected with a light bandage; your surgeon will give you instructions for caring for the new nipple until it completely heals in about six to eight weeks.

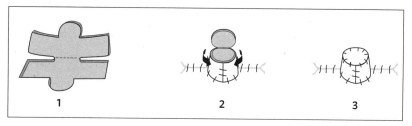

Figure 11.5. Creating a new nipple

A subsequent 30-minute tattooing session in your surgeon's office can add a more natural color to your new nipple and simulate the surrounding areola. It also camouflages mastectomy scars if your mastectomy incision was made around the areola. Nipple tattoos fade considerably, and they often disappear completely in a few years, so they're initially made darker. You may need two or three sessions to apply the full pigment—layering in multiple sessions provides longer-lasting color. Re-tattooing can also fine-tune pigment or improve splotchy or uneven areas.

Most plastic surgeons who perform breast reconstruction also provide nipple tattoos, but you might want to consult with a professional tattoo artist, especially if you prefer a more decorative tattoo. Before you schedule an appointment, call the studio or check the artist's website to be sure he or she has experience with the type of inking that you want. This is especially important if you'd like to have a *three-dimensional nipple* tattoo, which requires a special skill and experience. Call to set up a consultation appointment, then visit the studio to ensure that it's a sterile environment. Explain what you have in mind, review photos of the artist's work, and ask how many nipple tattoos the artist has performed. Request one or two client references before you leave. You may also want to ask for a list of ingredients in the pigments to be used, to be sure that you're not allergic to any ingredient in the ink.

Alternatively, if you decide not to have nipple reconstruction, you might want to consider 3-D tattoos that use subtle highlighting and shading to realistically simulate the look of areolas and protruding natural nipples. Temporary adhesive nipples are also available.

MAKING DECISIONS ABOUT RECONSTRUCTION

Studies show that women who have breast reconstruction consider it to be a quality-of-life option, and that most of them are satisfied with their decision. Your age, overall health, and how you view your breasts are important factors. You may feel strongly that reconstruction is well worth the effort and recovery, or that it's simply not that important to you, or you may prefer not to deal with any more surgery or recovery. Whether you ultimately choose to go flat or reconstruct, it's always a good idea to explore your options. You may find that breast reconstruction can provide more than you thought, or it may seem like too much time and trouble. Either way, the decision is yours.

Reconstruction is a personal decision that can be complex and stressful. You're more likely to be satisfied with your results if you take the time you need to thoroughly explore and understand all of your choices and get a second and third opinion. As you weigh each alternative, consider how many surgeries are involved, what to expect from recovery, and how long before you'll be able to resume your normal activities and routine at work or at home. Whatever you decide is right.

Answering the following five questions will help you make decisions that are best for you.

1. *Immediate or delayed reconstruction?* Immediate reconstruction isn't the right choice for every woman. Perhaps you'd rather avoid the added stress of researching options and making more decisions as you cope with a cancer diagnosis and treatment, or you prefer to keep reconstruction in mind as a future option. Adjuvant chemotherapy or radiation treatment may also postpone your reconstruction for 6 to 12 months.

2. *Implants or tissue flaps?* Choose a reconstructive method that matches your priorities. Do you want the least invasive reconstruction, the quickest recovery, or the most natural result? Does the idea of having a bonus tummy tuck along with your reconstruction appeal to you? You may not be a candidate for all reconstructive options, and some procedures may not be available in your area. That means settling for what's available locally or traveling to another city for your reconstruction.

3. *What size?* After mastectomy, you have an opportunity to have breasts that are smaller, larger, or the same size as your natural breasts. Think this through carefully, and make sure that you and your plastic surgeon are on the same page about size. Although reconstructed breasts can be reduced or made somewhat larger, you can avoid additional procedures if your surgeon gets it right the first time.

4. *Which surgeon?* Choosing the right surgeon is the most important part of breast reconstruction. More than anything else, it influences how your re-created breasts will look and your level of satisfaction with them. Surgeons have different qualifications, surgical training, and experience; they don't all perform the same procedures. Select a surgeon who is board certified with the American Board of Plastic Surgery or the American Society of Plastic Surgeons or both organizations. It's important to choose someone who is also experienced and skilled in the procedure you want. Your surgeon's priority should be your satisfaction and the best possible cosmetic result. Then get a second opinion from another surgeon; a third opinion is

even better. Talk to women who've had same type of reconstruction. Check with your health care insurer to determine whether you're restricted to surgeons within your plan.

5. *Modify your opposite breast?* If you have one breast removed, your surgeon can lift, reduce, or augment your opposite breast for a better match. This isn't required, but it's often the best way to achieve symmetry between your reconstructed breast and your natural breast.

Questions for Your Plastic Surgeon

- What procedure do you recommend for me and why?
- How many of these procedures do you perform monthly/annually?
- How many surgeries will I have and of what length and recovery?
- Realistically, what kind of result can I expect?
- What should I expect from surgery and recovery?
- What is the overall reconstructive time line from start to finish?
- What risks or complications may occur?
- How will you fix them?
- May I see before-and-after photos of your results for this procedure?
- Can you put me in touch with one or two of your patients who have had this same type of reconstruction?

CHAPTER 12

Treating Noninvasive Breast Cancer

DUCTAL CARCINOMA IN SITU

Most women with single, small areas of ductal carcinoma in situ can be treated successfully with breast-conserving surgery and radiation, followed by hormonal therapy. For a small group of women, surgery without radiation can also be considered.

Ductal carcinoma in situ (DCIS) is the diagnosis that is most likely to include "cancer" and "cure" in the same sentence. It's the earliest form of breast cancer; some experts consider it to be a precancerous condition. Almost all cases of DCIS are treated successfully. But not all cases of DCIS are alike, and there is no single approach to treatment. While virtually all invasive cancer begins as DCIS, not all DCIS will go on to become an invasive cancer.

A diagnosis of DCIS means that you have abnormal cells that are confined to the lining of a breast duct, and in their current state, they're unable to move into the fatty tissues of the breast. By itself, DCIS is noninvasive and not life threatening, but some types can come back after lumpectomy and radiation. About half of DCIS that returns after initial therapy recurs as DCIS; the other half that comes back does so as invasive breast cancer. Usually too small to be felt, DCIS was rarely diagnosed before screening mammography became widely available in the 1980s. More than three decades later, it now accounts for 20 percent of newly diagnosed breast cancers, not because it develops more often, but because routine screening with mammography is very good at finding it.

DCIS BASICS

DCIS affects an estimated 50,000 women in the United States each year, making it one of the most commonly diagnosed breast conditions. The name refers to abnormal cells in the epithelium, or the lining of the milk ducts (ductal carcinoma). The good news is that these cells are contained within the ducts (in situ) and have not spread to other organs. Without additional treatment following surgery, however, DCIS has the potential to evolve into invasive cancer.

The Appearance of DCIS Makes a Difference

Although DCIS doesn't usually form a lump or a tumor, a mass is occasionally identified by physical examination. More often, it shows up on a mammogram as microcalcifications, tiny clusters of white specks that are too small to be felt and that suggest an accumulation of abnormal cells inside a breast duct. To a radiologist's trained eye, these calcifications appear different than other benign calcifications. The radiologist also compares the current mammogram to previous mammograms, looking for the development of new calcifications and any other changes. If a needle biopsy fails to produce enough tissue to conclusively determine the nature of the calcification, a surgical biopsy is needed for a better sampling of the calcifications. If DCIS is diagnosed on a biopsy, surgery is then planned to ensure that all of the DCIS has been removed.

DCIS cells look like invasive breast cancer cells, but they behave differently. The basic difference is that they are unable to penetrate the duct walls and to metastasize elsewhere in the body. Low-grade DCIS cells look like healthy cells, but they're "lazy" and would require several years to become invasive breast cancer. Intermediate-grade cells appear somewhat different than healthy cells and grow faster. High-grade DCIS looks very different, divides more quickly, and is more likely to recur or become invasive cancer. Observing how the cells are grouped together is also important. DCIS may form certain telltale patterns: *cribiform*, low- to medium-grade cells with gaps between them, or *comedo necrosis*, which grows faster and plugs the center of the duct with dead DCIS cells. DCIS with comedo necrosis is more likely to recur or to transition to an invasive cancer and warrants more attention.

DCIS is considered to be stage 0 breast cancer. It's categorized as stage I when DCIS includes *microinvasion*, cells that are beginning to break through the ducts and enter the soft tissue of the breast. In some cases, DCIS is found alongside small areas of invasive breast cancer (figure 12.1), indicating that more aggressive treatment is necessary.

CUSTOMIZING TREATMENT CHOICES

The goal of treating DCIS is to eliminate it so that it doesn't become invasive or return. Thirty years ago, an unfounded belief held that DCIS was resistant to radiation, so women with DCIS frequently underwent mastectomy. Fortunately, over time, it became clear that most women with localized, small areas of DCIS can be treated successfully with breast-conserving surgery and radiation, followed by tamoxifen or an aromatase inhibitor if the DCIS is hormone sensitive (table 12.1).

Treatment options for DCIS are lumpectomy, lumpectomy and radiation, surgery followed by tamoxifen or an aromatase inhibitor if your DCIS is estrogen receptor positive, or mastectomy. Some older women who have very small areas of low-grade DCIS may have lumpectomy alone and then take hormonal therapy, either tamoxifen or an aromatase inhibitor, hormone-blocking therapies that reduce the risk of local recurrence. Chemotherapy isn't required for DCIS, because it isn't invasive, and the threat of metastasis is almost nonexistent. And because DCIS cells are confined to the ducts, a lymph node biopsy isn't usually needed. A sentinel node biopsy may be performed, however, when pathology shows DCIS cells that have made their way out of the ducts—this happens about 30 percent of the time; the diagnosis is then invasive ductal carcinoma. Sentinel node biopsy is also appropriate when invasive cancer and DCIS are found together, when DCIS is characterized by comedo necrosis, or when patients with DCIS have mastectomy.

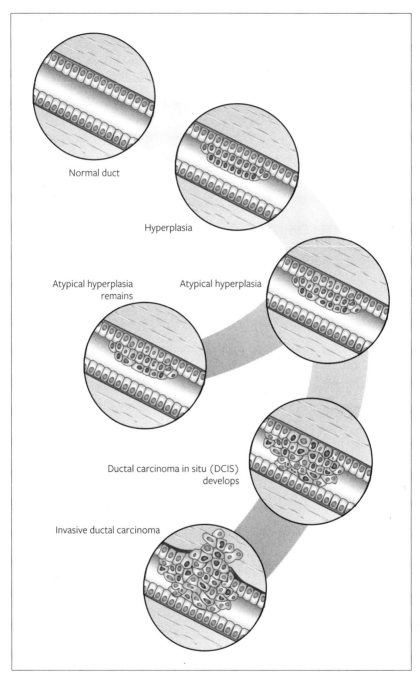

Normal duct

Hyperplasia

Atypical hyperplasia
remains

Atypical hyperplasia

Ductal carcinoma in situ (DCIS)
develops

Invasive ductal carcinoma

Figure 12.1. How healthy cells become ductal carcinoma in situ and invasive ductal carcinoma

Table 12.1. Comparing DCIS Treatment Options

	Laurie	Jan	Teri	Marie
Age	78	35	49	60
Size (cm)	0.7	1.2	2.5	2.0
Grade	Low	High	High	Intermediate
Biopsy margins	Clear	Clear	Close	Clear
Multifocal	No	No	Yes	No
Hormone status	ER+	ER+	ER–	ER+
Risk of recurrence	Low	Low	High	Low
Treatment choice	Lumpectomy + AI	Lumpectomy + brachytherapy + tamoxifen	Mastectomy	Lumpectomy + XRT + AI

Abbreviations are as follows: AI, aromatase inhibitor; ER, estrogen receptor; XRT, external radiation therapy.

Mastectomy

Mastectomy is more effective to remove lesions that are 5 centimeters or larger or for multiple areas of DCIS in different parts of the breast (table 12.1). If you have a family history of breast cancer and you're diagnosed with DCIS, a genetic counselor can explain how your history affects your risk for a recurrence and a future diagnosis and determine whether you might benefit from genetic testing. If you decide to be tested and you find that you have a genetic mutation that significantly raises the risk for a new breast cancer, your doctor will discuss the option of unilateral or bilateral mastectomy. After treatment with lumpectomy, routine follow-up should include a clinical breast exam every six months and an annual mammogram. If you have a mastectomy, you should continue to have an annual mammogram of your remaining healthy breast.

Even though DCIS doesn't meet the definition of invasive cancer, all cases are treated, although not necessarily in the same way. Postoperative therapy depends on the risk of recurrence, your tolerance of that risk, and your personal preference for treatment: survival is the same, regardless of the treatment. Several factors influence whether DCIS is more likely to return:

Lower Risk	Higher Risk
>age 40 at diagnosis	<age 40 diagnosis
postmenopausal	premenopausal
single, small area of DCIS	large or multiple areas of DCIS
low grade	intermediate or high grade
typical DCIS cell structure	comedo necrosis (dead cells)
ER+	ER–
clear margins	DCIS in margins

AN EXPERT'S VIEW

Assessing the Risk of Recurrence

Randomized trials have shown that radiation therapy reduces the risk of recurrence in the breast after lumpectomy for DCIS but it does not change long-term survival or risk of developing metastases. Two trials funded by the National Cancer Institute showed the risk of recurrence in the breast at 10 years in patients treated with lumpectomy without radiation is about 10–15 percent when the area of DCIS is less than 25 millimeters, has a nuclear grade of 1 or 2, and there is a tumor-free margin width of 3 millimeters or wider. Patients whose DCIS is larger or has nuclear grade 3, or who have narrow margins, have breast recurrence rates of 25 to 35 percent or higher at 10 years. Radiation therapy can reduce this risk to 5 to 10 percent at 10 years. Individuals diagnosed at age 40 or younger may also have increased risk of recurrence in the breast if they undergo lumpectomy without radiation therapy, even if the characteristics of the DCIS are favorable for omitting radiation in older women. But there is substantial disagreement among breast cancer specialists about the exact details of when it is reasonable to recommend not giving radiation therapy with regards to all these characteristics.

Genomic tests of DCIS may be able to help improve the ability to predict which patients may benefit least or most from radiation therapy. Many women with DCIS choose to have mastectomy, with or without reconstructive surgery. But breast cancer experts also disagree about which patients with DCIS should be treated with mastectomy instead of breast-conserving therapy. Individuals with DCIS larger than 3 to 4 centimeters with smaller breasts may develop substantial breast deformity after lumpectomy and hence have poor cosmetic results. Patients who have positive margins despite having more than one lumpectomy appear to have a high risk of recurrence in the breast despite radiation therapy and may be best treated with mastectomy.

—Abram Recht, MD

Radiation Therapy

Adjuvant radiation reduces the risk of DCIS coming back in the breast, either as another DCIS or as invasive breast cancer. Radiation therapy is almost always recommended after lumpectomy; it almost never follows mastectomy for DCIS because the chance of recurrence is quite small after the breast is removed (table 12.2). The decision to add adjuvant radiation is based on the grade of the DCIS, tumor size, and margin status. When treating DCIS, radiation oncologists may use Oncotype DX DCIS, a genomic test that analyzes the activity of several genes to predict whether your DCIS is more or less likely to respond to radiation with or without hormonal therapy after surgery.

Table 12.2. Ten-Year Risk of Recurrence after Treatment for DCIS

	Lumpectomy Alone (%)	Lumpectomy with Radiation (%)	Mastectomy (%)
Same breast	28.0*	13.0*	1–2

*Source: Early Breast Cancer Trialists' Collaborative Group, C. Correa, P. McGale, C. Taylor et al., "Overview of the Randomized Trials of Radiotherapy in Ductal Carcinoma in Situ of the Breast," *Journal of National Cancer Institute Monographs* 41 (2010): 162–77.

Tamoxifen and Aromatase Inhibitors

Most DCIS is estrogen and/or progesterone receptor positive and is treated after radiation with either tamoxifen or an aromatase inhibitor. Tamoxifen is a *selective estrogen-receptor modulator* (SERM), a type of drug that blocks estrogen from attaching to *hormone receptors* in cancer cells so that the cells can't grow. It's used for premenopausal and postmenopausal early-stage breast cancers. With an impressive track record for treating breast cancer and lowering recurrence, tamoxifen was the first breast cancer drug approved by the FDA and has been standard treatment for estrogen receptor–positive breast cancers since 1977.

Taking tamoxifen daily for five years reduces local recurrence in the affected breast and also cuts the risk of a new cancer developing in the opposite breast by more than 50 percent. These benefits persist for years after the medication is stopped. The National Surgical Adjuvant Breast and Bowel Project (NSABP) B-24 trial involving 1,804 DCIS patients who had breast-conserving therapy compared recurrence after taking tamoxifen or a *placebo* (a "fake" substance that has no therapeutic affect). Participants took the drug for five years, and after seven years of subsequent follow-up, tamoxifen significantly reduced recurrence (table 12.3).

Many women decline to use tamoxifen because of its side effects, including menopausal symptoms. The risk of endometrial cancer and blood clots is also increased, though the likelihood of developing these effects is small. Tamoxifen continues to be a workhorse in the

Table 12.3. DCIS Recurrence with and without Tamoxifen

	Placebo (%)	Tamoxifen (%)
Any recurrence	23	10
Same breast	13	7

treatment of DCIS and premenopausal breast cancers. Its side ef-fects continue to be studied, and researchers are looking for ways to create more patient-friendly versions of the drug. One trial is study-ing whether applying 4-hydroxytamoxifen, a tamoxifen gel, to both breasts once a day preserves tamoxifen's effectiveness while limit-ing absorption in the bloodstream, which may limit its side effects. Tamoxifen is currently given in pill form.

Aromatase inhibitors also treat postmenopausal, early-stage breast cancers that need estrogen to grow, including DCIS. The end result is the same—they reduce the stimulating influence of estrogen and progesterone on hormone receptors—but they do it differently than tamoxifen. Taken orally once daily, aromatase inhibitors stop the pro-duction of estrogen in postmenopausal women. Both tamoxifen and the aromatase inhibitor anastrozole are good treatment options for preventing breast cancer recurrence, but both have side effects that differ by age: younger women often experience more severe symp-toms. Since treatment benefits are similar for older women, treatment can be based on symptoms and tolerability. Anastrozole is more likely to cause *osteopenia* (thinning of the bones) or bone fractures, joint weakness, and vaginal symptoms, while tamoxifen is more frequently associated with increased hot flashes, blood clots, and stroke. Women under the age of 60 have more common and severe symptoms from either drug. If you become menopausal while taking tamoxifen, your oncologist may suggest that you switch to an aromatase inhibitor.

Tamoxifen is the hormone treatment choice for premenopausal women; aromatase inhibitors are prescribed for postmenopausal women. Tamoxifen is an alternative for postmenopausal women who can't tolerate the side effects of aromatase inhibitors. Chapter 13 has more information about the benefits and limitations of these medications.

How Research Has Influenced Treatment for Ductal Carcinoma In Situ

DCIS treatment has evolved considerably over the years. Lumpectomy with radiation is the gold standard treatment for most DCIS, but this wasn't always the case. In the 1980s, lumpectomy and radiation was recognized as successful treatment for invasive breast cancer, but radiation was thought to be less effective for DCIS, which was usually treated with mastectomy. A meta-analysis of four clinical trials involving more than 3,900 DCIS patients comparing lumpectomy with and without radiation showed that although radiation doesn't affect survival—which is already excellent for women with DCIS—it lowers the risk of DCIS coming back as invasive breast cancer by 50 percent. The National Surgical Adjuvant Breast and Bowel Project (NSABP) B-17 trial confirmed these results. Over the years, data from this and other NSABP trials have influenced how DCIS is treated. The B-24 trial established that adjuvant radiation decreases local recurrence by 50 percent; taking tamoxifen further lowers local recurrence by another 30 percent. Combined results of the NSABP B-17 and B-24 trials showed significant differences in recurrence five years after treatment: lumpectomy alone, 25 percent; lumpectomy and radiation, 13 percent; and lumpectomy, radiation, and tamoxifen, 8 percent.

IS DCIS OVERTREATED?

DCIS requires medical attention because it can return or develop into more worrisome invasive breast cancer. Removing the area of DCIS is important, as it sometimes reveals an associated invasive cancer that wasn't detected on a needle biopsy. Experts disagree about the best way to treat DCIS or whether it should be treated at all. Some research suggests that surgically removing low-grade DCIS with a wide rim of healthy tissue is adequate, and that additional treatment is unnecessary. This limited treatment is more likely to be recommended for an 80-year-old woman who has a tiny amount of low-grade, estrogen-positive DCIS than for a 40-year-old woman with a similar diagnosis. Some physicians and scientists believe, however, that surgery and radiation overtreat certain small areas of low-grade DCIS that remain dormant and are unlikely to become a significant problem during a woman's lifetime. (Several autopsy studies support this theory, finding more widespread DCIS than what is diagnosed in the general population.)

A conservative and somewhat controversial approach to DCIS is *watchful waiting*, close surveillance without treatment, or, alternatively, close surveillance with hormonal therapy. The Comparison of Operative to Monitoring and Endocrine Therapy (COMET) trial is investigating whether watchful waiting is a safe alternative for women who are at least 40 years old and have low-risk DCIS. This is similar to the preferred treatment approach for men who have low-risk prostate cancer.

Several trials are trying to establish a method of identifying which types of DCIS are harmless and which are potentially harmful. Until we have more answers, we can't reliably say how much treatment is too little or too much, and which women can safely skip surgery and/ or radiation.

MAKING TREATMENT DECISIONS

DCIS isn't an emergency, and it's not life threatening. You have time to understand and consider treatment options before making a decision (figure 12.2). Be an active participant in learning as much as possible about your diagnosis and your treatment options, including the success rates and side effects of each option, before deciding which one is best for you. Treatment decisions for women with DCIS should consider many factors, including your age, general health, and the specific characteristics of your DCIS. The process begins by understanding your risk for recurrence, your treatment choices, and your own priorities. You might choose lumpectomy and radiation over mastectomy if it's important to you that you keep your breast.

Another consideration is that if you have a recurrence after a lumpectomy and radiation, your breast cannot be radiated a second time, and a mastectomy would be required. Unilateral or bilateral mastectomy may be a better option if you already have an increased risk for breast cancer, including a strong family history or a mutation in a BRCA gene. Whether you choose lumpectomy with radiation or mastectomy, your survival afterward is the same as someone who has never had breast cancer. If you're having a difficult time deciding which surgery is best for you, reread chapter 9, especially "Choosing Lumpectomy or Mastectomy."

The decision to take tamoxifen is difficult for some women. Talking to your doctor about the results of your Oncotype DX DCIS test should help you decide about having radiation or hormonal therapy after surgery. Be sure to clearly understand your risk for recurrence and of losing your breast in the future if DCIS recurs, and then weigh the benefits and limitations of your options. Your doctor will help you make these important decisions.

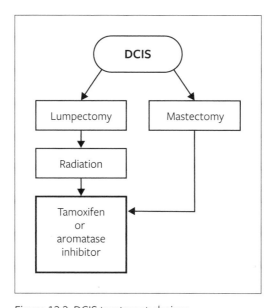

Figure 12.2. DCIS treatment choices

Susan's Story

I went to see two local oncologists, and I consulted with my gynecologist. I got different opinions about treatment, everything from doing nothing to prophylactic double mastectomy. It was quite confusing at the time. It was an extremely difficult decision, even though I was aggressive in finding out what I had to do, because I had to first admit to myself that I had a problem; it's easy to deny the fact that you do.

I didn't take tamoxifen right away, because it's difficult to go from being totally healthy to having to take what I felt was a very toxic medication. It puts you into chemically induced menopause, and I wasn't ready for that. I was young and full of life. I was afraid to take tamoxifen because I didn't know what it would do to me. Then I went for another opinion with a specialist at a well-known cancer center. He recommended increased vigilance and tamoxifen taken prophylactically. He was the first one to tell me, "You take tamoxifen because it could save your life. All of the side effects, the headaches, the vaginal dryness, I can treat." I think that was the turning point. I brought this information back to my doctor, a wonderful, intelligent man. He was the one who recommended mastectomy. I think he saw merit in both forms of treatment, but he left the decision up to me.

My fears were substantiated because I had every reaction in the book. I had severe headaches, trouble sleeping, and my stomach was upset. The vaginal dryness just hit from out of the blue. I went from being an active, energetic person to being exhausted all of the time. How did I get myself to stay on the tamoxifen? I told myself I was on a greater mission, and I knew that it was for five years, so I always felt that there was a light at the end of the tunnel. Some things did get better. The upset stomach was not as severe. I took sleeping pills so that I could sleep. My doctor was able to treat the vaginal dryness. Over the course of five years, I was able to separate the emotional strain of taking the tamoxifen from the actual physical effects. If I had to do it all over again, I would.

CHAPTER 13

Reducing the Risk
of Recurrence

SYSTEMIC THERAPIES FOR INVASIVE BREAST CANCER

Adjuvant therapy is given to women who have or have had breast cancer. This treatment "adds to" the efforts of their surgeons and radiation oncologists and increases the chance of cure. We have learned over the past 50 years that certain hormone therapy and chemotherapy can accomplish this successfully, and we're getting better at tailoring treatment to match each woman's risk of recurrence. Recurrence is still possible, but most women are cured and never have another breast cancer diagnosis after their initial treatment.

Scientific advances in the past decade have given doctors a medical insight they've never had before: the ability to identify the unique biology of an individual's tumor. Is it sensitive to hormones? Does it thrive on a particular protein? Is it slow growing or aggressive and more likely to return? With the ability to answer these questions for each patient, the traditional one-size-fits-all treatment model has shifted to *personalized medicine* that customizes the right treatment for the right patient. Personalized medicine doesn't just enhance the treatment arsenal—it redefines it.

Compared to just a few years ago, our understanding of breast cancer has expanded, and treatments are vastly improved. We've come a long way since surgeons could only remove a woman's breasts, send her home to recover, and hope for the best. We now have more treatment options than ever before. Even more treatments are in the development pipeline, and the number of long-term breast cancer survivors continues to grow.

Although surgery and radiation are intended to eliminate cancer in the breast and lymph nodes, the greatest danger of invasive cancer is the possibility that it might return in the lungs, liver, bone, or elsewhere. That's why *systemic therapy* is vital. Systemic drugs circulate throughout the bloodstream, destroying rogue cancer cells that may linger after surgery or radiation (figure 13.1). Hormone therapy and chemotherapy remain the primary systemic treatments used to reduce the risk of recurrence. Now oncologists also have numerous new medications that can be used alone or in combination with hormone therapy or chemotherapy for more effective treatment. Many of

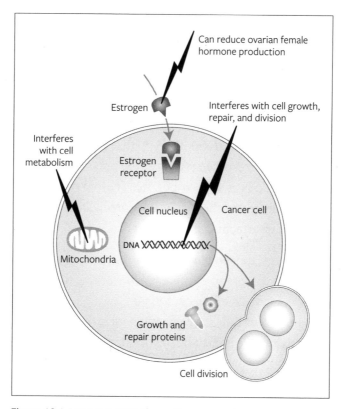

Figure 13.1. How systemic chemotherapy works

these drugs also have fewer side effects than chemotherapy, making them less likely to disrupt your daily life and normal activities.

Systemic treatments don't guarantee that cancer won't return, but they significantly improve the chance of living life without a distant recurrence elsewhere in the body. Unfortunately, systemic therapy doesn't always cure breast cancer, because even just a few remaining cancer cells can continue to multiply or lie dormant until something triggers them to "wake up" and begin reproducing.

NEOADJUVANT (PREOPERATIVE) AND ADJUVANT (POSTOPERATIVE) THERAPIES

Systemic medications used to reduce the risk of a distant recurrence are most often given as *adjuvant therapy* (after surgery)—they "add to" the benefit of surgery and other local therapy. For most people with invasive breast cancer, some type of adjuvant therapy is recommended to reduce the risk of their cancer returning.

Patients who have a high risk of recurrence, including individuals with locally advanced or inoperable large tumors, lymph node involvement, or inflammatory breast cancer, can benefit from neoadjuvant hormone therapy or chemotherapy that is given before surgery. *Neoadjuvant therapy* treats the cancer in the breast, lymph nodes, and other areas of the body as soon as possible (before surgery) to reduce the size of the cancer and the risk of it recurring later.

Neoadjuvant treatment can be used to:

- decrease large, inoperable tumors so that mastectomy is possible
- shrink large tumors so that breast-conserving therapy can be considered instead of mastectomy
- eliminate cancer cells in the lymph nodes, so that a less invasive sentinel node biopsy can be performed rather than a more invasive axillary dissection
- evaluate the effectiveness of a treatment before surgery; another type of chemotherapy can be tried if your tumor doesn't respond

- allow time for genetic testing, which can influence treatment decisions

Neoadjuvant treatment provides invaluable information about a patient's prognosis and also about the need for additional treatment. Research studies show that for women with HER2-positive or triple-negative breast cancer, a complete response (no evidence of residual cancer is found after treatment) is associated with an excellent prognosis. When neoadjuvant responses aren't optimal, however, women with HER2-positive breast cancer can then be treated with a drug called Kadcyla to improve their prognosis. Similarly, some women with triple-negative breast cancer can be treated with Xeloda (both drugs are discussed later in this chapter) if they don't have an optimal response to preoperative neoadjuvant therapy.

PREDICTING THE RISK OF RECURRENCE

The risk of recurrence is an important factor in treatment planning, although it can be confusing, and patients often misunderstand and overestimate it. When you consider your treatment options, it's important to understand how each one might affect your relative and absolute risks. Think of it this way: if your statistical risk of recurrence is 20 percent, and adjuvant therapy decreases that risk by 50 percent, and your risk then falls from 20 percent to 10 percent $(20 \times .5)$. In this situation, your relative risk reduction is 50 percent, but your absolute risk reduction is 10 percent. Your doctor can clarify how different treatments can affect your risk for recurrence. Despite recurrence statistics, many women are truly cured and never have another breast cancer diagnosis after their initial treatment.

The risk of a cancer recurring within five years of diagnosis is an important factor in treatment planning, because that's when most cancers that return are discovered. Overall, almost 90 percent of women diagnosed with early-stage breast cancer are alive at five years after treatment. Your oncologist will estimate your own risk based on your age, the characteristics of your tumor, and other predictive factors (table 13.1). Identifying your likelihood of having a recurrence helps to determine whether you need one or more of the systemic therapies discussed in this chapter.

The Difference between Remission and Being Cured

Discussions of cancer invariably involve the other "c" word: cure. "Can I be cured?" is the pressing question newly diagnosed patients want answered. Although most early-stage breast cancers are treated successfully and are truly cured, some resist treatment, and others disappear and seem to be cured, only to return later on. That's why physicians are hesitant to say that someone is cured. They often prefer instead to describe an initial absence of disease as *remission. Partial response/remission* means your cancer is still present, even though treatment has reduced your tumor. *Clinical complete response* or "no evidence of disease" means that physical examination, blood tests, and imaging scans find no detectable traces of your cancer. This is a good outcome, but even a complete remission doesn't guarantee that every cancer cell has been eradicated and won't return later on. Some women who have a clinical complete remission still have evidence of cancer cells in their breast or lymph nodes that is found during surgery. A *pathological complete response* (no evidence of cancer in tissue samples that are removed during surgery or biopsy after treatment) is the best possible result.

Several types of *genomic tests* have been developed to tell oncologists more about each woman's breast cancer. One test in particular, Oncotype DX, is standard of care for women with early-stage breast cancers that are hormone positive and HER2-Neu negative. It can help you and your doctor plan your treatment. (This test is different than genetic testing that looks for inherited mutations in a single gene like BRCA1 or BRCA2.) Oncotype DX is a classic example of personalized care because it identifies women who most need chemotherapy, while sparing thousands of women who can be safely treated instead with hormonal therapy alone. The test examines the activity of 21 genes in your breast tumor tissue. Based on changes in these genes, the software provides a Breast Recurrence Score from 0 to 100. This score reflects your chance of recurrence in the next 10 years and provides information of the risk reduction associated with adjuvant hormonal and chemotherapy (table 13.2). Medicare and most private health insurers cover the cost of Oncotype DX testing for eligible patients.

Table 13.1. Predictors of Recurrence

	Favorable	Less Favorable
Age at diagnosis	60	40
Tumor size	.2 cm	5 cm
Number of positive lymph nodes	0	All
Clear surgical margins	Yes	No
Hormone receptor status	ER/PR+	ER/PR−
HER2 status	Negative	Positive
Ki-67 status*	Low	High
Genomic test score	Low	High

Abbreviations are as follows: ER, estrogen receptor; PR, progesterone receptor.

*Ki-67 is a protein marker that can indicate rapidly growing cancer cells.

Table 13.2. American Society of Clinical Oncology Recommendations for Oncotype Testing

Age	Recurrence Score	Risk of Recurrence	Benefit of Adding Chemotherapy to Hormonal Therapy
≤50	0–15	Low	Little to no benefit*
	16–20	Low-medium	Some benefit but may not outweigh the risks and side effects#
	21–25	Medium	Benefit that is likely to be greater than risks of side effects#
	26–100	High	Benefit that is likely to be greater than risks of side effects^
>50	0–25	Low	Little to no benefit*
	26–100	High	Some benefit that is likely to be greater than the risks of side effects^

*May offer hormonal therapy alone.

#May offer hormonal therapy and chemotherapy.

^Patients with recurrence scores between 26 and 30 may be offered hormonal therapy and chemotherapy. Patients with recurrence scores greater than 30 should be considered for hormonal therapy and chemotherapy.

Aside from knowledge and experience, many oncologists use online computer programs to help predict the odds of a woman's breast cancer recurrence and to help inform treatment decisions. Although predictive programs are a major step forward, they describe the expected risk of recurrence and benefit of treatment for a group of women, rather than for an individual. These tools might estimate that 20 of 100 women with node-negative breast cancer will develop recurrent disease, but they don't tell us which 20 women are involved, so we end up treating all 100 with chemotherapy when only 20 will benefit. Other genomic tests, including Oncotype, MammaPrint, EndoPredict, Prosigna, and the Breast Cancer Index, help to further calculate a woman's recurrence based on the expression of certain genes in the tumor. These tests, however, are not standard for HER2-positive or triple-negative breast cancers. Researchers continue to develop tests with improved accuracy for estimating recurrence and whether chemotherapy or hormone therapy would be helpful.

Questions to Ask Your Doctor about Oncotype DX

- Is my breast cancer hormone receptor positive?
- Am I eligible for the Oncotype DX test?
- What stage is my breast cancer, and how likely is it to return based on this test?
- How long will it take to get the results?
- What does my recurrence score mean related to other information about my breast cancer?
- How will these test results influence my treatment plan?
- How can I get a copy of my test results?

REDUCING RECURRENCE WITH ADJUVANT HORMONE THERAPY

Before menopause, your ovaries produce *estrogen*, the primary female hormone, and *progesterone*. Both hormones are essential. They affect how you feel, how you look, and how you function. All cells in the body are exposed to these hormones as they circulate in the bloodstream, but not all cells react to them. Estrogen and progesterone trigger activity only in cells that have special proteins called *receptors* that act like antennae for these hormones. One or both hormones then attach to these receptors and stimulate cell growth, contributing to the health of your hair, skin, bones, and many other parts of your body. Some breast cancer cells also pick up these hormone signals and begin to multiply excessively. This abnormal growth results in tumors that need estrogen or progesterone to grow, just as a car needs fuel to run. These cells continue to divide as long as they're exposed to the hormone (figure 13.2).

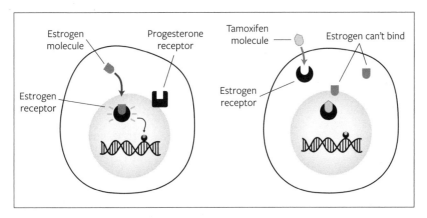

Figure 13.2. How tamoxifen works as a hormonal therapy

All breast tumors should be tested to determine their hormone receptor status. About 80 percent of breast cancers are *estrogen receptor positive* (ER positive); they have many receptors on the surface of the cells that make them sensitive to estrogen. ER-positive tumors are most common in women over age 50 and in women who have BRCA2 mutations, regardless of their age. Others tumors are *progesterone receptor positive* (PR positive). About 65 percent of breast cancers are "double positive" for both estrogen and progesterone. ER-positive tumors generally grow slowly and have a good prognosis when they're treated with medications that reduce levels of estrogen in the body or disable the tumor's ability to use this hormone. These tumors can return years after treatment, but adjuvant *hormone therapy* reduces this risk.

Hormone therapies that decrease the production of estrogen, block estrogen from attaching to receptors, or eliminate the estrogen receptors are the most important type of treatment for hormone-positive tumors. Even tumors that only partially express one of these hormones can benefit from this therapy. In addition, most hormone therapy drugs have a "legacy effect," meaning their benefits linger after treatment ends (table 13.3). (Hormone therapy isn't the same as menopausal hormone therapy that relieves menopausal symptoms by increasing hormone levels.)

Table 13.3. Common Antihormone Drugs for Hormone Receptor–Positive, Early-Stage Invasive Breast Cancer

Medication	Brand Name	Cancer Type
Tamoxifen	Nolvadex	Pre- and postmenopausal
Anastrozole	Arimidex	Postmenopausal
Exemestane	Aromasin	Postmenopausal
Letrozole	Femara	Postmenopausal
Goserelin	Zoladex	Premenopausal
Leuprolide	Lupron	Premenopausal

Breast cancers that lack hormone receptors are said to be *estrogen receptor negative* (ER negative) and *progesterone receptor negative* (PR negative). These are typically faster-growing cancers that tend to appear more often in premenopausal women. Hormone-negative tumors don't respond to hormone therapy and are generally treated with chemotherapy instead. Many tumors also express receptors for *androgen*, a primarily male hormone that women have in limited quantities. Treatment with "anti-androgens" isn't standard but is being studied to determine if it might be helpful.

The Role of Estrogen

Estrogen is primarily produced by the ovaries, although it's also made in smaller amounts by fat tissue and the adrenal glands. Because most cells in the female body have estrogen receptors, much of the body's systems are influenced by this hormone. Balanced levels of estrogen stabilize cholesterol levels, regulate mood, and promote healthy libido. Having too little or too much estrogen can create numerous health issues.

During puberty, estrogen changes girls into women. Breasts grow, hips widen, and by age 15, the menstrual cycle normally begins and prepares the body for pregnancy. Estrogen peaks midcycle and dips to its lowest levels during menstrual periods. Ovulation, when an egg is released from the ovaries, occurs at this time. (Birth control pills trigger the ovaries to produce less estrogen and forego monthly ovulation.) If the egg isn't fertilized, estrogen levels decrease and menstruation continues. When an egg is fertilized and pregnancy occurs, the combined effect of estrogen and progesterone stops ovulation. Estrogen levels peak around age 20, and by age 35, the steady production gradually declines. During their 40s or 50s, women might enter *perimenopause*—a transition phase between the childbearing years and menopause. Ovulation becomes irregular, which can cause heavy periods, cramping, and weight gain around the belly and buttocks.

Clinically, menopause begins when you haven't had a period for 12 consecutive months. During menopause, estrogen falls to its lowest level and the ovaries no longer release eggs. On average, women experience the onset of menopause at age 51. Coping with the characteristic hot flashes, mood swings, vaginal dryness, reduced energy, and other symptoms of "the change of life" can be difficult, although many women experience only mild symptoms or none at all. Menopausal hormone therapy can relieve these symptoms, but it also raises the risk for hormone-fueled breast tumors. Your doctor can recommend ways to alleviate menopausal symptoms and explain the benefits and risks of taking menopausal hormone therapy.

Tamoxifen

Initially approved in 1977 to treat metastatic breast cancer, tamoxifen was later recognized as an effective anti-estrogen therapy for women with hormone-positive breast cancers, and it's still the most widely used medication for premenopausal estrogen receptor–positive breast cancers. Less often, it's used to treat postmenopausal women. Tamoxifen is a *selective estrogen receptor modulator* (SERM), a class of drugs that bind to estrogen receptors, taking up space so that circulating estrogen can't attach and stimulate cancer growth, similar to a key that can't be pushed into a plugged lock.

Taken as a daily pill, tamoxifen (Nolvadex) is a medical workhorse with a favorable risk-to-benefit ratio, especially in premenopausal women.

- It decreases recurrence by up to 50 percent in premenopausal women.
- It lowers recurrence by up to 50 percent in postmenopausal women.
- It reduces the risk of a new cancer in the other breast by about 50 percent.
- It benefits women who have hormone receptor–positive tumors, regardless of age, tumor size, and lymph node involvement. It doesn't benefit women with ER-negative or PR-negative cancers.

These benefits continue for 5 to 10 years after treatment ends. Extending treatment for a total of 10 years is advised for premenopausal and postmenopausal women who have a higher risk of recurrence, including many women with stage II breast cancer and also those with stage III breast cancer. Women who become menopausal during treatment are usually switched to an aromatase inhibitor, a different kind of hormone therapy.

Side Effects of Tamoxifen

Tamoxifen is well studied, and its benefits and side effects are well documented. Unlike most breast cancer therapies, it provides beneficial effects that are unrelated to its effect on hormone-sensitive tumors. While tamoxifen acts as an anti-estrogen on some cells, it also has a favorable estrogen-like benefit that helps to prevent bone loss and lowers certain types of cholesterol.

Although the benefits of tamoxifen outweigh the risks for most women who take it, side effects can occur. Some women have no ill effects, while many others experience multiple undesirable conditions, including hot flashes, vaginal dryness or discharge, night sweats, and other menopause-like side effects that are usually mild and well tolerated. If these effects become too uncomfortable, they can be managed with over-the-counter or prescribed medications. Tamoxifen stops menstruation in some women, especially those who are over age 45 and who are already approaching menopause. Women treated with tamoxifen can have benign thickening of the lining of the uterus, and some studies have found an increase in hysterectomies in women who take it. With this in mind, it's important to alert your doctor of any abnormal spotting or bleeding, especially if you're menopausal and you take tamoxifen. You should also have regular gynecologic screenings.

Other more serious side effects are also possible. Tamoxifen somewhat increases the risk of stroke and blood clots in women who smoke or have a history of clotting. It also slightly raises the risk—less than 1 percent per year, according to the American Cancer Society—of developing endometrial cancer (in the lining of the uterus). This is because in addition to acting as an anti-estrogen in breast tissue, tamoxifen has an estrogen-like effect on the uterus, thus increasing slightly the risk of cancer in those tissues. In the National Surgical Adjuvant Breast and Bowel Project P-1 Study, women with a high risk for breast cancer who took tamoxifen preventively had double the risk of endometrial cancer compared to placebo; the absolute difference was very small, less than 1 percent in both groups. Most cases in the tamoxifen group were diagnosed early and cured with surgery, and deaths from uterine cancer occurred only in women who took the placebo. If you're treated with tamoxifen, you should have annual gynecologic exams and promptly inform your doctor of any spotting or abnormal bleeding, which can be signs of endometrial cancer.

Women who take tamoxifen also have a low risk of developing a uterine sarcoma, an unusual cancer of the uterus. Many women who take tamoxifen also believe that it is associated with weight gain, although well-conducted research suggests that such weight gain is more likely due to previous chemotherapy or the onset of menopause. Your oncologist can discuss these risk issues with you.

Aromatase Inhibitors

Although estrogen production dwindles after menopause, the adrenal glands produce small amounts of steroids that are converted into estrogen by an enzyme called aromatase. Fat cells also produce estrogen in small amounts that are enough to stimulate estrogen receptors in the breast—this is one reason why gaining weight after menopause raises breast cancer risk. *Aromatase inhibitors* (AIs), including anastrozole (Arimidex), letrozole (Femara), and exemestane (Aromasin), block most of this low-level estrogen production, further reducing estrogen levels after menopause (figure 13.3). Because AIs don't target estrogen production in the ovaries, they're not effective for premenopausal women.

For postmenopausal women with hormone receptor–positive breast cancers, aromatase inhibitors have more benefits and fewer serious side effects than tamoxifen. They reduce the risks of a local or metastatic recurrence and a new breast cancer in the opposite breast.

- AIs can be taken for five years instead of tamoxifen or as a five-year follow-up treatment after tamoxifen.
- Taking tamoxifen for two to three years and then switching to an AI (for a total of five years) is more beneficial than taking five years of tamoxifen.
- Five years of tamoxifen followed by five years of an AI continues to decrease the risk of recurrence, compared to no treatment after tamoxifen.
- Ten years of adjuvant treatment with an AI is recommended for women with lymph node–positive breast cancer. This extended regimen may also benefit many postmenopausal

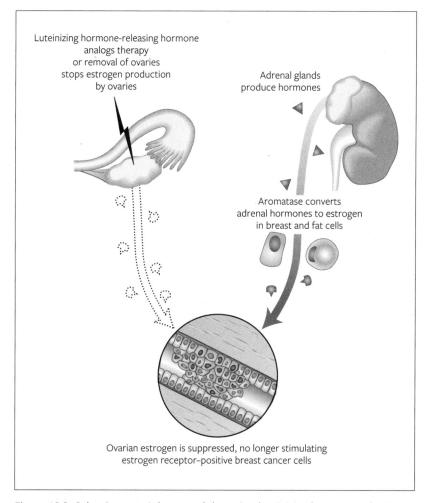

Figure 13.3. Other important hormonal therapies: luteinizing hormone-releasing hormone analogs and aromatase inhibitors

women with node-negative breast cancer, depending on their risk of recurrence.

- AIs are also effective against premenopausal ER-positive breast cancers in women whose ovarian function has been suppressed. Women who become menopausal while taking tamoxifen can switch to an AI for the remainder of their recommended regimen.

Postmenopausal women generally tolerate aromatase inhibitors as well as or better than tamoxifen and are less likely to experience vaginal bleeding or discharge, blood clots, or uterine cancer. Like tamoxifen, AIs can cause hot flashes, vaginal dryness, and stiff or aching joints (figure 13.4). Your doctor may recommend that you take a *bisphosphonate* (a bone-strengthening medication) to counteract the bone-weakening effect of aromatase inhibitors.

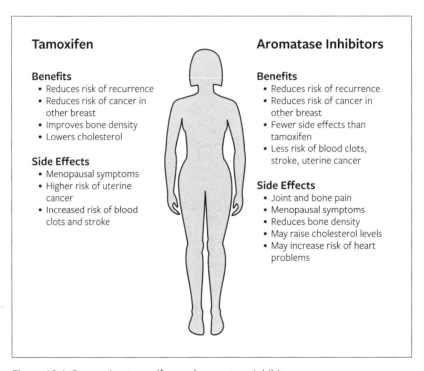

Tamoxifen

Benefits
- Reduces risk of recurrence
- Reduces risk of cancer in other breast
- Improves bone density
- Lowers cholesterol

Side Effects
- Menopausal symptoms
- Higher risk of uterine cancer
- Increased risk of blood clots and stroke

Aromatase Inhibitors

Benefits
- Reduces risk of recurrence
- Reduces risk of cancer in other breast
- Fewer side effects than tamoxifen
- Less risk of blood clots, stroke, uterine cancer

Side Effects
- Joint and bone pain
- Menopausal symptoms
- Reduces bone density
- May raise cholesterol levels
- May increase risk of heart problems

Figure 13.4. Comparing tamoxifen and aromatase inhibitors

Suppressing Ovarian Function

Therapy for premenopausal women with estrogen receptor–positive breast cancer who have a high risk for recurrence may include *ovarian suppression* to further reduce that risk. This can be accomplished with either goserelin (Zoladex) or leuprolide (Lupron), medications that stop estrogen production in the ovaries and cause temporary menopause until the medication is stopped. Ablation may also benefit younger premenopausal women who have already completed chemotherapy but are still menstruating; it may not be as beneficial for older premenopausal women. After a median follow-up of eight years, results from the TEXT and SOFT clinical trials showed that combining ovarian suppression with adjuvant tamoxifen or the aromatase inhibitor exemestane significantly reduced recurrence and disease-free survival compared to tamoxifen alone in some young women. Many women in the trial suffered from severe hot flashes, night sweats, and other side effects.

Two other methods of ovarian suppression are used less often. *Bilateral salpingo-oophorectomy*—surgical removal of both ovaries—is recommended for women who have a BRCA mutation and a high risk of breast and ovarian cancer. Otherwise, it's not often advised as an initial treatment option because it's irreversible and may not help to treat your cancer. With the availability of drugs that suppress ovarian function, it's also unnecessary. However, some patients prefer to have their ovaries removed rather than having monthly shots that are required to continue ovarian suppression until menopause. Radiating the ovaries is another, less common method of ablation, but it can be difficult to accurately target the ovaries without also radiating and damaging nearby organs.

REDUCING RECURRENCE
WITH CHEMOTHERAPY

Infused, injected, or taken orally, chemotherapy reduces recurrence for many women. The overall benefit is similar whether chemotherapy is given before or after surgery. Younger women seem to benefit more, perhaps because chemo indirectly suppresses their ovarian function. Chemo may be relatively less effective for women with small, node-negative tumors that are hormone receptor positive and don't have receptors for HER2, a protein that stimulates growth in 20 percent of breast cancers.

Chemotherapy is a common patient fear, but not every woman needs it. Its use for breast cancer has declined in recent years, and more than 70 percent of breast cancer patients are now treated with a different therapy. Chemotherapy may be recommended if you have a high risk of recurrence; it's less likely if your risk is low. For example, an aromatase inhibitor is typically the preferred treatment for post-menopausal women who have a small, estrogen receptor–positive tumor and no cancer in the sentinel lymph node; chemotherapy would add little benefit. In contrast, chemotherapy may substantially benefit premenopausal women with a large tumor that doesn't have estrogen or progesterone receptors but does have cancer in the lymph nodes. Your individual health, the characteristic of your breast cancer, and your personal preferences should also be considered.

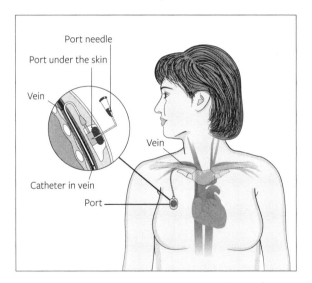

Figure 13.5. A chest port makes it easier to have infusions

Chemotherapy is given in cycles, often once every two to three weeks with a break in between to allow the body and blood counts to recover. Depending on the drugs used, it may be administered only on the first day of the treatment cycle. The entire treatment-recovery cycle for early-stage invasive breast cancer is then repeated usually four to eight times over three to six months. If you're at high risk for a recurrence, you may fare better with a higher dose of chemo that is given every two weeks instead of every three weeks.

If you have neoadjuvant chemotherapy (before surgery), you'll be carefully monitored throughout the course of your treatment to see how your cancer responds. Your first line of prescribed treatment is continued if the tumor responds; if your cancer progresses, the regimen may be modified. Most often, however, chemotherapy is given after surgery. In this case, your oncologist can monitor your tolerance of the chemotherapy but will have no way to objectively measure its effect because the tumor has already been removed.

What to Expect from a Chemotherapy Session

Walking into your first chemotherapy session can be intimidating, but knowing what to expect may help you feel better about what you'll experience. For most women, treatment with chemotherapy is easier than they expect; nausea and other commonly feared side effects can almost always be prevented. Oncology nurses and staff who treat patients are supportive and kind people who do their best to make you as comfortable as possible. Although patients aren't usually enthusiastic about chemotherapy, many are able to welcome treatment as life affirming and life saving, and their treatment turns out to be a more positive experience than they would have imagined.

A few days before your first treatment, you may have a minor procedure to have a small port implanted just beneath your skin (figure 13.5). The port is attached to a small catheter placed directly into a vein in your chest. Having the port in place avoids having to find a vein every time you have an infusion. Your chemotherapy will be given through the port, which doesn't interfere with exercise or normal activities, and it will be removed after you complete your final session.

When you arrive for your first infusion, a nurse will take a blood sample and send it to the lab. Your vital signs—pulse, blood pressure, and temperature—will then be taken, and your height and weight will be measured to ensure that the right dose is given. If your lab results show that you have no health issues that would interfere with treatment, your oncologist will order your chemotherapy and any steroids, anti-anxiety, or antinausea

(continued)

premedications prescribed for you. Your nurse will then place an IV tube in your arm or into your chest port, with the other end connected to a bag of chemotherapy on a rolling stand. You'll sit in a recliner as a slow drip of solutions is administered, beginning with saline, followed by any premedications, then chemotherapy, and ending with more saline.

Depending on your chemotherapy, a session may take several hours. You're free to watch television, work on your laptop, read, or talk to pass the time. You can also periodically get up and carefully walk around while you remain connected to your supply of chemotherapy. Women often bring their own blankets and snacks, as well as books, e-readers, or portable movie players to pass the time. It's a good idea to contact the treatment center before your first session to ask about the length of your chemo sessions, and what you should bring from home. You should also bring someone with you for your first treatment, until you know how the chemotherapy will affect you. When your session is finished, your nurse will remove your IV or disconnect your port, recheck your blood pressure, pulse, breathing, and temperature, and give you a list of posttreatment instructions.

Common Chemotherapy Drugs Used for Breast Cancer

Chemotherapy drugs destroy cancer cells in different ways. Some prevent cancer cells from dividing, while others interfere with cellular metabolism or repair processes. Common chemotherapy medications used for early-stage and locally advanced breast cancers are listed in table 13.4.

Combination chemotherapy includes treatment with two or more chemo drugs. It is usually more effective because it simultaneously targets different aspects of a cancer cell's growth, metabolism, or its ability to divide. Your doctor has many combinations to choose from, depending on the makeup of your tumor, your general health and preexisting conditions, and an understanding of possible side effects. If one drug or a combination of drugs is likely to be poorly tolerated, your oncologist can treat you with a different combination. For many women, several months of treatment with adjuvant chemotherapy reduces the risk of recurrence and breast cancer–related death. Your

**Table 13.4. Common Chemotherapy Drugs
for Early-Stage Invasive Breast Cancer**

Class of Drugs	Drug	Brand Name
Anthracyclines	Doxorubicin (A)	Adriamycin
	Epirubicin (E)	Ellence
Alkylating agents	Cyclophosphamide (C)	Cytoxan
Anti-metabolites	Methotrexate (M)	Mexate, Folex, Rheumatrex, Trexall
	Capecitabine	Xeloda
	5-fluorouracil (F)	Adrucil
Taxanes	Paclitaxel (T)	Taxol
	Albumin-bound paclitaxel	Abraxane
	Docetaxel (T)	Taxotere

reduced risk may be small or substantial depending on the exact nature of your breast cancer and how it responds to treatment.

Common chemotherapy combinations include:

AC: doxorubicin and cyclophosphamide
AC + paclitaxel: doxorubicin, cyclophosphamide, and then paclitaxel
AC + docetaxel: doxorubicin, cyclophosphamide, and then docetaxel
AC + docetaxel and carboplatin
EC: epirubicin and cyclophosphamide
TC: docetaxel and cyclophosphamide
CAF: cyclophosphamide, doxorubicin, and 5-fluorouracil
CEF: cyclophosphamide, epirubicin, and 5-fluorouracil
CMF: cyclophosphamide, methotrexate, and 5-fluorouracil
TAC: docetaxel, doxorubicin, and cyclophosphamide

Behaviors That Can Affect Chemotherapy

- Research shows that heavier women who receive the same dose of chemotherapy as their thinner counterparts may be underdosed if their oncologist uses their ideal weight rather than their actual weight. That can be harmful, because underdosing can reduce remission and disease-free intervals, which in turn affect survival. Clinical guidelines encourage oncologists to measure chemotherapy drugs based on a patient's actual size and weight, which doesn't appear to increase side effects.
- Smoking increases the chance of death from breast cancer or any cause. Nicotine can interfere with the effectiveness of chemotherapy. It also promotes infection, delays healing, and increases the chance for lung damage after radiation therapy. Smokers also have more side effects than nonsmokers, even months after treatment. Patients who stop smoking before treatment begins have no more side effects than nonsmokers.
- Some medications, vitamins, supplements, and herbs can intensify or weaken the effectiveness of your treatments. Let your doctor know about any and all that you take.
- Grapefruit pulp and juice, Seville oranges, pomegranates, and some other foods contain a substance that inhibits certain types of chemotherapy. Your doctor can advise how much of these you can safely consume during treatment or whether you should avoid them altogether.

Risks and Side Effects

Although chemotherapy is less toxic than it used to be and many women continue with their daily activities throughout the course of their treatment, some chemotherapy can be harsh, and patients must be healthy enough to withstand its toxicity and side effects. Your doctor may want you to undergo tests to be sure that your kidney, liver, and heart functions are strong enough. If you have certain health problems, your treatment may need to be changed or delayed.

Chemotherapy is *cytotoxic* treatment—it's harmful to cancer cells and normal cells alike, particularly those in the reproductive system, hair follicles, bone marrow, and the gastrointestinal tract.

Most chemo-related side effects involve these organs. Side effects differ in type and intensity depending on the drugs used and your own reaction to them. They're rarely life threatening or fatal, but when they occur, they can be a lot to deal with, especially if several develop simultaneously.

Common acute side effects can include fatigue, weight changes, temporary hair loss, mouth sores, changes in taste and sensation, and aching joints. Nausea and vomiting sometimes occur but aren't problematic for most women who are treated with anti-nausea medications. If you're treated with chemotherapy, you'll have periodic blood tests to monitor your blood counts. If needed, your doctor may recommend injections of growth factor proteins to increase your white blood count.

Other common side effects include cognitive lapses and memory problems known as "chemo brain." Some chemotherapy drugs induce early menopause, with hot flashes, vaginal dryness, and other symptoms that commonly occur with menopause. If you were taking hormone replacement therapy for the symptoms of natural menopause but stopped after being diagnosed with breast cancer, you may experience the same or similar symptoms with chemotherapy. Some drugs are associated with very low risk—less than .5 percent—of leukemia. Doxorubicin or epirubicin, which are anthracycline drugs, can weaken the heart muscle, so these drugs aren't ordinarily given to women who already have reduced heart function. Taxol and taxotere can cause *peripheral neuropathy* (numbness, tingling, or pain in the hands and feet). These side effects and others are discussed in more detail in chapter 18.

Many medications can reduce and sometimes eliminate the undesirable effects of chemotherapy. It's important to inform your health care team of any issues that develop during treatment so that they can be managed before they become more problematic. Having mouth sores, losing your hair, or feeling like you have the flu can make it difficult to continue with chemo, but most women, once they make the decision to have it, continue despite the difficulties.

Tips for Getting through Chemotherapy

- Get a flu shot before beginning chemotherapy.
- Schedule a dental hygiene appointment before your first round of chemo to ensure that you have no oral infections.
- Skip having your nails done in a salon because the risk of infection is high.
- Consider shopping for a wig or learning how to use head scarves if your chemo will cause you to lose your hair.
- Ask your spouse, partner, or a close friend to keep you company during infusions.
- Make getting through chemo and caring for yourself your priority.
- Eat nutritionally balanced meals.
- Stay active and exercise to the best of your ability.
- Find ways to stay motivated and stay positive.
- Talk to someone about your feelings, fears, and thoughts as you go through treatment.
- Be patient with your body when it needs time to heal.

REDUCING RECURRENCE WITH HER2 INHIBITORS

Human epidermal growth factor 2 (HER2) is a protein involved in normal cell growth. While healthy cells have about 20,000 receptors for HER2, one in five breast cancers, especially among young women, have up to two million of these receptors, which overamplify the number of signals cells receive to divide and grow. HER2-positive cancer cells develop faster because they're constantly bombarded with an overload of these messages. This makes them more aggressive and more likely to metastasize and recur. Until the advent of anti-HER2 drugs, these breast cancers had a poor prognosis. They now have one of the best breast cancer prognoses.

HER2-positive breast cancers were traditionally treated with chemotherapy, but with discouraging results. They went from barely treatable to very treatable with the development of trastuzumab (Herceptin), and the prognosis for women with these breast cancers is now quite good. Trastuzumab is a type of *targeted therapy*, a drug that's engineered to disable or block specific molecular characteristics of a tumor, rather than attacking all of a person's cells as chemotherapy can do. Some targeted medications work by impeding the cells' ability to form new blood vessels or to continue dividing. Others shut down the cells' self-repair mechanism. Trastuzumab is a special type of targeted therapy known as a *monoclonal antibody*. (Medications in this class of drugs always end with "mab," short for monoclonal antibody.) It binds to HER2 receptors on breast cancer cells—like putting a lid on a jar—so that growth signals are unable to transmit and cell division slows or stops.

Early-stage HER2 breast cancers are usually treated with a combination of chemotherapy and trastuzumab. This is followed by a total of one year of trastuzumab alone, which is infused in 30- to 90-minute sessions before surgery, after surgery, or a combination of both. A longer regimen doesn't improve disease-free survival, and for women with small HER2-amplified tumors, a shorter course is sometimes possible. Most women with early-stage HER2-positive breast cancer do very well with trastuzumab and chemotherapy followed by trastuzumab alone, with excellent seven-year disease-free survival rates. For women with tumors that are smaller than 1 centimeter, some physicians prefer less intense adjuvant treatment with paclitaxel plus trastuzumab for 12 weeks, followed by trastuzumab alone for a total treatment period of one year.

Despite the success of trastuzumab, some HER2 breast cancers become resistant to its effects. Another monoclonal antibody, pertuzumab (Perjeta), blocks HER2 from sending signals to other proteins that encourage cell growth and reproduction. For women with early-stage HER2-positive breast cancer, a combination of trastuzumab, pertuzumab, and chemotherapy can be considered before or after lumpectomy or mastectomy. Depending on the nature of your breast cancer, your oncologist may consider one of the following regimens:

- paclitaxel and trastuzumab
- paclitaxel and trastuzumab with either paclitaxel or docetaxel

- trastuzumab, pertuzumab, and either paclitaxel or docetaxel with carboplatin
- docetaxel, carboplatin, and trastuzumab, with or without pertuzumab
- doxorubicin and cyclophosphamide, then paclitaxel and trastuzumab
- doxorubicin and cyclophosphamide, then paclitaxel, trastuzumab, and pertuzumab

For most women with HER2-positive breast cancers, a combination of chemotherapy, trastuzumab, and pertuzumab is standard. About 60 percent of women who receive this regimen preoperatively have no residual cancer when lumpectomy or mastectomy is later performed. Some women with HER2-positive tumors can be treated postoperatively with Herceptin HYLECTA, a medication that combines trastuzumab and hyaluronidase-oysk, an enzyme that allows Herceptin to be administered by injection rather than infused. This two-in-one drug is usually injected under the skin for two to five minutes once every three weeks. Talk to your doctor about this option if Herceptin is recommended for you and you prefer injections over infusion.

Herceptin: Building a Gamechanger

How do you develop a specific medicine for a hard-to-treat cancer when you don't understand how it works or what makes it grow? That was the challenge taken up by Dr. Dennis Slamon and colleagues at the University of California, Los Angeles (UCLA), in the 1980s. Ten years earlier, molecular scientists had discovered oncogenes, genes that overexpress proteins and fuel tumor growth. That clue inspired the UCLA researchers' hypothesis: if they could find a specific oncogene in breast cancer tumors, they could then explore ways to dismantle or disrupt it. They subsequently found that 20 percent of breast cancers had too many copies of the HER2 oncogene, which overproduced the protein that instructed cancer cells to grow. HER2 breast cancer was a worthy starting place: it was resistant to many types of chemotherapy, often recurred and metastasized, and carried a poor prognosis for survival. With the molecular culprit identified, a large part of the problem was solved. The next step was to find a way to block HER2 signals.

Around the same time, scientists at the biopharmaceutical company Genentech were working to develop monoclonal antibodies—man-made copies of natural immune system proteins that fight off bacteria and viruses. Progress against HER2 cancers took a giant leap forward when UCLA and Genentech researchers collaborated to create a monoclonal antibody that could suppress the growth of HER2-positive tumors in mice. When they injected lab mice with HER2, the mouse immune systems responded by making multiple antibodies against the protein, in the same way the flu vaccine prompts your body to produce antibodies. Researchers then selected the antibody that most efficiently bound to the HER2 protein and disrupted its function. This was the point where previous trials of antibodies had failed, because the human immune system recognized mouse antibodies as foreign objects and rejected them. This time, the scientists spliced sections of the mouse HER2 antibody onto a human antibody. They hoped this cleverly disguised "humanized antibody" would fool the immune system into accepting it. The new antibody, named trastuzumab (Herceptin), worked on HER2 breast cancer cells in the lab, but would it work as well in people?

Clinical trials of women with metastatic HER2-positive breast cancer showed that trastuzumab combined with chemotherapy dramatically slowed tumor growth, reduced tumor size, and improved survival. As a result, Herceptin became the first antibody to target a specific component of a tumor's unique biology, and in 1998, it received FDA approval to treat advanced HER2-positive breast cancer. More trials followed, and in 2006, Herceptin in combination with chemotherapy became standard of care for adjuvant treatment of early-stage, HER2-positive tumors. This pioneering research changed the outlook for HER2 diagnoses from very poor to very treatable, and it has since saved thousands of lives. It also paved the way for other targeted cancer therapies that have since been developed.

Side Effects

Cells in the heart muscle have HER2 receptors that are unintentionally targeted by trastuzumab and pertuzumab. Of women who take these drugs, 2 to 4 percent develop reduced heart muscle function. The risk is greater when either drug is combined with doxorubicin or epirubicin, which can also cause heart damage. Most women who are affected improve when they stop these medications; some women must delay treatment or switch to another treatment. You'll need to have heart tests before you begin this medication and periodically during and after treatment.

If you could become pregnant, it's important to use a reliable method of contraception while taking trastuzumab and pertuzumab, because they can be fatal to a fetus. They can also be toxic to infants, so you shouldn't breastfeed while you take either drug. Because most women who are treated with trastuzumab are also given chemotherapy, side effects from both treatments may develop.

Other Anti-HER2 Medications

Since the success of trastuzumab, other drugs have been created to specifically target HER2 receptors. Ado-trastuzumab emtansine, or T-DM1 (Kadcyla), is an adjuvant targeted treatment for some women with early-stage HER2-positive breast cancer. It's a "smart drug," meaning that it consists of trastuzumab attached to a small dose of emtansine, a strong chemotherapy medicine. Ado-trastuzumab emtansine delivers chemotherapy directly to the receptors of HER2 cells. It's given intravenously every three weeks for women who were neoadjuvantly treated before surgery with trastuzumab and paclitaxel or docetaxel and then had breast cancer surgery that discovered that a portion of the tumor still remained. An FDA-approved companion test can determine if you're eligible for this medication. Another targeted medication, neratinib maleate (Nerlynx), treats early-stage, HER2-positive breast cancer that is likely to recur. It's a daily pill that is taken for one year, after one year of trastuzumab.

Like other chemotherapy medicines, the emtansine portion of this drug disrupts the way cancer cells grow, but it can also affect healthy cells. It doesn't usually cause hair loss or vomiting, as many other chemotherapy drugs do, but headache, nausea, fatigue, muscle and joint pain, and low *platelet* (small particles involved with blood clotting) counts may occur. Infusion-related reactions, including skin redness, tenderness, or swelling, may also develop. If you take this medication, you must be closely monitored because, less frequently, it can cause severe and even life-threatening liver and heart problems. You shouldn't take Kadcyla if you're premenopausal, sexually active, and not using birth control or if you're already pregnant, because it can cause birth defects and can be fatal for embryos.

Generics and Biosimilars: Alternatives to Brand Name Drugs

Pharmaceutical companies spend billions of dollars researching, developing, and testing new cancer drugs, which they patent and sell under their brand name. When a patent for a company's drug expires, other companies can manufacture a copy of the drug and then sell it if approved by the FDA. Because the makeup and clinical utility of the original drug have already been tested and approved, manufacturers of *generic* and *biosimilar* drugs don't incur the same costs of research, development, and clinical trials. In many cases, this cost savings is passed along to the consumer. Both types of medications share other similarities, but they also have important differences.

Generics are made by synthesizing chemical drugs, while biosimilars are biological treatments (proteins) that are made from living organisms. Both generic drugs and biosimilars have the same active ingredients as their brand name counterparts. They must be identical in quality, dose, strength, the way they're administered, and intended use. Prescribing guidelines differ, however. Generics are interchangeable with brand name drugs—they can be substituted for the brand name drug by the pharmacist. Biosimilars require a specific prescription from your health care provider unless the FDA makes a specific determination that they are interchangeable. Generic drugs are approved with little more than a chemical analysis and a demonstration that they are distributed similarly in the bloodstream as the brand drug (this is called "bioequivalence"). Although biosimilar drugs must also pass human clinical trials, and in some cases nonclinical studies in animals, development and approval are abbreviated compared to the standard FDA drug approval process.

A biosimilar drug is a copycat of an existing biologic medication. It must be "highly similar" to its brand name counterpart and offer "nearly identical" safety, purity, and clinical effectiveness with the same side

(continued)

effects, although it can contain somewhat different product stabilizers and other inactive ingredients. Biosimilar drugs must also be delivered in the same way: if the original drug is given intravenously, the biosimilar drug must also be given intravenously. Some biosimilar drugs treat breast cancer. Trastuzumab-dkst (Ogivri) and trastuzumab-pkrb (Herzuma), for example, are FDA-approved biosimilars of Herceptin, which is a monoclonal antibody that treats early-stage, HER2-positive breast cancer. Other biosimilars relieve side effects. Filgrastim-sndz (Zarxio) and filgrastim-aafi (Nivestym) are biosimilar forms of filgrastim (Neupogen), a drug that helps to maintain white blood cells counts during chemotherapy.

Your oncologist can explain whether a generic or biosimilar drug might offer you reduced cost or easier administration, or whether brand name drugs are a better treatment choice.

TREATING TRIPLE-NEGATIVE BREAST CANCER

Most breast cancers are classified by the characteristics of the tumor: they have receptors for estrogen, progesterone, or HER2. *Triple-negative breast cancers* (TNBCs) are defined by the characteristics they lack: they don't have receptors for estrogen, progesterone, or HER2, and they don't respond to hormone or anti-HER therapies (figure 13.6). While anyone can develop triple-negative breast cancer, it's more common in African Americans, younger women, and individuals who carry a BRCA gene mutation; about 75 percent of breast cancers in people with a BRCA1 mutation are TNBC. If you're diagnosed with TNBC before age 60 and/or have blood relatives with breast or ovarian cancer, a genetic counselor can determine whether you might benefit from genetic testing. This is an important step, because having a BRCA mutation can change your treatment recommendations.

Mammograms can detect most TNBC tumors, which tend to be more aggressive, making treatment more challenging. So it's critically important to have a multidisciplinary health care team with experience in treating these difficult cancers. Most cases are treated with a combination of surgery and chemotherapy, and some women also have radiation. Lumpectomy can remove the tumor if it's small

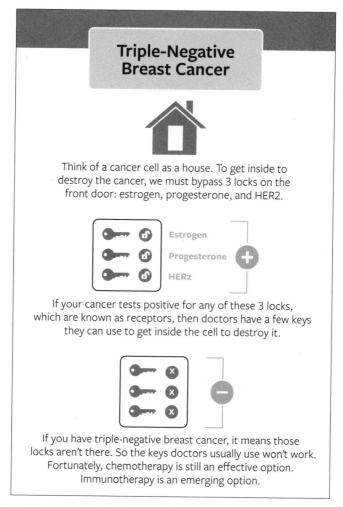

Figure 13.6. Standard therapies don't target triple-negative breast cancers. https://www.cdc.gov/cancer/breast/triple-negative.htm

enough. Larger tumors that respond to neoadjuvant chemotherapy may be reduced sufficiently for lumpectomy. Some women with TNBC who are treated with neoadjuvant chemotherapy achieve a pathologic complete response: their posttreatment tissue samples show no evidence of breast cancer. For women with TNBC who do not achieve a complete remission from preoperative chemotherapy, an oral chemotherapy may be recommended after surgery to further reduce the risk of recurrence.

TNBC often responds well to chemotherapy, which can be given postoperatively but which may not be needed after surgery for extremely small tumors (5 millimeters or less). A common approach is to give four doses of adriamycin and cytoxan given together every 2 weeks, followed by 12 weeks of taxol. Your doctor will explain why you might not need chemotherapy or which regimen is the best for you and why. Compared to women with hormone receptor–positive breast cancers, prognosis with TNBC is less favorable during the first five years after diagnosis, but it's good if those years are free of recurrence, because a recurrence after five years is uncommon. Several studies have shown that moderate exercise for two or more hours a week reduces the risk of recurrence for women with TNBC. This reduction in risk may be equal to that of women with hormone receptor–positive breast cancer who take tamoxifen to reduce their risk of recurrence.

If your TNBC is large or cannot be removed initially with surgery or if it has reoccurred or metastasized, your doctor may recommend clinical trials of new treatments for which you may be eligible. Breast cancer drugs, including those that are used to treat TNBC, that are

Questions to Ask Your Doctor about Treatment

- Do I need chemotherapy, hormonal therapy, HER2 therapy, or a combination?
- How soon do I need to begin treatment?
- How often will I take treatment, and for how long?
- When will we know whether my treatment is working?
- What short- and long-term benefits and side effects can I expect?
- How will the recommended treatment affect my ability to continue my daily activities?
- What is the best and worst outcome I could experience?
- What if my cancer doesn't respond?
- What are the short- and long-term risks of a recurrence elsewhere in my body? How can I reduce those risks?
- Am I eligible for any clinical trials?

successful in clinical trials are first approved for metastatic therapy before they're eventually approved for early-stage TNBC. One immunotherapy, atezolizumab (Tecentriq), is FDA approved for women with metastatic triple-negative breast cancer that is positive for PD-L1, a protein that helps some cancer cells to evade the immune system. Atezolizumab stimulates the immune system and allows *lymphocytes*, cells that are part of the immune system, to attack breast cancer cells. Intriguing results of the Impassion130 trial suggest that combining atezolizumab with the chemotherapy drug nab-paclitaxel produces an effective first-line therapy for women who are newly diagnosed with TNBC.

Dealing with the Uncertainty of Triple-Negative Breast Cancer

Having triple-negative breast cancer can make you feel isolated and alone, because fewer women have this diagnosis. A support group can help you understand and cope with issues you may experience with TNBC, but if you join a general breast cancer group, you might find that you're the only woman there with this diagnosis. It may be more helpful to seek out a group that is specifically for women with TNBC, as they will have a better understanding of what you're going through. Another support option is "Talk to Someone," a free online and mobile app developed by the US Centers for Disease Control for TNBC patients.

MAKING TREATMENT DECISIONS

Chemotherapy, hormone therapy, and anti-HER2 treatments save lives, but they require difficult decisions. If you're newly diagnosed with early-stage, estrogen receptor–positive breast cancer with no lymph node involvement, hormone therapy may be the only adjuvant treatment you need. Conversely, if you have several positive lymph nodes or other factors that indicate a moderate to high risk of recurrence, your oncologist may recommend that you receive chemotherapy followed by a hormone medication. To make this decision, your oncologist will typically discuss three factors with you, including (figure 13.7):

1. Your age and general health
2. Your risk of recurrence
3. The expected level of risk reduction as well as the risks of therapy

Predictive testing can help you make decisions about chemotherapy and hormone therapy, based on the likely benefits of each treatment. Your attitude is also a crucial factor when making these significant decisions. If you're health focused and particular about what you put in your body, the idea of taking one or more toxic drugs can be difficult. You may feel strongly about doing anything you can for even a small increase in survival, or you may decide that the side effects of a particular treatment don't offset its potential benefit. A preexisting health condition may also lead you away from some options. Chemotherapies that cause neuropathy would be a poor choice if you're diabetic and you already have nerve damage, for example. Similarly, some hormone therapy might not be your best treatment alternative if you already have bone loss, though this can usually be treated.

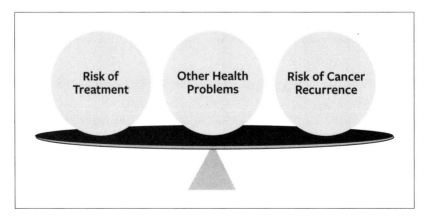

Figure 13.7. Balancing risks and benefits

Should You Consider Genetic Testing before You're Treated?

Many experts, including the American Society of Breast Surgeons, urge genetic testing for all breast cancer patients. Although most women with breast cancer don't have an inherited genetic mutation, you might consider being tested because your test results can influence your treatment decisions. Being tested before you have surgery gives you the opportunity to use your test results to help you decide whether lumpectomy or mastectomy would be best for you. If you test positive for a mutation, your treatment and follow-up may need to be more aggressive, because having a mutation in a BRCA1, BRCA2, or TP53 gene increases the risk for a future diagnosis of breast cancer in your opposite breast. If you're concerned or have reason to suspect that your cancer may be caused by an inherited mutation, a genetic counselor can determine if genetic testing is right for you. If you previously tested negative for a single mutation in a risk-raising gene such BRCA1 or BRCA2, a genetic counselor can tell you whether you should be retested with a newer multigene panel.

Although many side effects can be managed, most treatments involve taking the bad with the good, and the priority of any treatment is always to provide you with the best possible outcome. While the unpleasant nature of side effects may be hard to accept, a cancer that returns can be life threatening. These are important considerations when you weigh your treatment alternatives.

Your age can also influence your treatment decisions. Many breast cancer diagnoses occur in older women, who more often have heart disease, hypertension, or other chronic ailments that can affect treatment and prognosis. While these conditions don't preclude successful adjuvant therapy, some older women may be too ill or too frail to withstand side effects or complications that can occur from treatment. Elderly women with preexisting health conditions are more likely to have a recurrence and poorer prognosis than someone without those same conditions. Most women who develop breast cancer in their 70s and 80s have estrogen receptor–positive tumors that can be treated with hormone medications rather than chemotherapy.

Women in their mid- to late 80s who have slow-growing breast cancers may choose to forego treatment beyond lumpectomy. If you're over age 70, a geriatric assessment can identify any age-related factors to determine whether you're sufficiently fit for chemotherapy.

When it's time to make your decisions, you'll likely have multiple, equally effective choices, although in some cases, you may have only one truly good treatment option. Helping you to sort through various treatment options is a part of your oncologist's role. You may also want to seek a second opinion before deciding on treatment. Cancer experts don't always agree about specific treatment protocols, and getting another physician's input can inform you of treatment alternatives that you're unaware of or can reassure you by confirming that the choice you're making is best. Most patients who get a second opinion ultimately follow their first doctor's advice, but it's always a good idea to hear another professional's view. Many women testify to the power of making positive, active decisions with their treatment team.

Davi's Story

When my doctor called to tell me I had breast cancer, I almost dropped the phone. It was just .6 centimeter of infiltrating carcinoma, and my sentinel lymph node biopsy was clear. We had hoped that I could take tamoxifen, but the tumor wasn't estrogen sensitive, so that wasn't an option. Chemotherapy would reduce the risk of the cancer coming back, but my tumor was very small, and the risk of recurrence was very low. My oncologist is a firm believer in being aggressive, and I am too. He sent me to another oncologist, who said that chemo was a no-brainer; even though I had a tiny cancer, it was like a dandelion. A seed could have blown around and be somewhere in my body just waiting to hatch. So he strongly advised chemotherapy.

I had chemo once every three weeks. I lost a lot of weight. I weighed probably 108 on a good day, and I dropped to 92 pounds on my worst day. I had no appetite whatsoever. I was nauseous. I knew my hair was going to fall out, and I had it cut short. I recommend that if you're going to have chemo, go get your head shaved, because when your hair starts to come out, it's frightening. You wake up and it's in your bed and all over your clothes. I didn't get a wig. I made scarves that I painted and bejeweled. To this day, my youngest son says, "Mom, you looked so glamorous in the scarves, why don't you wear them now?" Now I have my hair back in abundance. With chemotherapy, there is a light at the end of the tunnel. You know it's not forever. You know how many weeks and months it's going to be, and you get your hair back, you get your strength back, and you put weight back on. I'm so glad I did chemotherapy, and even while I was doing it, it never entered my mind to stop. After the chemotherapy, there was a one-month break, and then I started radiation. I'm normally hyper, with tons of energy, and I was a little tired with radiation, but it wasn't bad. I didn't feel any pain. Compared to the chemo, it was a piece of cake, so I wasn't complaining. I knew I would just bite the bullet and, as the Nike ad says, "Just do it."

Eva's Story

When I found a pea-sized lump in my breast while showering, I had nagging thoughts about why this was happening to me. I did all the right things: lived a healthy lifestyle, ate lots of broccoli, nursed our sons, and exercised. I didn't have breast cancer in my family. A biopsy showed that I had a small invasive lobular cancer. Fortunately, my lymph nodes weren't affected; the cancer had not spread. My surgeon explained that I had the choice of lumpectomy or mastectomy, and that some women even have double mastectomies because this type of cancer can recur in the other breast. He suggested that after surgery, I should have radiation and/or chemotherapy. He said to get other opinions.

My mother died of ovarian cancer when she was only 46. I didn't want to suffer and die as she had. Even as I was facing breast cancer, I knew I didn't have a death sentence. There were treatments, and I was going to do everything possible to get through this. As a librarian and curious person, I researched treatment options. I perfectly fit the profile of a person who could and should have a lumpectomy. Because of my general good health, I had no complications and recovered swiftly.

When I met the oncologist, we had an instant rapport. This was important to me because I would be in his hands from now on. I had complete faith and trust in him. He explained the medication, radiation, and chemotherapy. Radiation wasn't stressful. True, it was a daily routine and I had to drive to a hospital for treatment, but then I drove straight to work. The

(continued)

young man who administered the minute-long laser beam was friendly, and we clicked right away. Then came chemotherapy. I remember the tingly feeling as the medicine flowed through my body, uncomfortable at first but then painless. With the support of a friend who had gone through breast cancer, my family, and my doctor, I felt very strong. I believed, and still do, that I am a survivor, a strong individual, determined to conquer—with help—this chapter of my story and move on. Months went by, almost uneventfully, and fortunately I didn't feel tired or nauseated.

Then my treatments were over. My hair gradually grew back in lovely, soft curls. I was happy. Little did I know that in the new year, I would get another surprise. As I was dressing, I felt a pea-sized lump in my other breast. This time the biopsy showed that cancer had spread into the lymph nodes and treatment had to be stronger. Still, I wasn't frightened because of my oncologist's supportive care. Radiation wasn't noticeably different this time, but the more aggressive chemo was. My hair fell out after the first treatment, but I was ready with my wigs.

More than 10 years have gone by since I was treated. I learned to see what's important in life. I spend time with my family and friends, doing the things I enjoy or always wanted to do before but didn't have the time or opportunity. I take care of myself physically, intellectually, and emotionally. I exercise almost every day. I take classes at a local college, play with my grandchildren, and see my girlfriends. And I count my blessings often.

CHAPTER 14

Cancer Again

TREATING A LOCAL OR REGIONAL RECURRENCE

After mastectomy or lumpectomy, the majority of breast cancer survivors never develop a recurrence in the same breast or where their breast was. A small percentage of women, however, develop a local or regional recurrence, which can usually be treated effectively. Routine mammography can often detect a post-lumpectomy recurrence, but it is sometimes found by women or their doctors when the breast looks or feels differently.

A common fear for anyone who has breast cancer is that it will return after treatment. Although the majority of breast cancer survivors never again hear, "You have breast cancer," some women do have a *recurrence*; their breast cancer comes back, even years or decades after treatment. Breast cancer can recur when even a few microscopic cancer cells somehow avoid the effects of treatment, remain in the breast, and then start to grow again. Although any breast cancer can come back, most don't return after initial treatment.

A recurrence can be:

- *local*, occurring at the site of the original cancer or in the surgery scar;
- *regional*, appearing in the chest skin or fat, or in the lymph nodes under the arm, under the breastbone and between the ribs, or above the collarbone;
- *locoregional*, or a regional recurrence that is diagnosed at the same time as a local recurrence; or
- *distant*, meaning anywhere else in the body (chapter 15).

Learning that you have breast cancer again can be disheartening and scary. You may feel that your body is betraying you or that you previously had the wrong treatment, but neither is true. In fact, your previous treatment probably delayed your recurrence. A recurrence develops for reasons we don't fully understand and can't yet prevent, but it doesn't happen because of anything that you do or don't do. Your risk of a recurrence is influenced by the subtype of your original breast cancer. Estrogen receptor–positive and triple-negative tumors, for example, tend to recur more than tumors that are hormone negative or HER2 sensitive. The type of surgery and other treatment that you had may also influence whether you have a recurrence.

Your oncology team will review with you many of the same details that were discussed with your initial diagnosis, such as the size and location of the new tumor, the hormone receptors and HER2 status, as well as the amount of time that has elapsed since your initial diagnosis. This information will help your team discuss prognosis and treatment recommendations with you.

Understandably, your new diagnosis may make you feel exceptionally vulnerable. It can be difficult to accept that you need to go through treatment again when you assumed that part of your life was behind you. But most breast cancers that come back can be treated, and having been through treatment before, you'll know what to expect this time around, and you may be treated with newer medications that have fewer side effects. Many factors affect overall prognosis, which is generally better if your recurrence is limited to the breast and not found in the chest, in the lymph nodes, or elsewhere.

Compared to someone who has never had breast cancer, if you're a breast cancer survivor, you have a higher risk for another diagnosis in either breast. Most breast cancers that return are found within five years of primary treatment. But recurrence can develop many years later, so it's important to remain vigilant. The longer you're free of breast cancer, the less likely it is to return. When your treatment is over, continue doing monthly self-exams to look for any changes in your breasts and have posttreatment screenings and follow-up appointments, so if a recurrence develops, it can be identified and treated as soon as possible. If you still have one or both of your breasts, you still need routine mammograms and other follow-up imaging or testing that your doctor recommends.

Questions to Ask Your Doctor about Recurrence

- What kind of recurrence do I have?
- What are my treatment options?
- What are the benefits and side effects of these treatments?
- What follow-up care will I need?
- Am I likely to have another recurrence?
- Should I enroll in a clinical trial?
- What support groups can help me?

FINDING AND TREATING A LOCAL RECURRENCE

Most breast cancers that recur are found in the same area as the original tumor. If you have a recurrence, you may have no symptoms or you might have one or more of the following signs, which you should discuss with your doctor as soon as possible. Some of these same symptoms can develop with arthritis, infectious conditions, or inflammatory problems, so it's important to have testing that determines the exact cause.

- a lump or a swollen area on your chest, in your armpit, or above your collarbone
- a change in the shape or size of your breast
- dimpling, puckering, or other change in the breast skin
- a discharge from the nipple
- redness or a rash on or around the nipple or on the breast skin
- a nipple that becomes inverted or looks different

To identify a recurrence, your doctor will integrate the results of a carefully taken medical history, a physical examination, and many of the same tests that were used to diagnose and stage your previous diagnosis. The first step is a mammogram (if you still have your breast), followed by an ultrasound or MRI if the mammography result is unclear or finds a suspicious area. If these test results suggest a recurrence, a tissue biopsy is then performed to determine whether the cancer has recurred. Most often, the original tumor and the recurrence are the same type of breast cancer, but they can also be different—a recurrent cancer may be estrogen receptor negative even though the original tumor was estrogen receptor positive. Performing a biopsy is an important diagnostic step to be certain of the recurrent tumor's biologic "personality" so that the best treatment plan can be defined. Additional x-rays and scans may follow to determine whether cancer cells have spread beyond the breast.

A local or regional recurrence is not immediately life threatening; you and your doctor have time to thoroughly evaluate and restage your cancer before making treatment choices. Treating this type of recurrence focuses on removing the new tumor and preventing the cancer from reappearing in that location or elsewhere. Treatment can eliminate all evidence of a breast cancer recurrence if the tumor can be removed and if you don't have a distant metastasis. The likelihood of controlling recurrent breast cancer depends on several different circumstances, including the following important characteristics:

- The size of the tumor.
- Whether the tumor is confined to the breast or has progressed to the lymph nodes or beyond.
- Whether the entire tumor can be removed.
- Whether the recurrence is inflammatory breast cancer (cancer cells have spread into the lymphatic system under the skin).
- Whether the tumor is hormone receptor negative or hormone receptor positive.
- Whether the tumor is HER2 positive.
- The number of tumors.
- The extent to which the cancer cells have mutated and are resistant to treatment.

- Whether the recurrence has already spread to other parts of the body (*distant metastasis*).
- The length of time since the initial breast cancer diagnosis. Breast cancer that returns several years after original treatment can be more difficult to treat.

Recurrence after Lumpectomy

Breast cancer doesn't usually recur after lumpectomy and radiation, but it can sometimes return in the area of the original tumor. Among 100 breast cancer survivors, up to 10 will have a local or locoregional recurrence after lumpectomy and radiation within 10 years of their first diagnosis. A post-lumpectomy recurrence can often be detected by routine mammography, but it can also be found by women or their doctors when they notice that the breast looks or feels differently.

If you previously had ductal carcinoma in situ (DCIS) that was treated with lumpectomy and radiation, you have a slightly higher risk of recurrence compared to women who were treated with mastectomy; your probability of survival is the same, however. If you were originally treated for DCIS, a recurrence may be DCIS or invasive. Although you'll need to go through treatment again, DCIS is less serious than a recurrence of invasive breast cancer, which is more aggressive and can spread to other areas of the body. Most invasive breast cancers that recur are also invasive, although infrequently they return as noninvasive DCIS.

Another lumpectomy with or without radiation may be an option for a small recurrent tumor that is confined to the breast. More commonly, a local recurrence after lumpectomy is treated with mastectomy to remove the cancer and reduce the likelihood of having yet another recurrence. Any abnormal or cancerous lymph nodes are also removed.

Postoperative radiation may also be advised if your breast wasn't previously radiated. Because a local or regional recurrence increases your risk of later developing a distant recurrence, systemic therapy is often also recommended. It may also be advised depending on your previous treatment, your menopausal status, and whether your tumor is sensitive to hormones or HER2. If your new tumor is hormone sensitive and you previously took tamoxifen, it's reasonable for you to now take an aromatase inhibitor, or vice versa. Hormonal therapy with or without chemotherapy may also be used preoperatively in an attempt to shrink the tumor if it's extensive and inoperable. Chemotherapy may be recommended if your cancer is a more aggressive type, such as triple-negative breast cancer.

Recurrence after Mastectomy

You may wonder how breast cancer can come back if your breast was previously removed. Even though surgeons remove all of the visible breast tissue during a mastectomy, it's not possible to remove every breast cell. A recurrence may still develop in the few remaining breast cells in the thin layer of fatty tissue under the skin, on the chest wall, in nearby lymph nodes, or in the breast skin. The risk of this happening is greater if you had cancerous lymph nodes at the time of your mastectomy, especially if several nodes were positive. A recurrence after mastectomy is often found when a pea-sized lump appears on or under the original incision scar or in the nearby skin, which may become red and swollen. Approximately 5 to 10 percent of women who have a mastectomy to treat breast cancer have a recurrence in the chest wall (or underarm lymph nodes) within 10 years.

The lump is surgically removed, and unless your initial treatment included radiation, the chest wall is radiated. In rare cases, parts of the breastbone and ribs may be removed if the cancer has spread further. Systemic therapy is also ordinarily advised, because some women who develop a local recurrence after surgery and radiation eventually also develop distant metastasis. Chemotherapy may be recommended if the recurrence is aggressive; otherwise, a common approach is to offer hormonal therapy if the tumor is hormone receptor positive, because the benefit may be substantial with fewer side effects.

If you had breast reconstruction after your mastectomy, rest assured that it doesn't affect your risk of recurrence. Nor does it hide a recurrence should one develop. It's important to be aware that a recurrence is always a possibility and that you should routinely examine your breasts for any changes and be monitored as recommended by your doctor.

Treating New Primary Tumors

If you develop a tumor in your breast after treatment, a biopsy is performed to determine whether it's a recurrence or an unrelated *new primary cancer*. Your risk for a new primary cancer is higher if you have an inherited mutation in a BRCA gene or another gene that is known to increase the risk of breast cancer.

After lumpectomy, a new primary cancer can occur in either of your breasts. If a mastectomy removed one of your breasts, a new cancer may develop in your remaining breast. The chance of another breast cancer increases over time after either type of surgery. About 5 percent of women are diagnosed with a new primary tumor within 8 years of their original diagnosis, while up to 14 percent have another breast cancer after 25 years. The risk may be higher if your initial tumor was hormone receptor negative.

Treatment for a new primary cancer depends on which breast is affected. If it's in the same breast as your previous cancer and you were treated with breast-conserving therapy, you'll likely need a mastectomy, because radiating the same breast twice can cause extensive tissue damage. A new tumor in the opposite breast is treated as a new case of breast cancer, with lumpectomy and radiation or mastectomy. Systemic therapy may also be recommended, depending on the pathology of the cancer cells.

FINDING AND TREATING
A REGIONAL RECURRENCE

A regional recurrence in the lymph nodes or chest wall is uncommon, but it's more serious than a local recurrence because it's a sign that the cancer has progressed beyond the breast and that it could enter the blood or lymph vessels to migrate elsewhere in the body.

Although a regional recurrence doesn't always produce symptoms, a lump or swollen area in the underarm or near the collarbone, or persistent pain in the arm or shoulder may appear. Diagnosis is usually made with ultrasound, MRI, CT or PET scan, and biopsy. A complete medical workup is often done again to determine whether the cancer has spread anywhere else in the body.

Treating a Recurrence in the Lymph Nodes

A recurrence can involve lymph nodes in one or multiple locations, including axillary nodes under the arm and internal mammary nodes under the ribs near the breastbone. More aggressive breast cancers may also spread to the supraclavicular lymph nodes in the neck or above the collarbone. If a recurrence is confirmed, the lymph nodes are surgically removed (if feasible), and the area is then radiated. Recurrence in the axillary lymph nodes is typically addressed with an axillary lymph node dissection followed by radiation. Surgical removal of lymph nodes is generally not recommended for recurrence in the supraclavicular (near the collarbone) or internal mammary lymph nodes due to increased risks associated with surgery in these locations. Because a regional recurrence indicates a greater risk of distant metastasis, systemic therapy that is tailored to the characteristics of the recurrence and your past medical history may also be recommended. If your original tumor was estrogen receptor positive and treated with adjuvant hormonal therapy, for example, and it recurs as an estrogen receptor–negative tumor, you might now be treated with a course of chemotherapy.

Treating a Recurrence on the Chest Wall

A recurrence on the scar line is considered to be a local recurrence. But a recurrence elsewhere on the chest wall is considered to be *advanced breast cancer*, even though it may not appear elsewhere in the body. This type of chest wall recurrence may involve skin, muscle, and the fascia (the sheath-like covering over the muscle) below the area of the original breast tumor. Symptoms may include a pain or pulling sensation in the chest on the side that was previously treated or a sore area that doesn't heal.

If the area of recurrence is too large to be completely removed, neoadjuvant chemotherapy may sufficiently shrink the tumor so that surgery can be performed. Obtaining negative surgical margins is critical. If your initial treatment didn't include radiation therapy, the area of recurrence is then radiated to reduce the likelihood of any cancer cells surviving. Even if you were treated before with radiation, or if your new tumor can't be surgically removed, your radiation oncologist may suggest another round of radiation but at a lower dose, depending on your circumstances and the length of time since your initial treatment.

CHAPTER 15

Treating Metastatic Breast Cancer

Oncologists hope that their patients with metastatic breast cancer will have a complete remission and that they can live without breast cancer. At the same time, their work focuses on helping women to live with metastatic breast cancer as a chronic disease, as new therapies are developed.

Although most women with early-stage breast cancer never have another diagnosis, unfortunately, some women eventually develop *metastatic breast cancer* (MBC), which is a recurrence that appears beyond the breast and lymph nodes. About 6 to 10 percent of women have breast cancer that has already metastasized when they are first diagnosed. In contrast, most metastases occur in women who were initially treated for breast cancer that was confined to the breast, or in the breast and one or more lymph nodes. Metastatic breast cancer (also called distant recurrence or stage IV breast cancer) most often appears in the liver, lungs, or bone. Breast cancer cells that are found anywhere in the body are still breast cancer—not brain, lung, or bone cancer—and are treated accordingly.

UNDERSTANDING YOUR PROGNOSIS

Stage IV breast cancer is life threatening, and except for a small number of patients, it is not cured. But it can often be managed, sometimes for many years. More women with metastatic breast cancer are living better and living longer because of improving treatments for these hard-to-treat cancers. A small group of women who have a limited recurrence in a single spot and have no other evidence of disease after surgery, radiation, and chemotherapy or hormone therapy may continue to be in remission. Among the estimated 150,000 individuals with metastatic breast cancer in the United States, 36 percent have lived at least five years beyond their diagnosis. Some live many years beyond their treatment and continue to do well. Meanwhile, detecting breast cancer earlier and having more effective treatments continue to reduce the number of women who have a distant recurrence and improve survival for those who do.

Generally, the outlook is better for women who have metastasis that is confined to bone, which often responds to localized radiation and hormone therapy and is easier to treat than breast cancer that has spread to the brain or to the lungs. Women who tend to do better are typically older, postmenopausal, and have estrogen receptor–positive, "bone only" recurrent cancer that develops many years after their initial treatment. The specific type of breast cancer is also important. Women with HER2-positive MBC often have an excellent treatment response with therapy that is targeted against HER2/neu. Some of these women do well for years or decades after diagnosis of recurrent cancer. In contrast, women who have a recurrence of triple-negative breast cancer tend to have more aggressive cancers and poorer prognoses. Overall, the chance of living five or more years beyond the diagnosis of metastatic breast cancer has doubled during the past two decades (figure 15.1).

While it's important to be realistic about your prognosis, metastatic breast cancer is different for every patient. For the most part, survival statistics are too impersonal to be helpful or meaningful for an individual. They

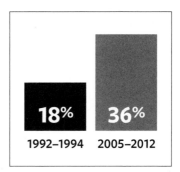

Figure 15.1. Metastatic breast cancer five-year survival trends for women under age 50

are numbers that reflect average survival for the overall population of women who have MBC, but they don't realistically reflect your own circumstances, overall health, or outlook. Nor do they reflect new treatments that have become available since the last statistics were published. Your doctor can give you more information about your own circumstances and prognosis.

When Others Don't Understand

While uplifting, sometimes the oft-repeated public announcements that we are "curing" breast cancer and "winning the war on breast cancer" may make people wonder why you can't be cured too. Most people have a family member, friend, or coworker who has been diagnosed with early-stage breast cancer. For the most part, they've probably seen those people treated and then go on with their lives. Even so, many people are unaware that metastatic breast cancer (MBC) is not the same situation. In fact, in a survey of 2,000 people, 60 percent of respondents knew little to nothing about MBC, and 72 percent believed that it was curable as long as it was diagnosed early. Half of the people who were surveyed thought that breast cancer progressed because patients either didn't take appropriate preventive measures or have the right treatment. Some people may find it hard to understand that the metastasis in your lung isn't because of a previous behavior, or they may be unaware that someone who has been treated successfully can be diagnosed again years later, and these misunderstandings can lead to unintentionally insensitive comments. Much of the time, people don't know how to deal with this information or what to say to you. You may find yourself ignoring remarks like this or educating others about MBC, especially when they don't understand why you'll continue to have imaging, exams, tests, and various therapies. You are not obligated to share any or all of the details of your diagnosis. You may choose what you want to share, with whom, when, and at what pace. Similarly, you can decide about sharing your feelings, worries, and hopes.

Coping with Uncertainty

Any cancer diagnosis can be difficult to accept. Knowing that you're dealing with an unpredictable and incurable disease, with no clear idea of what lies ahead, can be especially overwhelming. You shouldn't blame yourself for your diagnosis. Your breast cancer didn't develop and spread because of something you did or didn't do or because your primary treatment was wrong.

Facing metastatic breast cancer is a difficult, ongoing battle that can be physically, mentally, and emotionally draining. You'll need all of your strength, stamina, and hope to face challenges that are a part of living with MBC. It helps to keep two things in mind. First, while you may feel isolated and afraid, you never have to be alone. An army of individuals and organizations is ready, willing, and able to compassionately support you by lending an ear, sharing experiences, and gladly providing physical and mental hugs. Second, while it may sound cliché, staying positive is important. It may be easier at some times than others, perhaps when a particular treatment works well and your life goes on as if you had never been diagnosed. It's the down times that can be hard, when you feel unwell or when a treatment fails and your life is once again in limbo. During these uncertain periods, it helps to turn to family, friends, or faith for help and hope. Your doctor or nurse can suggest a cancer counselor or a support group. Whether one-on-one or group support works better for you, having the support you need when you need it will help you to regroup, face MBC head on, and live your life.

DIAGNOSING METASTASIS

Metastasis is a multistep process (figure 15.2):
- Cancer cells invade nearby healthy cells, which can then replicate more abnormal cells.
- Cancer cells penetrate the circulatory or lymph system and are carried to other parts of the body.
- Cancer cells stop moving as they are lodged in capillaries at a distant location, and then divide and migrate into the surrounding tissue.
- Cancer cells form small tumors at the new location (called micrometastases).

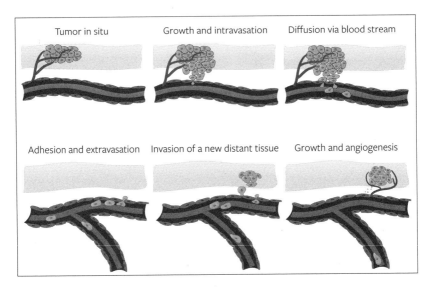

Figure 15.2. How breast cancer metastasizes

Malignant cells must first invade through the walls of the ducts or lobules of the breast into the surrounding soft tissues. Cells that drain from the breast and reach the lymphatic system or blood vessels are swept along to nearby lymph nodes or veins. Some are destroyed by the immune system. Others may make their way into the bloodstream, which provides a "highway" that carries them to distant sites and into surrounding tissues. Cancer cells often die at some point in the process, but when favorable conditions exist at every step, surviving cells can evade the immune system and "hide out" for months or years without symptoms until something triggers them to begin growing and reproducing until tumors form.

Metastases elsewhere in the body eventually cause symptoms that may include fatigue, poor appetite, weight loss, a general feeling of being unwell, a persistent and progressive pain, and fractures. Symptoms can differ depending on the location of the metastasis:

- Bone metastases can result in bone pain or fracture.
- Metastasis to the lung can cause a chronic cough, chest pain, and shortness of breath.

- Signs of liver metastasis include abdominal pain, nausea and vomiting, and loss of appetite.
- Brain metastasis can cause nausea, vomiting, dizziness, changes in vision, persistent headaches that progressively become worse, and personality changes.

Metastatic breast cancer is usually diagnosed after one or more of these symptoms develop.

X-rays, ultrasound, or an MRI usually follow and reveal a suspicious area. A biopsy is then performed to determine with certainty whether the area is benign or malignant. It will show whether the cancer found is indeed breast cancer and if the biology of the recurrence is similar or different from the original diagnosis. Most often it's the same, though breast cancer cells can recur as a different subtype than the original diagnosis and require a different systemic regimen. An estrogen receptor–positive breast cancer may recur as estrogen receptor negative, or a tumor that was negative for HER2 may be positive, for example. This doesn't necessarily mean that the tumor cells changed or mutated. Rather, the original cancer may have had several populations of cancer cells, and one population was able to resist the original therapy and recur.

After MBC is diagnosed, careful *restaging studies* that often include CT scans or a PET scan follow to determine where the breast cancer has recurred. Tumor marker tests look for proteins that are made by the cancer and released into the bloodstream. These tests (typically CEA, CA27-29, or CA15-3) can provide additional information about MBC, but they can also produce false positive or false negative results. High levels of these serum marker proteins may indicate a recurrence, but a confirming biopsy is needed to be sure. A positive blood test can be influenced by some noncancerous conditions, and it isn't necessarily evidence of cancer. A negative test doesn't necessarily mean that there's no cancer, because some tumors don't produce higher levels of tumor markers. *Tumor markers* can be one indication of cancer, but it's a limited observation because some cells produce large amounts of these proteins, even when the extent of the recurrence is small. National guidelines don't recommend using tumor marker studies to identify evidence of a breast cancer recurrence; they are more useful in monitoring treatment response or progression in women with MBC.

If you're diagnosed with metastatic breast cancer, you may have one or more of the following secondary tests to determine the extent of your cancer.

- Blood tests include a complete blood count (CBC), a common test that measures the number of red blood cells that carry oxygen throughout the body, white blood cells that fight infection, and platelets, which help to clot blood during bleeding. Other blood tests measure whether the kidneys, liver, and other organs are functioning properly.
- A chest x-ray looks for indications that the tumor has metastasized to the lungs.
- An MRI can provide additional information about the area and extent of the cancer.
- During a bone scan, a small amount of material is injected and images of the bone are reviewed for evidence of metastasis.
- A PET/CT scan checks for breast cancer in other parts of the body by measuring changes in your metabolic rate. The PET scan measures how a small amount of injected radioactive dye is absorbed as it passes through the body. Breast cancer cells, which have a somewhat higher metabolic rate than healthy cells, "light up" areas that may indicate malignant cells. The CT scan uses x-rays from different angles to create computerized images of the chest and/or abdomen. The combined scan results produce detailed, three-dimensional images of abnormalities, including tumors in the body.

TREATMENT STRATEGIES

Breast cancer is a treatable disease. Oncologists hope that their patients with metastatic breast cancer will have a complete pathological response. This is the ideal response to treatment: you have no evidence of cancer, your symptoms are alleviated, and your quality of life improves. But no treatment is likely to eliminate a metastasized cancer completely and permanently. Still, it is important to know that countless cancer researchers continue working to find new and better therapies. Treatment can hopefully give you months or years, or perhaps even a decade or more of remission or stability when your cancer doesn't grow. Treatment relieves symptoms and enormously improves quality of life. It keeps you feeling as good as you can for as long as you can. It also prolongs life, often substantially. This is the fundamental goal of personalized MBC therapy, to give you the maximum benefit with the least side effects over a long period of time.

Treatment may produce one of several responses:
- a *complete pathological response* (disease free), where all symptoms, physical findings, and evidence of cancer disappear, if only for a while
- a *partial response*, such as when some improvement occurs but isn't a complete response
- *stable disease*, whereby the cancer doesn't grow or shrink
- *no response* (progressive disease), when the tumor grows and progresses

Oncologists typically think about breast cancer treatment as a marathon rather than a sprint. Treating metastatic disease requires a long-term approach that may allow for more conservative, less aggressive treatment. It can be a rollercoaster of repeated treatment and remission. You may feel good as your symptoms recede and your cancer stabilizes or disappears, but if your treatment stops working, your cancer may return or progress. It is important to keep in mind that during your breast cancer treatment, you may also have ongoing treatment for other underlying health issues like diabetes or rheumatoid arthritis that may also affect your quality of life. Depending on your symptoms and your response to treatment, you likely can continue your normal daily activities, but you may need to adjust what and how much you do.

Doctors don't have a simple or standard equation for designing MBC treatment plans. Everyone is unique and has different circumstances, and treatments are customized for each patient. Your own plan will consider several factors, including:

- The type of your primary cancer and your previous treatment.
- The size, location, and number of metastatic tumors.
- The molecular characteristics of your tumors.
- Your symptoms.
- Your age and overall health.
- Available treatment options.
- Treatment risks and side effects.
- How much certain treatments can be expected to help you and for how long.

A particular treatment is continued as long as it works and while side effects are tolerable. If you feel well and your physical exam and x-rays show that your MBC is stable, your treatment will probably remain unchanged, and you may continue on it for months or years. When one treatment stops working or you develop intolerable side effects, another one can be tried. Some women are willing to accept more side effects and discomfort to have extra time, while for others quality of life is more important than the number of weeks, months, and years of life. Your doctor will help you to weigh the risks and benefits of different options and consider the quality of life you'll have with each choice. When talking to your doctor about potential treatment, ask if you have time for reflection and for additional research before you decide which regimen is best for you. These complex topics are often difficult for oncologists and patients to discuss, but it's these challenging discussions that make for the best decisions and for the strongest connection between doctor and patient.

Monitoring Changes in Treatment

The important indication that palliation (relief from symptoms) is being achieved is that the patient says she feels better. Yet symptoms often vary from day to day and may be due to treatment, disease, or other nonmalignant causes such as arthritis. So more objective means are helpful to avoid making inappropriate changes in therapy. Physical examination can help identify lesions in the skin, chest wall, and lymph nodes. Most metastatic lesions are in nonpalpable organs, such as bone, liver, and lung. In these cases, physical examination may be of little value.

X-rays and scans evaluate internal metastases and provide precise measurements of the cancer's size before and after treatment. But these tests are inconvenient and expensive, and they can be misleading if they aren't carefully interpreted. Many clinicians follow serially performed blood tests at each follow-up period (roughly every three to four weeks). For example, decreased levels of circulating liver enzyme in a patient with liver metastasis is a good sign. The most commonly used tumor markers in breast cancer are CA15-3 or CA27-29 and carcinoembryonic antigen (CEA). The CellSearch circulating tumor cell test is FDA approved to detect tumor cells that float in the bloodstream (figure 15.3). Some physicians monitor the quantity of circulating tumor cells to look for evidence of response to treatment.

Together, the results of four measures (history, physical exam, scans, and blood tests) help shape the decision of whether a patient with metastatic disease should stay on the therapy she has started or whether she should switch to another therapy for better symptom relief. The results of these tests must be used together with the physician's judgment. Any one of these tests may be falsely positive or negative, and therefore treatment should rarely be changed based on the results of one of the evaluations if everything else is equal and the patient is doing well. If the history and physical exam suggest that the patient's condition might be getting worse but they aren't definitive, however, a tumor marker that is rising significantly might be helpful in confirming the physician's suspicion that it's time to change therapy.

—*Daniel F. Hayes, MD*

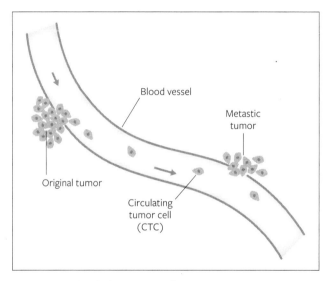

Figure 15.3. Circulating tumor cells

Although surgery and radiation are first-line treatments for early-stage breast cancers, they are typically less useful for advanced disease because distant metastases are the greatest threat to life. Sometimes a specific problematic site—brain metastases, fluid in the space around the lung, a tumor in the spinal cord, or cancer that threatens to fracture a bone—can be treated locally with surgery or radiation. Systemic medications are the primary treatment for patients with MBC, who usually have multiple sites of metastases that can be simultaneously treated to disrupt or destroy one or more vulnerabilities of cancer cells:

- Receptors on the surface of cancer cells for estrogen, progesterone, or androgens (male hormones).
- DNA and other genetic material that form the core of cancer cells.
- The HER2 protein on the surface of the cancer cells that can be attacked with antibodies.
- Specific proteins on the surface of cells or within cells that control cell growth.
- "Signaling pathways" that regulate the metabolism, growth, and division of breast cancer cells.

> **Questions to Ask Your Doctor**
> **about Metastatic Breast Cancer**
>
> - What treatment or combination of treatments are best for me?
> - How will this treatment improve my quality of life?
> - What side effects should I expect?
> - Will I need more tests?
> - How will we know whether treatment is working?
> - What will happen with treatment that stops working?
> - Will I be able to live my normal life?
> - How long can I live with this disease?
> - Am I eligible for a clinical trial?
> - Can you recommend a counselor and/or an MBC support group?

Chemotherapy

Chemotherapy is a first-line treatment for women who have hormone receptor–negative, metastatic breast cancer and won't benefit from hormone therapy. Chemotherapy works quickly, and it typically shrinks tumors faster than hormone therapy. In addition, chemotherapy is often also used as a second-line therapy for women who no longer respond to hormone therapy. Your doctor may prescribe a chemotherapy that is used for early-stage breast cancer, one that specifically targets MBC, or a combination of both (table 15.1). One chemotherapy drug is usually given at a time, because there is little evidence that combining two or more drugs is more effective against metastatic breast cancer than a single chemotherapy approach. There is no reliable way to predict which one will be most effective for a woman who is being treated, although oncologists have good information on which chemotherapy drugs are most likely to help.

Table 15.1. Chemotherapy Options for Metastatic Breast Cancer

Chemotherapy Drugs for Early-Stage and MBC	MBC-Specific Chemotherapy Drugs
Paclitaxel (Taxol)	Gemcitabine (Gemzar)
Capecitabine (Xeloda)	Vinorelbine (Navelbine)
Albumin-bound paclitaxel (Abraxane)	Ixabepilone (Ixempra)
Docetaxel (Taxotere)	Erubilin (Halaven)
Doxorubicin (Adriamycin)	Mitoxantrone (Novantrone)
Epirubicin (Ellence)	Pegylated liposomal doxorubicin (Doxil, Caelyx)
5-fluorouracil (Adrucil)	
Methotrexate (Maxtrex)	
Carboplatin (Paraplatin)	
Platinol (Cisplatin)	

Oncologists observe certain cancer care principles to improve the chance and the duration of response to breast cancer treatment with chemotherapy:

- A single chemotherapy agent may prove effective while limiting side effects if you've previously been treated with chemotherapy.
- A combination of certain chemotherapies may improve the chance of responding, but it doesn't typically result in longer survival than treatment with a single chemotherapy drug.
- If your cancer didn't respond to a previous chemotherapy regimen or it recurred, you'll be treated with a different chemotherapy drug or combination.

More Isn't Necessarily Better

In the 1990s, patients with leukemia, multiple myeloma, and lymphoma were being successfully treated with high-dose chemotherapy. Believing that this regimen would do the same for their breast cancer patients, oncologists began recommending this intense regimen for all women with breast cancer who had four or more positive lymph nodes. The idea was that if some chemotherapy was good, massive doses would be even more effective. And in fact, higher doses of certain chemo drugs did benefit some women with breast cancer. But the ultra-high-dose regimen didn't effectively destroy more cancer cells, and it damaged immature stem cells in the bone marrow. This was a serious problem because these are the same cells that ordinarily mature into healthy red blood cells that carry oxygen to tissues, white blood cells that fight infection, and platelets that help to clot blood.

To counteract this collateral damage, women who had ultra-high-dose chemo also underwent stem cell transplants—a procedure that can cause a variety of complications—to replace the patient's own bone marrow with stem cells. Eventually, large studies proved this treatment to be no more advantageous than standard-dose chemotherapy for breast cancer; for some women, it was fatal. Although high-dose chemotherapy with stem cell transplant continues to be the standard of care for many cancers, it's no longer used for breast cancer. Many more advanced and effective therapies are now available to treat women with metastatic breast cancer.

- A specific chemotherapy is ordinarily used until it's no longer effective or until side effects become intolerable.

If you have a limited amount of metastatic breast cancer and you're feeling well but you aren't a candidate for hormone therapy, treatment with capecitabine, a drug that is generally well tolerated, might be a good option until the cancer progresses. This might be followed by treatment with taxol or taxotere, and then doxil, gemcitabine, eribulin, or other single chemotherapy drug. If you have a good response to chemotherapy but your blood counts are unacceptably low, treatment can continue with lower doses of chemotherapy to restore healthy blood levels.

Despite diligent efforts, the percentage of women who improve or remain stable during treatment with any single chemotherapy drug is generally moderate, from 30 to 60 percent. Few of these responses are complete remissions, but many women have significant responses to chemotherapy. If an initial chemotherapy regimen stops working and the cancer begins to progress, a different drug can be substituted. Multiple lines of treatment, sometimes four or more, may be given sequentially in an effort to prolong life and maintain quality of life while living with metastatic breast cancer.

Understandably, anyone who is going to receive chemotherapy thinks about the possible side effects. Fortunately, most chemotherapy for breast cancer is outpatient therapy that is relatively well tolerated. Doses are customized to each woman's height and weight and are sometimes modified based on a woman's underlying health condition and tolerance of these medications. Chemotherapy drugs for metastatic breast cancer can cause the same short-term side effects as drugs that are used for early-stage breast cancer, including fatigue, nausea, diarrhea, flu-like symptoms, decreased appetite, muscle or joint pain, hair loss, rash, low blood counts, and others. Some chemotherapy drugs have other side effects that are listed below.

> *doxorubicin*: missed menstrual periods, darkening of skin or nails, weakening of the heart muscle
> *epirubicin*: change in urine color, mouth sores or ulcers, weakening of the heart muscle, and less commonly shortness of breath
> *paclitaxel*: mouth sores and neuropathy (numbness or tingling of the fingers and toes), allergic reaction during infusion
> *docetaxel*: mouth sores, fluid retention with weight gain, swelling of the ankles or abdominal area, nail changes, neuropathy
> *gemcitabine*: skin rash, decreased appetite
> *capecitabine*: itching or peeling, or darkening of the skin on feet or hands
> *vinorelbine*: muscle weakness, neuropathy
> *ixabepilone*: drowsiness, dizziness, finger and toenail changes

eribulin: shortness of breath, neuropathy, constipation, mouth
    sores

cisplatin: kidney problems, ringing in ears or hearing loss,
    metallic taste in mouth

carboplatin: allergic reactions to the infusion, kidney problems,
    change in hearing

mitoxantrone: low blood pressure, abnormal EKG, heart rhythm
    abnormalities, discoloration of the whites of eyes and/or urine

Hormone Therapy

Women with metastatic breast cancer often expect to be treated with chemotherapy. Yet hormone therapy, one of the oldest treatment approaches for this disease, is still one of the most straightforward, effective, and well-tolerated treatments for women with metastatic hormone-positive cancer. In many cases, the same hormone therapies that are used for early-stage breast cancers are preferable as a first line of therapy because they often produce remission that continues for several years or longer with minimal side effects. Hormone therapies are usually continued for as long as they relieve symptoms and stabilize tumors, even though in most cases they typically stop working. When one hormone therapy no longer works for you, your doctor may recommend another or the addition of a targeted agent. At some point, chemotherapy is often recommended.

Treatment for hormone-driven metastatic breast cancers depends on your menopausal status, your general health when diagnosed with MBC, the hormone therapy you initially had, the length of time since your initial diagnosis, and the extent of the metastases. If you're premenopausal, your treatment might begin with tamoxifen alone or in combination with either oophorectomy (removal of your ovaries) to stop estrogen production or goserelin (Zoladex) or a similar medication to suppress ovarian function, followed by an aromatase inhibitor. If you were previously treated with tamoxifen, your doctor will suggest trying a different hormone therapy. If you're postmenopausal, treatment will ordinarily include an aromatase inhibitor (anastrozole, exemestrane, or letrozole) or fulvestrant (Faslodex), an antiestrogen that is given by monthly injection into the muscle to degrade the estrogen receptor. Fulvestrant is generally as effective as an aromatase inhibitor if you're postmenopausal and have MBC. If a hormone therapy is helpful and results in a response that lasts one, two, or more years, then a second or third hormone therapy is often recommended if the disease progresses.

Hormone therapies are not a good choice if you:
- have estrogen and progesterone receptor–negative breast cancer
- have hormone-sensitive MBC that has already been treated with hormone therapy and no longer responds
- have a very aggressive cancer or a large amount of metastatic disease
- are very ill and need a therapy that will provide you with the quickest response

Breast Cancer That Responds to Male Hormones

It seems odd that what is primarily a female cancer could be driven by a predominantly male hormone. Yet many breast cancer cells have receptors for androgens, hormones that influence male traits and reproductive activity. (Testosterone, the primary male hormone, is one example of an androgen.) Androgen is expected to be found in prostate cancer in men, but not so much in female breast cancer. Women have small amounts of androgen, just as men have small amounts of estrogen. In women, androgen is made by the adrenal glands and converted into estrogen by the aromatase enzyme. Androgens can help promote tumor growth in some hormone receptor–positive tumors, some HER2-positive tumors, and an estimated one-third of triple-negative breast cancers. Some studies have shown that "anti-androgens" that reduce the level of androgens in the bloodstream can be helpful for women whose breast cancers respond to androgens. Similarly, drugs that block or destroy the androgen receptors on breast cancer cells can benefit some women with metastatic breast cancer. Prostate cancers are already successfully treated with a variety of anti-androgen drugs, and clinical trials are now exploring whether they may work as well for androgen receptor–positive breast cancers.

Targeted Therapies

Researchers are always working to develop new medications that meet or exceed the effectiveness of chemotherapy without its toxic side effects. Rather than attacking all of a person's cells, as chemotherapy does, these engineered drugs selectively disable or block the specific molecular characteristics that fuel individual breast cancers. Unlike chemotherapy, which attacks both malignant and healthy cells, targeted drugs can slow or stop the signals that tell cancer cells to grow and multiply.

Targeted drugs are powerful weapons against cancer cells. Some impede the cells' ability to form new blood vessels or to continue dividing. Others shut down the cells' ability to repair their own DNA damage. Some targeted medications consist of molecules that are small enough to enter and take direct aim at cancer cells. But cells can become resistant if the targeted gene, protein, or receptor mutates and is no longer affected by the drug. To avoid this problem, targeted therapies can be combined with one or more hormone or chemotherapy drugs.

Tamoxifen, aromatase inhibitors, and fulvestrant have been used for many years to treat women with metastatic estrogen receptor–positive breast cancer. Newer targeted drugs that work by blocking substances that help cancer cells to survive and grow now give women improved and longer response to treatment (table 15.2).

CDK4/6 inhibitors, including abemaciclib (Verzenio), palbociclib (Ibrance), and ribociclib (Kisqali), prevent cancer cells from multiplying. These are ordinarily given with an aromatase inhibitor or tamoxifen, though one of these drugs, abemaciclib, can be used as a single treatment. These CDK4/6 inhibitors lead to better outcomes for many postmenopausal women with metastatic hormone-driven, HER2-negative breast cancers. The aromatase inhibitors reduce estrogen levels, while the CDK4/6 inhibitors slow the growth of cancer cells. Multiple clinical trials found that adding one of these drugs to hormone therapy significantly prolongs the time patients remain in remission and improves overall survival. If you are premenopausal, your oncologist might recommend ovarian ablation or suppression before taking a CDK4/6 inhibitor and an aromatase inhibitor.

Side effects may include fatigue, headaches, and nausea, and gastrointestinal issues. Diarrhea can be severe but subsides when the dose is adjusted. The most common side effect is neutropenia (low white blood cell count), which can increase the chance of infection; white cell levels typically return to normal when the dose is adjusted or temporarily stopped. Neutropenia is less common, and gastrointestinal issues develop more frequently with abemaciclib. Some patients experience thinning hair while taking these drugs. More serious effects are liver problems and blood clots. Additionally, ribociclib may also cause a change in heart rhythm that can be serious. If you take this medicine, your heart function will be tested before and during your treatment. CDK4/6 inhibitors can rarely cause severe lung inflammation. If you're treated with one of these medications, you should be routinely monitored for signs of lung disease and/or pneumonitis. If you develop symptoms, your doctor may recommend that you suspend or discontinue treatment. The FDA states that "the

Table 15.2. Treatment Options for Hormone-Positive, HER-Negative Metastatic Breast Cancer

Early-Stage Hormone Drugs That May Be Used for MBC	MBC-Specific Hormone Drugs (with or without chemotherapy)	Appropriate Uses
Tamoxifen (Nolvadex)	Megestrol acetate (Megace)	Pre- and postmenopausal
Goserelin (Zoladex)		Premenopausal
Leuprolide (Lupron)		Premenopausal
Anastrozole (Arimidex)	Fulvestrant (Faslodex)	Postmenopausal
Exemestane (Aromasin)	Alpelisib (Piqray)	Postmenopausal
Letrozole (Femara)	Ribociclib (Kisqali)	Postmenopausal
	Palbociclib (Ibrance)	Postmenopausal
	Abemaciclib (Verzenio)	Postmenopausal
	Everolimus (Afinitor)	Postmenopausal

overall benefit of CDK4/6 inhibitors is still greater than the risks when used as prescribed."

Mammalian target of rapamycin (mTOR) pathway inhibitors were developed when researchers discovered that certain tumors that become resistant to hormone therapy can be treated by blocking the mTOR pathway, which signals cancer cell growth. Everolimus (Afinitor) given with the aromatase inhibitor exemestane (Aromasin) is the first mTOR pathway inhibitor approved by the FDA to treat postmenopausal women who have already been treated with the aromatase inhibitors letrozole (Femara) or anastrozole (Arimidex). In clinical trials, everolimus combined with exemestane more than doubled progression-free survival in postmenopausal patients, compared to exemestane alone. Side effects can include fatigue, diarrhea, vomiting, nausea, elevated blood sugar and cholesterol, rash, mouth sores, and less frequently pneumonitis (inflammation of the lung).

PI3K inhibitors target the PIK3CA gene, which is important for the health of normal and cancer cells. Mutations in this gene may allow it to be overactivated and fuel cancer growth and resistance to hormone therapy. The oral drug alpelisib (Piqray) given with fulvestrant has been shown to almost double progression-free survival—compared to fulvestrant alone in men and postmenopausal women with metastatic PIK3CA-mutated, hormone receptor–positive, HER2-negative tumors that grew or spread during or after treatment with an aromatase inhibitor. Alpelisib (Piqray) is the first FDA-approved treatment that specifically targets the PIK3CA pathway for these advanced breast cancers. Common side effects of alpelisib include nausea; diarrhea; fatigue; rash; elevated levels of blood sugar, creatinine, and liver enzymes; decreased levels of calcium and lymphocyte count; reduced appetite and weight loss; delayed blood clotting; and hair loss (figure 15.4).

Anti-HER2 medications. One result of many years of research is targeted therapy directed against the HER2 protein that is on the surface of some breast cancer cells. These proteins act as receivers (receptors) that bind to certain substances called ligands, and then signal the cell to grow and divide.

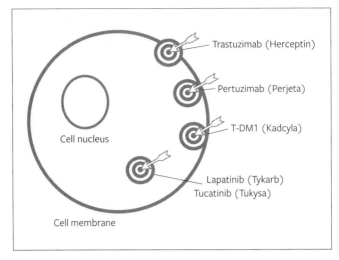

Figure 15.4. Multiple new medications target specific proteins and genes to treat breast cancer

Targeted medications for HER2-positive metastatic breast cancer. Trastuzumab (Herceptin) and pertuzumab (Perjeta) belong to a class of targeted drugs known as *monoclonal antibodies* that are specifically engineered to slow the growth of HER2-positive metastatic breast cancers. Women who receive these medications as a first-line treatment may obtain complete remission, sometimes for many years. Combining trastuzumab with chemotherapy drugs, including taxol, taxotere, navelbine, or platinum drugs typically improves its effectiveness. Pertuzumab (Perjeta) given with trastuzumab and chemotherapy increases survival more effectively than trastuzumab and chemotherapy alone. Although trastuzumab doesn't affect bone marrow or cause hair loss as chemotherapy often does, in rare cases it can cause headache, fever, chills, and nausea or vomiting, which can be managed with other medications. In some women, trastuzumab can affect the strength of the heart muscle, and monitoring is advised to ensure that the heart remains healthy. Because of this small risk of heart damage, trastuzumab is not usually combined with the chemotherapy drug doxorubicin. Possible side effects of pertuzumab include diarrhea, rash, vomiting, headache, and dry skin.

Another drug called Ado-trastuzumab emtansine (Kadcyla) is trastuzumab that has been attached to a potent chemotherapy drug called emtansine. Trastuzumab targets HER2 molecules in a tumor, enabling the direct delivery of emtansine's toxic payload directly to the cancer cells. This drug is given intravenously every three weeks unless the tumor continues to grow or intolerable side effects develop. Like other chemotherapy medicines, the emtansine portion of this drug disrupts the way cancer cells grow.

Some highly effective drugs don't bind to the HER2 protein but instead work within the cell to disrupt the activity of the HER2. The HER2 inhibitor lapatinib (Tykerb) is for women who have already had chemotherapy and trastuzumab. Combined with certain chemotherapy, trastuzumab, or hormone therapy drugs, lapatinib inhibits enzymes that the HER2 protein uses to signal cancer cells to grow. It may shrink the tumors, slow their growth, and extend the time before HER2-positive metastatic breast cancer progresses. Possible side effects include fatigue, nausea, severe diarrhea, vomiting, and rash. Some women who take lapatinib have developed hand-foot syndrome, which causes the hands and feet to become sore and red, and may include blistering and peeling. Some clinical trials show that a similar drug, neratinib (Nerlynx), which is used for early-stage breast cancers after a year of trastuzumab, may also be effective (figure 15.5).

PARP inhibitors for inherited breast cancers. In women who have a BRCA gene mutation, breast cancer cells have an already impaired ability to repair themselves when DNA damage occurs. A class of drugs called *PARP inhibitors* further impairs the ability of breast cancer cells to repair themselves and survive. Olaparib (Lynparza) and talazoparib (Talzenna) are PARP inhibitors that are approved to treat metastatic, HER2-negative breast cancer in men and women who have a mutation in a BRCA1 or BRCA2 gene. PARP inhibitors block the PARP enzyme (poly ADP-ribose polymerase) that cancer cells use to repair their DNA damage. Compared to chemotherapy alone, olaparib and talazoparib may give women who have BRCA-related, HER2-negative metastatic breast cancer more time before

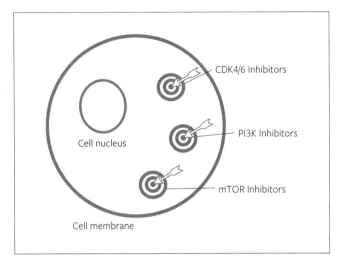

Figure 15.5. For women with HER2-positive breast cancer, multiple medications target the HER2 and related proteins

their cancer progresses. If you have metastatic breast cancer, your doctor can tell you whether you meet guidelines for genetic counseling and genetic testing to see if you would benefit from adding a PARP inhibitor to your treatment regimen. Some non-BRCA triple-negative cancers have the same underlying DNA repair problem and may also be susceptible to PARP inhibitors, but this is an area of ongoing research.

Although PARP inhibitors have side effects, they're often better tolerated than chemotherapy drugs. Headache, diarrhea, low white and red blood cell counts, nausea, vomiting, and fatigue are common. In rare cases, PARP inhibitors can increase the risk of developing acute myeloid leukemia, cancer that starts in the blood-forming cells of the bone marrow.

Immunotherapy

Although our immune systems defend against viruses, bacteria, and other foreign invaders, they don't always have an automatic response to cancer. Tumor cells can be good at adapting and disguising

Bone-Protective Medications

Your body continually breaks down and rebuilds your bones to keep them strong. Bone metastasis or treatment with an aromatase inhibitor can weaken this process, increasing susceptibility to fractures and leading to significant bone loss, especially in the hip, lower back, and upper thigh. *Bisphosphonates*, medicines that prevent or treat postmenopausal osteoporosis, can reduce fractures in women who have metastatic breast cancer in the bone (table 15.3). Research also suggests that these drugs may reduce the risk of postmenopausal cancers from spreading to the bones, but these findings remain controversial. Intravenous bisphosphonates, such as zoledronic acid and pamidronate, are more effective than oral bisphosphonates. A newer class of drugs called Rank-ligand inhibitors (Xgeva) also reduces the risk of fractures, but in a different way. Denosumab (Prolia, Xgeva) can increase bone mass in women who are treated with an aromatase inhibitor. A small group of women who take bisphosphonates or Rank-ligand inhibitors develop bone pain, and even fewer women develop an unusual disease of the jaw or femur.

themselves. Taking advantage of immune system "checkpoints" is one example of how cancer cells find ways to evade an immune system's best efforts so that they can continue to divide and grow. Checkpoints are proteins in immune system cells that need to be turned on or off to start an immune system response. They act as a built-in safety mechanism to keep the immune system from attacking healthy cells. It's a biologically smart maneuver, but it's one that some breast cancer cells can use to trick the immune system into leaving them alone.

Priming a patient's immune system to defeat cancer has long been a dream of researchers, and immunotherapy drugs are the first step in the realization of that dream. These "checkpoint inhibitors" target immune system checkpoints and restore the body's natural response against cancer cells. They trigger a proactive immune system response, similar to the way a measles or tetanus vaccine works: injecting you with a vaccine that contains a small amount of the measles or tetanus prompts your immune system to create antibodies against these diseases. Immunotherapies are an inspiring example of personalized medicine. They stimulate your own immune system to better recognize and kill cancer cells.

Since 2011, immunotherapy drugs have been used successfully to treat advanced melanoma, Hodgkin lymphoma, and some lung cancers. In 2019, atezolizumab (Tecentriq) became the first FDA-approved checkpoint inhibitor for breast cancer. Specifically, it's approved in combination with nab-paclitaxel to treat metastatic triple-negative breast cancer, which can be especially resistant to treatment. Previously, chemotherapy was the only available therapy for this hard-to-treat type of breast cancer, but it wasn't very successful.

Given intravenously every two weeks, atezolizumab given with the chemotherapy drug nab-paclitaxel (Abraxane) can be used as part of a first-line treatment for triple-negative tumors that are positive for PD-L1, a protein that falsely signals the immune system that everything is normal. Used alone, atezolizumab produces low response rates, but pairing it with chemotherapy produces a much stronger response. Atezolizumab attacks PD-L1-positive MBC with a two-punch approach: the antibody blocks PD-L1 proteins, prompting the immune system to recognize cancer cells as abnormal and hopefully begin to fight them while the chemotherapy destroys tumor cells. Side effects may include fatigue, nausea, loss of appetite, a persistent cough, neuropathy in the feet and hands, anemia, neutropenia, constipation or diarrhea, and hair loss in some women.

While immunotherapy holds great promise, it's a new frontier in medicine, and there is still much about it that we don't yet know. It doesn't work for everyone, although researchers aren't sure why. It's not recommended if you have an autoimmune condition or if you take steroids to treat a condition other than cancer.

WHEN TREATMENT STOPS WORKING

When do you decide that you no longer want to fight your disease? For many patients, it's when continuing treatment is unlikely to prolong life. It may be when chemotherapy is your only recourse after

Table 15.3. Medications That Protect or Strengthen Bones

Drug	Type	How It's Given
Alendronate sodium (Fosamax)	Bisphosphonate	Daily or weekly (pill)
Risedronate (Actonel)	Bisphosphonate	Daily or weekly (pill)
Ibandronate (Boniva)	Bisphosphonate	Monthly or every three months (pill)
Zoledronic acid (Reclast)	Bisphosphonate	Once annually (intravenously)
Zoledronic acid (Zometa)	Bisphosphonate	Monthly* (intravenously)
Clodronate (Bonefos)	Bisphosphonate	Once daily (pill)
Pamidronate (Aredia)	Bisphosphonate	Monthly (intravenously)
Denosumab (Xgeva)	Monoclonal antibody	Monthly (injection)
Denosumab (Prolia)	Monoclonal antibody	Biannual (injection)

*Quarterly infusions may be as effective.

other therapies have failed, and your quality of life will be better without additional treatment. Some women say that they reach a point when they're ready to let go of the difficulties of living with metastatic breast cancer and their worry and fear of the future. Only you will know when the time is right for you, and only you can make that decision.

Making the decision may be emotionally difficult, and your family may want you to continue with treatment. Deciding to discontinue treatment doesn't mean you're giving up or giving into your cancer. It means that you've made the choice to prioritize feeling as comfortable as possible for as long as possible. Transitioning from treatment to palliative care and hospice care can help you with this new goal and make your life easier. You can read more about these important options in chapter 23.

The Metastatic Breast Cancer Project

The Metastatic Breast Cancer Project provides an opportunity to be a part of ongoing international research to accelerate understanding and treatment of MBC. The innovative project connects metastatic breast cancer patients with scientists to expand understanding of this disease and develop new therapies. It's a unique approach to getting answers faster. Participation is quick, easy, and won't take much of your time. Once you enroll (www.mbcproject.org), you'll receive a kit to return a sample of your blood or saliva. You'll also be asked for permission to access your medical records and have a small tissue sample taken from your previous biopsy. Your data, without any identifying information, will be added to a global metastatic breast cancer database that can be freely accessed by the research community. There's no cost to you, and the project is broadly supported by the breast cancer and research communities. It's an opportunity to help others who will develop MBC to live better and longer.

Yvonne's Story

One evening I went home and found a card in the mail from my health insurer that read, "When you are 40 you need to have an annual mammogram." I was 47 at the time, and that was where my journey into the world of breast cancer began. After my first mammogram showed a suspicious area, my family physician, who is small in stature but has the biggest heart, looked for the best surgeon he could find and made the appointment for me himself. The surgeon was reassuring and kind. I'll always remember what he said to me on my first visit: "If this area is what they're concerned about, I wouldn't worry too much, but let's do a biopsy and see." The next week was unbearable. I went alone to get the results. My surgeon said, "This has bowled me over." I felt sick. I knew what was going to be said next. I wept. The tears just came rolling down like an overflowing dam. I asked, "Why now? Why now?" He responded, "I don't know what else is going on, but this is major stuff."

I then visited my family doctor, who said, "Yvonne, I have the very best oncologists for you. They are very, very good." I put together my small group of supporters before my mastectomy and breast reconstruction. My daughter, Trudy, and three other close friends would accompany me on doctors' visits and have input in every aspect of my treatment.

They became my ears, my brain, and my memory. My small prayer group became my family. Karen, a trusted friend (you always need one of those), was my encourager, my prayer partner, and the one who saw to it that my faith was intact and my spirit was lifted high.

When it was time for my chemotherapy, thank God I didn't have the dreaded nausea or any of those horrible experiences. My friend Max was a tower of strength. Because he had personal experience with chemotherapy and its effect on the body, his support was invaluable. Whether it was the tamoxifen or the chemotherapy, I went spiraling into menopause. That was rough. It took three years for my body to settle down and for the cancer to give me a break.

Then I started to feel severe pain in my right leg. In spite of radiation treatments to my lower femur, six months later, the pain was escalating and my gait was abnormal. After more radiation for the upper part of my femur, the pain got worse, and I had to use a cane. My quality of life was now reduced to a bare minimum, and my situation seemed dire. I then saw an orthopedic oncologist, who told me that my pain was caused by my breast cancer, which had returned in my bone. He recommended surgery to place pins in the femur to stabilize it. Once again, I called upon my faith to sustain me and give me the strength to face yet another period of pain and difficulty while the healing process took its course.

I refuse to let cancer win the fight. I can proudly state that I'm now in my 11th year of survivorship, although I can't say that I'm cancer free or that I'm in remission. Breast cancer changed my life. Every day of my life is a day of celebration, another day that I have survived breast cancer, and I now live each day as if it were the very last one. When those cancer cells metastasize wherever and whenever they choose, my oncologists and I deal with them and see them as bumps along the road.

CHAPTER 16

Considering Breast Cancer Clinical Trials

Participating in a clinical trial can be both exciting and frightening, like taking part in an experiment. Yet clinical trials in cancer care are carefully designed and supervised by physicians, scientists, and hospital and university review boards to ensure that each participant receives excellent treatment. Clinical trials are the key to making progress against cancer. They may provide women with the ability to receive new treatments that are hoped to improve the prognosis and lives of women with breast cancer.

Every new cancer drug and treatment we have came about because people were willing to participate in a *clinical trial*, research that finds new ways of preventing, detecting, and treating cancer and other diseases. Past trials are the basis of our practice of medicine today, and the trials of today will improve treatment for women in the future. These objective and comprehensive studies answer basic questions to improve health. Is a newly developed medication more effective than standard treatments? Is a shorter or longer regimen more beneficial? Is a larger dose more beneficial without more intense side effects?

Some clinical trials are funded by the US government, while others are sponsored by cancer centers, hospitals, teaching universities, or pharmaceutical companies who make the drugs. Trials may be conducted across the United States or in several international locations. All US clinical trials require approval from the Institutional Review Board (IRB), an independent committee of physicians, statisticians, health care advocates, and others who ensure that trials are conducted ethically and that your rights as a participant are protected. The IRB also verifies that the risks of a trial are as low as possible and that they don't offset the potential benefits. Researchers must follow a specific protocol that describes precisely how the trial is to be conducted. They report interim results to various government agencies, in peer-reviewed publications, and at scientific meetings.

TYPES OF TRIALS

Different types of trials are used to further research and provide more effective treatments:

- *Observational studies* follow the same group of people over time to determine how their health changes. One example of an observational clinical trial is the Women's Health Initiative, a groundbreaking study launched in 1993 that continues to provide information about health issues that affect postmenopausal women.
- *Epidemiological studies* look for patterns that answer where, when, and how diseases occur among large groups of people. The goal of one such study might be to identify the rate of triple-negative breast cancer in African American women, for instance, while another might attempt to identify specific risk factors for breast cancer.
- *Prevention studies* look for better ways to prevent a disease in people who have never had it or to prevent the disease from returning. Tamoxifen and raloxifene were subjected to this type of study before being approved as preventive breast cancer medications.
- *Intervention studies* identify behaviors that can improve health, such as studies that examine the benefits of exercise. A study to determine how mindfulness affects well-being during treatment would be one example.

All drugs and treatments must pass a series of tests that prove their safety and effectiveness before receiving FDA approval (table 16.1). After new drugs are tested in the laboratory, researchers use clinical trials to observe how well they work in people.

Table 16.1. Clinical Trial Phases

Phase	Purpose	Participants	Length
0	How does the body react?	10 to 15	Several months
I	Is it safe?	20 to 100	Several months
II	Does it work?	40 to several hundred	Up to two years
III	Is it more effective than standard treatment?	Up to 3,000	One to four years
	FDA Approval or Disapproval		
IV	Long-term safety and effectiveness	Several thousand	Several years

- Phase 0 trials are the first step to try new drugs on patients. These are very small trials to initially learn how people react to the drug.
- Phase I trials involve a small group of participants to determine the highest dose that can be given safely and with the least toxicity.
- Phase II trials often includes hundreds of people to determine whether the new drug or treatment produces the desired response.
- Phase III trials can involve thousands of people in different locations. Participants are randomly assigned to receive either new treatment or to the control group that receives standard treatment or a placebo.
- Phase IV trials can involve several thousand participants to gather more information about safety and side effects over a

longer time. This level of study also observes how the cost and effectiveness of the new treatment compare to standard treatment. Some Phase IV trials are conducted after the FDA has approved a drug or treatment.

Questions to Ask Your Doctor and the Trial Coordinator

- How is the new drug or treatment better than the current treatment?
- What are the possible benefits, side effects, or risks of the new treatment?
- How often will I receive treatment?
- What kinds of tests and treatments are involved?
- How will the doctor know if the treatment is working?
- Will I stay on my current medication?
- How long do I have to make up my mind about joining this trial?
- What happens if I decide to leave the trial?
- How will I be told about the trial's results?
- May I speak to someone who is already in the trial?

FINDING A CLINICAL TRIAL

Many women appreciate the opportunity to participate in a clinical trial, even if they ultimately choose not to do so. Your doctor may be aware of clinical trials related to your diagnosis and can provide you with information and answer your questions. If your doctor is unaware of clinical trials that may be in your best interest, you can use the searchable database of the National Institutes of Health to find a trial for which you're eligible (www.clinicaltrials.gov). The National Cancer Institute suggests that you prepare a Cancer Details Checklist before registering for participation. (Download the form at www.cancer.gov.) Ask your doctor to help you fill out the form if you don't have all of the information.

For more information about participating in a particular trial, contact the trial coordinator at the telephone number in the trial listing. Have a prepared list of questions that you want to ask. The researcher will ask you some questions to determine your eligibility. If you meet all of the requirements for participation and you want to join, the researcher will enroll you. Alternatively, you can ask your doctor to contact the trial coordinator on your behalf. If you decide that you'd like to take part in a particular trial that you find on your own, be sure to discuss your participation with your doctor before you enroll.

> **To find trials that may be helpful for you, look for information about the following:**
> - What is the trial's objective?
> - Is the trial still enrolling participants?
> - What are the eligibility requirements?
> - Does the trial offer you an opportunity to obtain treatment that would otherwise not be available?
> - If this is a trial of a new drug, are you one of the first patients to experience it? If so, will you possibly receive a low starting dose or a dose that isn't effective? Or will you receive a high dose, which may mean more side effects?
> - Is the trial location somewhere convenient or where you're willing to travel?
> - Are you willing and able to meet the time requirements for monitoring, testing, and follow-up that will be required?
> - How long will the trial run?

WHAT TO EXPECT FROM ELIGIBILITY, ENROLLMENT, AND PARTICIPATION

Multiple clinical trials are conducted to increase our knowledge about surgery, radiation, and systemic therapies to treat breast cancer. Each trial has criteria for eligibility and participation. Participants must meet requirements for age, gender, type and stage of cancer, previous treatment, general health, and other requirements. A trial that is testing a new drug for metastatic breast cancer, for example, may enroll only patients who have HER2-positive or triple-negative breast cancer that no longer responds to chemotherapy. Another trial may be looking only for women who have had a recurrence of hormone receptor–positive breast cancer. Some trials for newly diagnosed patients limit participation to women who have had no prior treatment.

Before participating, you'll be required to sign an informed consent document to show that you understand the purpose of the trial, its benefits and risks, what will be expected of you during the trial, and your patient rights. In no case should an informed consent request that you waive your legal rights or the legal responsibility of anyone affiliated with the trial. Your name, personal data, and other information regarding your participation is protected and confidential.

Clinical trials often, but not always, provide all drugs and treatments that are being studied and any related monitoring or follow-up at no cost. Before enrolling, ask the trial coordinator for a list of all of the costs that the trial sponsor pays for and any expenses that will be your responsibility. Also ask your health insurance company to clarify what trial-related costs it will and won't pay for or reimburse. Health insurance often covers the cost of hospital stays, outpatient appointments, testing, and other trial-related costs, for example, but rarely pays for travel or lodging expenses associated with participation in research.

If you decide to take part in a clinical trial, you may need to travel to a trial center for your treatment, periodic testing, and doctor visits. If a trial location isn't convenient, you'll need to decide whether you want to travel to the site as necessary for the duration of the trial. Some trial sponsors—the people, agencies, organizations, or companies who finance the clinical trial—may provide travel to the trial site or reimburse travel costs, but many do not.

After You Join

You may join a trial at its beginning or while it is ongoing—clinical trials often last several years. Taking part in a clinical trial provides you with a high standard of care. Your medical history will be reviewed, and you'll have a physical examination. You may also have a blood test to determine how much of the medication you should receive. During the trial, your health will be monitored with diagnostic tests, doctor visits, and exams to determine how well the treatment is going and how you're doing. The trial consent form will outline the details of how this will occur.

A clinical trial may provide you with access to an experimental drug, but even when early research data are promising, there's no guarantee that the drug will or won't work as hoped. It's always possible that a drug you're given as a trial participant may be ineffective or have unintended serious side effects. It's important to let the trial team know about any side effects that you experience or if you notice or feel anything out of the ordinary. Depending on which phase of a trial you participate in, you may not know whether you received the new drug, a standard of care medication, or a placebo until the trial is over.

Your participation is voluntary, and you can withdraw from a clinical trial at any time if you don't get the answers you need, you're concerned about some aspect of the trial that isn't resolved, or your personal circumstances change.

Your Health Insurer's Responsibilities while You're a Participant

The Affordable Care Act, a federal law that regulates health insurance plans, requires that health plans created since March 23, 2010 (when the law took effect), provide routine health care while you participate in a clinical trial. Some restrictions may limit which trials are covered. The law also prohibits health insurers from denying or limiting coverage for routine health care—office visits, lab tests, medicine, or treatment—for health issues that are unrelated to the trial. For example, if you're diabetic and participate in a trial of breast cancer treatment, the costs of blood tests, doctor visits, and insulin related to the treatment of your diabetes are still covered by your insurance, as they were before you became a clinical trial participant. The law also prohibits health insurers from increasing your health care premiums or deductibles because you join a clinical trial or from otherwise trying to keep you from participating in it.

When the Trial Is Over

If the trial successfully tests a new medication, the drug will continue to the next clinical trial phase or move to request FDA approval. In most cases, new groups of people are selected for the next phase. Study results are usually published online or in a published article, but you usually don't receive feedback about your individual participation or results.

Clinical trials are the key to making progress against cancer. Without them, we would be unable to move forward with newer and better treatments. Participating may or may not improve your quality of life and/or survival after other therapies fail, but it will help to move science forward to help others.

Regina's Story

My surgeon described my tumor as invasive carcinoma, a fast, aggressive cancer that develops in the mammary duct. He said that it literally just "bursts out," and that, in terms of timing, I was fortunate that I had reacted to the lump I had found right away. My oncologist talked about the whole process of chemotherapy, what goes on, and he asked me if I would be interested in participating in a clinical trial. I said yes. He explained the drugs that would be used and how my treatments might differ by being part of the trial.

I got all this paperwork, some seven or eight pages about the trial. I read through it, and I decided, yeah. I would be part of group A, B, or C, and I wouldn't know what group I would be part of. I looked at it this way: no matter whether I became part of the group that received the trial drug or I just received regular treatment, based on my diagnosis, I'd be getting the best treatment, no matter what. I also thought that my participation might help someone else—maybe someone younger or somebody older.

I had several tests before starting treatment in the trial. Having the treatments on Friday, I was sick on Saturday and Sunday. On Monday, I would get up because my son was going to school, and I tried to keep to my same routine—getting him up and ready. One day, my nurse asked if I would mind sharing the room with a new patient who was anxious about her treatment. The treatment area was a big room with two large recliners and a sofa, so two people could easily share it, and I said, "No problem."

(continued)

My mom was with me and the new patient's friend was with her; her anxieties were extreme. She got sick when they hooked her up to the IV anti-nausea medication. We became friends, exchanged phone numbers, and she still calls me now and then.

The trial staff was very sensitive to our personalities, to the manner in which people came in, and how they were relating. A psychiatric nurse was available twice a week.

CHAPTER 17

Treating Less Common Types of Breast Cancers and Male Breast Cancer

The majority of breast cancer diagnoses are infiltrating ductal or intraductal breast cancer, but other subtypes can also develop. The knowledge that oncologists have gained about these less common breast cancers has helped to improve care for individuals with all types of this disease. Men can also develop breast cancer, especially those who are carriers for a BRCA gene mutation. Male breast cancer in men is a treatable and curable disease.

Any cancer diagnosis is frightening. Dealing with unusual breast cancers that occur only rarely and may be unfamiliar to your oncologist can be even more unsettling. The cancers in this chapter are less common, and some are rarely seen. If you're diagnosed with one of these, ask if your oncologist has experience treating it. You may want to pursue a second opinion at a teaching university or a large medical center that has physicians who have treated people with your specific diagnosis.

INFLAMMATORY BREAST CANCER

Inflammatory breast cancer (IBC) accounts for just 1 to 3 percent of breast cancers. Most IBCs are a type of invasive ductal carcinoma that develops in the breast ducts before spreading beyond into breast tissue. IBC develops when cancer cells accumulate in the lymph vessels under the skin, causing lymph fluid to build up in the breast skin. As a result, the skin may appear to be inflamed, though despite its name, this breast cancer doesn't involve inflammation or infection. Symptoms appear when lymph fluid builds up in the breast skin. Lymph nodes in the underarm and above or below the collarbone may be swollen. There may also be itching and redness in much of the breast; a pink, purple, or bruised appearance; burning or tenderness; a heaviness or swelling that increases breast size; or nipples that are inverted (figure 17.1). A classic sign of IBC is dimpling or rippling that is sometimes referred to as *peau d'orange* (skin of the orange). IBC develops more often in young white women, especially those who are obese, in young African American women, and in older men.

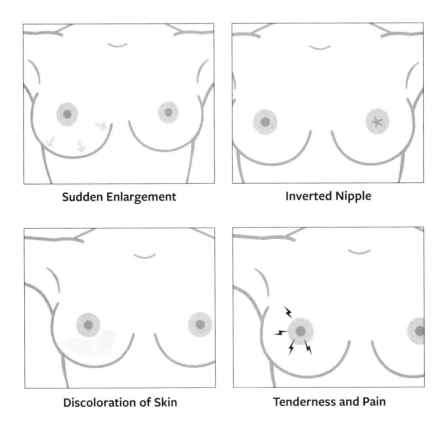

Sudden Enlargement

Inverted Nipple

Discoloration of Skin

Tenderness and Pain

Figure 17.1. Inflammatory breast cancer

Diagnosing IBC can be challenging because it doesn't always form a palpable tumor. Symptoms mimic *mastitis*, a breast infection that's treated with antibiotics, and can lead to a misdiagnosis. Adding even more diagnostic confusion, blocked lymph channels, swelling, and pinkness in the breast can also be caused by previous breast surgery or radiation to the breast or underarm. Most women who develop IBC have dense breasts, which makes mammography difficult. IBC can develop and progress between annual mammograms and advance quickly; symptoms may worsen in days or weeks rather than months or years. Ultrasound, a CT scan, PET scan, or bone scan can determine whether it has spread.

Prompt treatment is critical because IBC has usually already advanced to nearby lymph nodes (stage III) or into the body (stage IV) by the time it's found. Once confirmed by biopsy, IBC is often treated with an aggressive multistep approach that includes preoperative chemotherapy to shrink the tumor, followed by mastectomy, axillary lymph node dissection, and radiation. Hormonal therapy, such as an aromatase inhibitor, may be recommended if the IBC is hormone receptor positive. Similarly, if the tumor is HER2 positive, then HER2 targeted therapy will be included.

LOCALLY ADVANCED BREAST CANCER

Breast tumors occasionally become large before they're discovered. *Locally advanced breast cancers* can develop when a woman doesn't tell her doctor about a breast lump or abnormality, doesn't have routine mammograms, or when a mammogram or physical exam fails to detect breast cancer while it's small. One study found that most locally advanced breast cancers are discovered in the year or two between routine mammograms, when they've already spread into the breast tissue and/or lymph nodes. This type of breast cancer is usually stage III when detected and includes:

- tumors that are larger than 5 centimeters (about 2 inches) in diameter

- tumors that have grown into the chest wall muscle or the breast skin
- cancers that involve four or more lymph nodes under the arm or near the collarbone
- lymph nodes that are "matted" (attached) to one another or "fixed" to other structures and the cancer has spread to the underarm lymph nodes
- inflammatory breast cancer

Locally advanced breast cancers are generally more difficult to treat and have a poorer prognosis than early-stage tumors. Aggressive treatment usually includes neoadjuvant chemotherapy to shrink the tumor, followed by surgery with lymph node sampling, radiation therapy, and chemotherapy or hormonal therapy if the tumor is sensitive to estrogen or progesterone. Herceptin is also advised if the tumor is HER2 positive. For women who would be unable to tolerate chemotherapy because of their age or other health issues, preoperative hormonal therapy is sometimes considered if the tumor is hormone positive.

BILATERAL BREAST CANCER

Bilateral breast cancer—cancer in both breasts at the same time—is an unusual occurrence that accounts for just 2 to 5 percent of all diagnoses. Cancer in the second breast is usually detected by a routine screening mammogram or sometimes on an MRI that was ordered to evaluate the first breast cancer. Bilateral breast cancers are sometimes similar in origin (both ductal or both lobular), or they may be different subtypes in both breasts. Hormone receptor and HER2 receptor status of bilateral breast cancers may be similar or completely different. In either case, both cancers need to be evaluated and treated vigorously.

Although two simultaneous diagnoses sound doubly frightening, prognosis isn't necessarily worse than it is with a single breast cancer. Bilateral tumors develop independently and are staged separately; one might be stage 0 while the other is stage I or stage II. Treatment can be different, depending on the nature of each tumor. One breast may be treated with lumpectomy and radiation and the other with mastectomy, for example. Prognosis is good if the cancers are caught early and haven't metastasized.

Postmenopausal women or younger women who have BRCA mutations or a strong family history of breast cancer are especially susceptible to bilateral breast cancer. Younger women who are diagnosed with breast cancer are encouraged to have genetic testing and are treated more aggressively if they're found to have a mutation in BRCA1, BRCA2, or other predisposing gene. A genetic component is not as common for women who are 70 or older, because women with inherited genetic syndromes tend to develop breast cancer at a younger age.

HEREDITARY BREAST CANCER

If you have a risk-increasing genetic mutation, any breast cancer you develop is considered to be hereditary, and treatment may differ from other *sporadic* (nonhereditary) breast cancers. Hereditary breast cancers tend to occur at a younger age, behave more aggressively, and more often develop in both breasts. Your treatment plan should address these special circumstances and can sometimes mean more difficult decision-making. If you're considering treatment alternatives for hereditary breast cancer, ask your doctor if you're eligible to participate in any studies that specifically focus on your type of cancer. You can also search for clinical trials at clinicaltrials.gov.

Treatment considerations for hereditary breast cancer may include the following:
- Bilateral mastectomy is often considered or recommended, depending on the type of mutation you have. People with mutations in the BRCA1 gene, for instance, have a high risk of developing aggressive cancers and have a better prognosis after mastectomy than women with slow-growing, PTEN gene–related tumors that don't necessarily require mastectomy.

Removing the breast tissue greatly reduces the risk of developing another breast cancer or having a recurrence. If you choose to have your breasts reconstructed, it can be done at the same time as your mastectomies.

- Reducing estrogen levels as much as possible is recommended, because BRCA mutation carriers, especially those with a BRCA2 mutation, have greater risk of developing estrogen-fueled breast and ovarian cancers. Estrogen production can be stopped with bilateral oophorectomy to remove both ovaries or suppressed with injections of estrogen-blocking drugs like goserelin (Zoladex) and leuprolide (Lupron). Both approaches significantly lower the risk for another breast cancer and ovarian cancer, but they also induce menopause and eliminate fertility.
- Some type of chemotherapy is ordinarily prescribed for hereditary breast cancers, which tend to be more aggressive than sporadic breast cancers, especially in women who have a mutation in BRCA1. Some research suggests that BRCA-related triple-negative breast cancer also responds well to platinum-based chemotherapy.
- Poly ADP-ribose polymerase (PARP) inhibitors are especially effective against hereditary breast cancers. They're drugs that are engineered to block an enzyme that cancer cells need to repair DNA damage; without the enzyme, the cells don't survive. The PARP inhibitor talazoparib (Talzenna) treats locally advanced or metastatic HER2-negative breast cancer. Side effects include hair loss, headache, and reduced appetite. Talazoparib can reduce red and white blood cell counts, and increases the risk of acute myeloid leukemia and bone marrow failure. You shouldn't take this drug if you're pregnant or breastfeeding.

BREAST CANCER DURING PREGNANCY OR LACTATION

You may be surprised to learn that breast cancer during pregnancy is not that unusual. One diagnosis is made for every 3,000 pregnancies, most often in women in their 30s. Identifying breast cancer while you're expecting can be difficult, because changes in the breast can mimic swelling, tenderness, lumps, and other common side effects of pregnancy. Breast density also increases during pregnancy, making mammography less effective. Because tumors are more difficult to detect during pregnancy, breast cancers may be more advanced when diagnosed. For these reasons, your doctor should perform a careful clinical exam of your breasts at your first prenatal visit to be aware of any changes that occur while you're pregnant. Always tell your doctor about any unusual changes in your breasts, regardless of how small or insignificant they may seem.

Learning that you have a potentially life-threatening disease during such a meaningful time in your life can be overwhelming and disappointing, especially if you find that you need chemotherapy while you're carrying your baby. Your doctor will quickly outline a plan that focuses on treating you while allowing your baby to fully develop. If diagnosed, your doctor may also recommend that you see a *perinatologist*, an obstetrician who specializes in complicated pregnancies. Most importantly, breast cancer can be treated safely during pregnancy while taking precautions to protect your baby.

During your first trimester: Mastectomy (with either sentinel lymph node biopsy or axillary lymph node dissection, depending on the presence or absence of lymph node involvement) is generally preferable over breast-conserving therapy, because radiation isn't safe for your fetus. Certain chemotherapies, if needed, can be started during the second trimester, but radiation, hormonal therapy, and targeted therapies must wait until your baby is born.

During your second or third trimesters: Mastectomy or lumpectomy (with sentinel lymph node biopsy or axillary lymph node dissection, depending on the presence or absence of lymph node involvement) can be performed at this time, and if necessary, neoadjuvant or adjuvant chemotherapy can be started as well. At this stage, these treatments aren't harmful for your baby, whose organs are fully developed. Hormonal and targeted therapies are delayed until you give birth.

If you're diagnosed after your baby is born, you'll need to stop breastfeeding because some therapies can be passed to the baby through breast milk. Biopsy or lumpectomy can damage milk ducts in the breast, so ideally, your surgeon should have experience operating on lactating breasts.

Becoming Pregnant after Treatment

If you have early-stage breast cancer before becoming pregnant, some experts recommend waiting for at least two years after treatment before trying for a child—early-stage tumors that recur ordinarily do so within this time frame. Deciding to get pregnant while you're being treated for advanced breast cancer is more challenging, because treatment often continues indefinitely and may have effects on a developing fetus. Your doctor can help you work through these issues and make the best decision.

PAGET'S DISEASE

Paget's disease of the breast is an uncommon and aggressive form of DCIS that develops in the ducts at the base of the nipple and then spreads into the nipple and the areola. Symptoms may include inflammation, crusty or scaly nipple skin, or a clear or bloody discharge that doesn't improve. These signs are sometimes misdiagnosed as eczema or dermatitis. In about 10 percent of cases, women don't have any symptoms.

Because Paget's disease cells are typically large and high grade and most women diagnosed also have DCIS or invasive breast cancer, early diagnosis is important, and prompt treatment is critical. About half of women with Paget's disease have cancer in the underlying breast tissue that can be detected by mammography; in this case, the entire breast, including the nipple and areola, may need to be removed. If the cancer in the underlying breast tissue isn't extensive and it is close to the nipple, removing the nipple, areola, and a small portion of the underlying breast tissue, followed by radiation, will suffice. The nipple and areola must be removed if malignant cells are found there; clinical trials show a very high rate of recurrence otherwise. Optional nipple reconstruction is then a relatively quick and straightforward option.

UNCOMMON INVASIVE BREAST CANCERS

Medullary carcinoma is an unusual breast cancer that occurs most frequently in women with BRCA1 mutations. The term "medullary" is used because these tumors look similar to the medulla, the soft, gray tissue of the brain stem. Medullary tumors have the appearance of high-grade, aggressive tumors, but they behave more like low-grade, slow-growing breast cancer that typically remains in the breast and doesn't involve lymph nodes. Medullary tumors respond well to treatment and have a better prognosis than other types of invasive ductal cancers. Local therapy includes surgery with or without radiation, followed by chemotherapy, hormonal therapy, and trastuzumab (Herceptin) if the tumor is positive for the HER2 protein.

Tubular carcinomas are often discovered early. These tumors appear on mammography or breast ultrasound as irregularly shaped masses and may have nearby calcifications. Under the microscope, the cells look like small tubes about the size of a pea. They're typically slow growing and have a good prognosis. The five-year survival rate exceeds 90 percent, and at 10 years without a recurrence, the survival rate is almost the same as it is for women who have never had tubular cancer. The survival rate is even higher when the cells appear without other types of breast cancer cells. Tubular tumors are more common in women aged 50 and older. Because tubular breast cancer is often estrogen receptor positive, treatment usually begins with lumpectomy and radiation, followed by hormonal therapy. Women with smaller tumors may do well with surgery alone. Chemotherapy isn't usually necessary because these tumors don't typically spread to the lymph nodes; it is recommended, however, when more than one lymph node is positive. Women with this type of cancer have a higher-than-average likelihood of developing cancer in the opposite breast, so close surveillance is important.

Mucinous carcinoma is another rare subtype of invasive ductal breast cancer. Characterized by a gelatinous tumor suspended in a component of mucus called mucin, it's a slow-growing, low- to medium-grade breast cancer that sometimes develops near or mixed with DCIS or invasive ductal carcinoma in older women. When these tumors are large enough to feel, they're bumpy and spongy, similar to a fluid-filled cyst. Symptoms may include thickening or swelling of the breast, a change in breast shape or size, or an irritated, scaly, reddened, or dimpled nipple or breast skin. A nipple that develops a discharge should also be checked by your doctor. Some women develop tender underarm lumps. Treatment includes surgery; surgeons sometimes recommend a sentinel node biopsy as well, although this type of breast cancer rarely spreads to the lymph nodes. Radiation and hormone therapy are also recommended, since mucinous carcinoma is normally hormone sensitive. Prognosis of this cancer is most often better than other invasive breast cancers.

The cancer cells of *papillary carcinoma* develop in fingerlike projections called papules. Under a microscope, the cells are quite small and arranged in patterns like the fronds of a fern. When papillary carcinoma is discovered early and while it's still noninvasive, it's treated as DCIS. Normally, however, it's invasive by the time it's found, and it's then treated as invasive ductal carcinoma, usually with a good outcome. Treatment includes a combination of surgery, radiation, chemotherapy, hormonal therapy, and Herceptin if the tumor is HER2 positive.

Metaplastic carcinoma of the breast is one of the rarest of all breast cancers. It may cause breast pain, changes in the nipple, a lump, or other symptoms that are common to other breast cancers. Lumpectomy or mastectomy is the first line of treatment. A sentinel node biopsy is typically performed, even though metaplastic breast cancer is less likely to spread to the lymph nodes than other invasive breast cancers. If one or more nodes contain cancer cells, the remaining nodes are removed or radiated to reduce the chance of a recurrence. Metaplastic breast cancers are often triple negative, in which case they're treated with surgery and a combination of radiation and chemotherapy. Other cancers of this type that are estrogen or progesterone driven are treated with hormonal therapy, and with HER2 targeted therapy if the tumor is HER2 positive.

Phyllodes tumors develop in the connective tissue of the breast and grow in patterns that resemble leaves—*phyllodes* is Greek for "leaflike." These fast-growing tumors normally remain within the breast. They're most often discovered in women who are in their 30s and 40s, although women of any age can be affected. Most phyllodes tumors are benign; about 1 in 10 are malignant. Lumpectomy with a wide margin is recommended in either case because both benign and malignant phyllodes tumors tend to return in the same location when not enough surrounding tissue is removed. Malignant phyllodes tumors have a higher risk of recurrence than benign phyllodes tumors, and borderline phyllodes tumors fall somewhere in between. A partial or total mastectomy may be recommended if the tumor is large in relation to the breast. Phyllodes tumors don't ordinarily respond significantly to radiation, chemotherapy, or hormonal therapy. Close follow-up with frequent breast examinations is advised, especially when the tumors are malignant.

LYMPHOMAS AND SARCOMAS

Breast lymphoma is a malignancy in the lymph system of the breast. It's not breast cancer by definition, but because the lymphocytes (the cells that are in the lymph nodes) circulate throughout the body, women who have non-Hodgkin lymphoma in the breast often have lymphoma elsewhere. It's quite rare; less than .5 percent of malignant breast tumors are lymphomas. Most cases are stage I or II tumors that are found more often in women with autoimmune disorders—the average age at diagnosis is 55 to 60. The prognosis for early-stage lymphoma of the breast is generally good.

Breast implant–associated anaplastic large cell lymphoma (BIA-ALCL) is a rare condition that can develop in women who have breast implants with a textured surface. The most common presentation of BIA-ALCL is a fluid collection around the implant that develops at least 1 year, and on average 8 to 10 years, after the implant was placed. Other symptoms include breast swelling, enlarged lymph nodes in the underarm or in the neck, or a mass in the breast or the implant capsule (the scar tissue that naturally forms around the implant). Approximately 80 percent of BIA-ALCL cases are diagnosed at an early stage, treated with surgery alone, and have a good prognosis. Optimal surgical treatment includes removal of the implant, the implant capsule, any masses associated with the implant capsule, and any involved lymph nodes. Treatment with chemotherapy and radiation is only recommended for more advanced disease.

Breast sarcomas are tumors that begin in fat, blood vessels, nerves, and other soft tissues that support the ducts and lobules of the breast. Sarcomas may develop in the blood or lymph vessels after radiation therapy. Left untreated, sarcomas can metastasize, particularly to the lungs. Smaller, low-grade sarcomas may be removed with lumpectomy with a wide margin, though total mastectomy (without removing any lymph nodes) is more common. Radical mastectomy may be recommended for sarcomas that are discovered at an advanced stage, followed by radiation and/or chemotherapy. Sarcomas in the breast don't respond to hormonal therapy. Rarely, a special type of sarcoma called an angiosarcoma can develop in breast cancer patients 7 to 10 years after radiation therapy. Unfortunately, angiosarcomas are often difficult to treat.

CANCER OF UNKNOWN PRIMARY

In rare instances, a *cancer of unknown primary* (CUP) forms when a malignant tumor elsewhere in the body metastasizes to the breast but can't be identified. Sometimes the cause is never found. CUPs may be symptomless or cause symptoms that are common to other conditions, including a palpable lump or persistent pain in one area of the breast. Sometimes additional symptoms may develop, including:

- a persistent cough or fever
- abnormal bleeding
- a change in bladder or bowel habits

- sudden weight loss or loss of appetite for no apparent reason
- night sweats

Diagnosis may be made with physical exam, urinalysis and stool tests, and bloodwork, followed by a biopsy. If the cells can be identified, the diagnosis is made and treated accordingly. When the biopsied cells aren't what is expected (that is, malignant cells that clearly are not breast cancer cells), then the diagnosis is CUP. Sometimes, however, even a variety of scans, screening, and lab tests can't identify the primary cancer because it's small and slow growing or it's been destroyed by the immune system. It may have also been unknowingly removed during surgery for a different condition. Treatment is then based on the pathologist's best guess as to the most likely type of cancer. CUPs are becoming less common as diagnostic testing is improved. Because they're not breast cancers, CUPs aren't addressed with breast cancer treatments, although surgery, radiation, and other types of chemotherapy may still be required. If you're diagnosed with a CUP, speak to your doctor about participating in a clinical trial that is investigating this type of malignancy.

MALE BREAST CANCER

Men have breast tissue, estrogen, and progesterone, and they too can develop breast cancer. It doesn't happen often, although men who have a BRCA mutation are more at risk. (Any man who develops breast cancer should consider genetic testing to see if he has a predisposing mutation.) Malignancies in the small amount of breast tissue behind a man's nipples account for about 2,600 breast cancer diagnoses annually. In the United States, a man's risk for a diagnosis is 1 in 883, compared to 1 in 8 for women: one man is diagnosed for every 100 women with breast cancer. Most cases develop between ages 60 and 70, but men of any age can be affected. Overall, prognosis is similar when men and women are diagnosed at the same stage. Men, however, don't often check their breasts, don't have clinical breast exams as part of their annual physicals, don't have mammograms, and their tumors are more often advanced at the time of diagnosis. Male cancers have less room to grow in the breast, and they spread more quickly to nearby tissues. About 40 percent of men with breast cancer are diagnosed with stage III or IV breast cancer that has already metastasized, and as a result, overall survival rates are lower for men than for women.

Symptoms of Male Breast Cancer

- A painful or painless lump, swelling, or thickening in the breast.
- A lump or swelling under the arm or around the collarbone.
- Dimpling, puckering, redness, or scaling of the breast skin.
- Redness or scaling of the breast skin or of the nipple.
- A nipple becomes inverted or secretes a discharge.

Monthly self-exams are recommended, especially for men with a strong family history of breast cancer; certain other cancer—genetic counseling and testing are advised for men who have such a family history—or a mutation in a BRCA, CHEK2, PALB2, or other mutation that is related to male breast cancer. Men with Klinefelter syndrome, a rare genetic disorder, have a much greater risk of breast cancer. Having previous radiation to the chest can also increase a man's risk.

Invasive ductal carcinoma is the most common breast cancer in men. Lobular cancer rarely develops, because men have few lobules. Less often, men are diagnosed with inflammatory breast cancer or Paget's disease. Treatment includes mastectomy—neoadjuvant radiation may be used to shrink the tumor—followed by chemotherapy if the tumor has metastasized and/or tamoxifen (most male breast cancers are estrogen receptor positive). Fat grafting to replace lost tissue or a customized prosthesis are options if the removed area of tissue is large.

PART FOUR

Finding Answers

CHAPTER 18

Managing Breast Cancer Treatment Side Effects

Treatment for breast cancer continues to become more effective, and we have made tremendous progress in reducing the side effects. Many side effects can now be prevented, and others can be successfully treated. If a symptom persists, don't give up on finding relief. You may need to try several approaches before finding one that works well for you.

Breast cancer treatments save lives, but they also have the potential to cause unwanted side effects. Depending on the type of treatment, these reactions can affect women differently. Ranging from mild to miserable and acute to intense, temporary or long-lasting side effects are the emotional and physical downsides of treatment. Some effects decline or resolve on their own as your body adjusts to a medication. Not all of them can be eliminated, but most can be managed to varying degrees so that you don't suffer unnecessarily.

When your doctor prescribes a medication or treatment, ask about side effects that you should expect and what you should do if and when they appear. It's important to listen to your body during treatment, and to let your doctor know about any symptoms or side effects that cause discomfort or pain or interfere with your ability to eat, sleep, or function. Your oncology team is there to support you and to help identify ways to manage side effects as you complete your prescribed therapy.

FATIGUE

Fatigue is the most common side effect of cancer therapy. More than feeling tired now and then, fatigue is an utter lack of energy, a relentless exhaustion that can affect your ability to feel and function normally, even after a good night's sleep. If your treatment includes chemotherapy, you may experience fatigue, especially for a few days after the first day of each treatment. After a cycle or two of treatment, you'll know when to expect this cyclical fatigue; you can then plan to do more on your "good days" and not as much on days when you feel less energetic. Physical activity is one of the best antidotes for fatigue. It may sound odd to recommend activity for women who experience fatigue, but regular physical activity can in fact improve your stamina and sense of well-being.

- Talk to your doctor about other factors that can contribute to your fatigue, including medications that treat nausea, diarrhea, or heartburn; an underactive thyroid; chronic pain, stress, or depression. Ask if you should be tested for anemia, a lack of red blood cells that saps energy and can be corrected with transfusions if necessary. *Psychostimulants*, medications that stimulate certain parts of the brain, are only occasionally prescribed for women who experience ongoing problems with cancer-related fatigue.
- Eat whole grains, fruits and vegetables, lean protein, and nutrient-dense, iron-rich foods.
- Exercise every day. People often think that the remedy for fatigue is rest, but the opposite is true, and a lack of physical activity can cause or aggravate fatigue. Even walking around the house or around the block can help you feel more energetic. Include movements that will improve strength and flexibility.
- Accept that you may not yet be able to accomplish all that you did before treatment.

Questions to Ask Your Doctor about Side Effects

- What side effects should I expect from this treatment?
- Can these effects be prevented?
- Are there other treatments with fewer or less intense side effects?
- What do you recommend to relieve my side effects?
- What complementary therapies, if any, may be helpful?
- How soon should I see a response? How long will it last?

NAUSEA AND VOMITING

Chemotherapy drugs for breast cancer, especially cyclophosphamide, cisplatin, and doxorubicin, are among the most likely to cause nausea and vomiting. Some chemotherapy drugs cause this by affecting receptors in the gastrointestinal tract. Others affect specific areas in the brain that trigger nausea and vomiting to rid the body of toxins. These unpleasant effects aren't only uncomfortable; they can also contribute to weight loss, nutritional deficiencies, dehydration, and fatigue, making it more difficult for your body to fight the effects of cancer and toxic treatments.

Before the 1980s, few patients who were treated with chemotherapy were spared nausea and vomiting. Fortunately, preventive *antiemetic* drugs used alone or combined with a corticosteroid are now effective for most patients. The trick is to proactively match the right antinausea drug to the specific chemotherapy drug used. If one antiemetic medication doesn't work well, your doctor can choose a different one. Odansetron (Zofran), palonosetron hydrochloride (Aloxi), and aprepitant (Emend) are frequently used to prevent or treat nausea. Dronabinol (Marinol) and nabilone (Cesamet) are also FDA approved for chemotherapy-induced nausea and vomiting but are prescribed less often.

Try these tips to minimize the nausea you experience. Let your doctor know if you can't keep fluids down or you throw up for 24 hours or longer.

- Breathe through your mouth when you feel nauseated.
- Avoid eating greasy, fatty, or strong-smelling foods, like onion and garlic.
- Eat several small meals rather than fewer large meals.
- Stay hydrated. If plain water doesn't appeal, add the juice of a half lemon, orange, or lime.
- Choose cool or cold foods, rather than warm or hot foods.
- Suck on hard candy or ice.
- Season your food with ginger or drink ginger tea.
- Don't lie flat for an hour or two after eating.
- Wear loose clothing.
- Practice mind-body and relaxation techniques (chapter 19).

HAIR LOSS

Hair loss is probably the best-known side effect of chemotherapy and one of the most dreaded. It can be distressing because it's such a visible part of a woman's persona. Yet not all chemotherapy drugs cause hair loss, and not all women who are treated with chemotherapy lose their hair. Those that do lose hair not just on their head, but also on their face (including eyebrows and eyelashes), arms and legs, and the pubic area. That's because many chemotherapies, including doxorubicin, paclitaxel, and docetaxel, damage rapidly growing cells, including hair follicles. Hair loss can occur immediately after starting treatment, or it may gradually fall out after two to four weeks. If you cut your hair short or shave it off, you'll avoid finding clumps of it on your brush, on your pillow, or in the shower. An experienced professional stylist may be able to help with a shorter hairstyle. It's an emotionally difficult action to take, but doing so can help you to feel a sense of control.

If you plan to wear a wig, choose one before you begin chemotherapy, so you'll have it when you need it. Visit a wig shop where a professional can help you match your natural color and style, or try different styles, lengths, or colors. Most health insurers cover all or

Nail and Skin Changes

Radiation therapy can cause the skin of the treated area to become red and sensitive, as if it were sunburned, and certain chemotherapies can thin and dry the skin. Taking a few precautions a week or two before you begin treatment and until your skin heals can help. Bathe or shower using lukewarm water and a baby soap or other mild, unscented moisturizing soap or cleansing cream. While your skin is still damp, gently rub in a fragrance-free cream or ointment, which moisturizes more effectively than lotion. Keep your skin well lubricated throughout the day, especially after washing your hands. If your skin becomes itchy, try not to rub or scratch; your doctor can prescribe a soothing topical medication. When outdoors, protect your skin with sunscreen that has an SPF of 30 or higher and protects against both UVA and UVB rays.

Chemotherapy can also cause temporary changes to your nails that resolve after treatment. They may get darker, become brittle, or develop indentations, and in some cases, they may lift from the nail bed. Wear gloves when you wash dishes, and try to keep your hands dry and well moisturized. Keep your nails short, and don't file any spots or grooves that appear. Prevent dry cuticles with a generous application of a cuticle cream or a moisturizer that doesn't contain alpha or beta hydroxy acid. If you polish your nails, use a formaldehyde-free light shade and add a top coat. Avoid artificial nails until your treatment is over, and if you have professional manicures or pedicures, bring your own sterilized tools to protect against infection. Let your doctor know right away if you develop any signs of infection or inflammation.

part of the cost of treatment-related wigs with a doctor's prescription for a "cranial prosthesis." If a wig is beyond your financial means, contact the American Cancer Society or Ebeauty (www.ebeauty.com) for information on a donated wig. The Look Good Feel Better program (www.lookgoodfeelbetter.org) provides free information about selecting wigs, fitting turbans, and tying scarves. Hats or artfully tied scarves are also options to protect your head from the sun.

Hair begins to regrow a few weeks after treatment ends, sometimes in a different color or texture—for example, if your hair was light and straight before treatment, it may be dark and curly when it grows back. New growth may be gray until the cells that produce pigment begin functioning again. Avoid hair color, bleaching, or perms for at least six months after treatment until your hair follicles fully recover.

Caps That Reduce Hair Loss

Scalp cooling and *cold caps* can reduce treatment-related hair loss. Worn before, during, and after each chemotherapy session, both methods apply frigid temperatures to the scalp to constrict blood vessels in the head and lessen the amount of chemotherapy that damages hair follicles (figure 18.1). The Dignicap system and the Paxman Scalp Cooling System are essentially ice packs for the head. Both use a cap filled with silicone gel that is chilled to –15 to –40 degrees Fahrenheit before it's applied to your scalp. Treatment centers that have these devices typically make them available for a fee. Cold caps (Arctic Cold Caps, Chemo Cold Caps, Penguin Cold Caps) work differently. They need to be replaced periodically as the cap thaws and the temperature drops. If you choose this method, you're responsible for renting the cap and refrigeration unit, applying the cap, and replacing it when needed.

Studies show that, overall, cold caps and scalp cooling systems work well in more than half of women who use them. Depending on the type and dose of your systemic treatment, these methods can save 50 to 90 percent of your hair. Women who are treated only with taxane chemotherapy appear to have better results than those who are treated with just anthracycline chemotherapy. Your oncologist can discuss which types of chemotherapy are good treatment options for you and how well they might work with these hair-preserving therapies. Headaches can occur with either procedure, and the experience is chilling, so you'll need to bring a blanket to your chemo session. Your health insurance may cover a portion of the cost if you have a prescription for a cranial prosthesis. The nonprofit organization HairToStay (www.hairtostay.org) helps women pay for cold caps and scalp cooling.

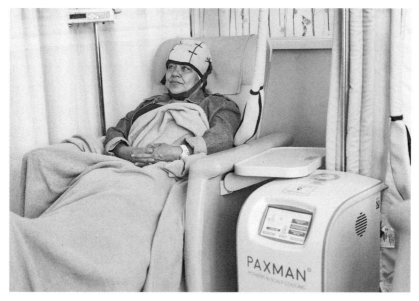

Figure 18.1. Scalp cooling or cold caps may save some or most of your hair. Used with permission from Paxman

PREMATURE MENOPAUSE

Menopause naturally occurs after age 50 when the ovaries stop making estrogen. For many younger women, early menopause is caused by breast cancer treatment. Whether it occurs naturally or is induced by treatment, the "change of life" experience is different for every woman. Some have numerous uncomfortable side effects, while others have almost none.

Symptoms of sudden, treatment-related menopause can be more intense than the symptoms of natural menopause, which develop gradually. *Menopausal hormone therapy*—supplemental estrogen with or without progestin—that reduces the effects of natural menopause isn't recommended for breast cancer patients or survivors, because it can stimulate breast cancer cells and cause a recurrence or a second breast cancer. If needed, your oncologist can prescribe medications or suggest other ways to ease your symptoms. Below are some things you can do reduce the most common symptoms.

Hot Flashes

A sudden feeling of intense heat in the face, neck, and chest, sometimes accompanied by flushed skin and sweating, is the most common symptom of menopause. A *hot flash* suddenly appears for no apparent reason. It might be gone in 30 seconds or last 10 minutes. Some women continue to have hot flashes for a few months or several years, although they tend to eventually fade away with or without treatment. Experts aren't quite sure what causes these episodes, but the most common theory is that the brain detects too much body heat when estrogen declines and responds by releasing hormones that dilate blood vessels. This allows for more blood flow to dissipate heat, but it also raises the heart rate and produces sweat.

Smoking and obesity increase the likelihood of hot flashes. Avoiding alcohol, caffeine, and spicy foods that can trigger a hot flash can reduce the frequency and intensity of episodes. When a hot flash begins, do something to cool your body: drink a cold beverage, take a tepid shower, or wash your face with cool water. Dress in layers, so that you can cool off in a hurry when you need to. Keep your bedroom cool, use cotton sheets, and avoid caffeinated beverages before bedtime to reduce *night sweats*, hot flashes that occur while you sleep. Meditation and mind-body practices like yoga or tai chi can also help. If your hot flashes are unbearable and frequent, consider acupuncture or hypnosis, or ask your doctor about prescribing antidepressants, antiseizure medications, or blood pressure drugs that may reduce the frequency and severity of this symptom.

Vaginal Atrophy

Female genitals, which are extremely sensitive to estrogen, can become dry and atrophied without it. Over-the-counter moisturizers (K-Y and Replens) help to temporarily replace lost moisture and restore elasticity to vaginal tissues. Avoid douching, which can further irritate the vagina. For persistent atrophy, some doctors may recommend low-dose estrogen cream, a dispensing ring, or tablets that are placed in the vagina and release minimal doses of estrogen that remain in the vagina and don't appear to increase the risk of a recurrence if you're being treated for breast cancer or have had it previously.

Painful Intercourse

Estrogen-reducing therapies can affect blood flow to the vagina, thinning the tissue and causing *dyspareunia*, dryness and irritation that make intercourse painful. Water-based lubricants (Astroglide, Silk-E, and others) replace natural secretions and make intercourse easier, while oil-based lubricants or products that aren't specifically designed to be used on the vagina may further irritate sensitive tissue. Ask your doctor if you would benefit from using a lubricated vaginal dilator for 10 to 15 minutes every other day to gradually stretch your vagina, making intercourse less painful. The dilators can also improve *vaginismus*, an involuntary tightening of the vaginal muscles that makes penetration impossible. Strengthening your pelvic floor, the muscles that support organs in the pelvis, can also reduce sexual discomfort. Regular sexual activity also promotes blood flow to vaginal tissues.

Three Ways to Strengthen Your Pelvic Floor

1. *Kegel exercises.* With your bladder empty, contract the muscles you use to stop urination. Hold the contraction for two to three seconds, then release. Do 5 sets of 10 repetitions per day. You can perform Kegels just about anywhere: while you drive, shower, or watch TV.
2. *Pelvic floor therapy.* A specially trained physical therapist can help you stretch and strengthen your pelvic muscles with massage or mild electrical stimulation that releases the connective tissue in your pelvic region. She may place biofeedback sensors on your vaginal wall to measure the strength of your muscle contractions or manipulate your pelvic floor muscles by massaging inside and outside your vagina.
3. *Yoga.* Regularly practicing yoga provides a variety of benefits, including relaxation, and that often improves the discomfort caused by *dyspareunia* or *vaginismus*. Some poses, including cobra, child's pose, and happy baby, strengthen the pelvic and abdominal muscles, which can also ease pelvic pain during sex (figure 18.2).

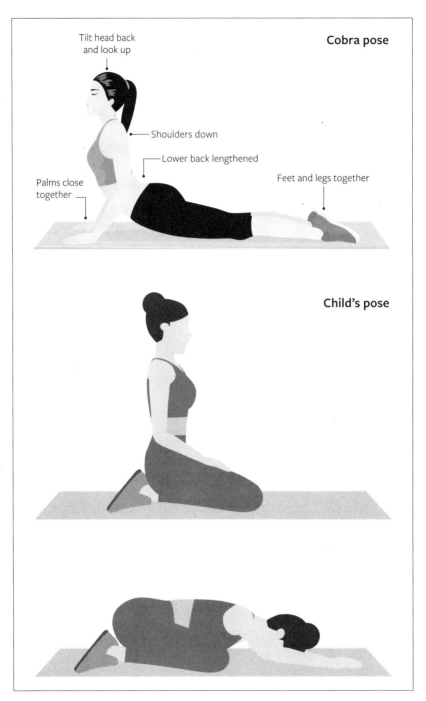

Figure 18.2. Cobra and child's pose

Treatments That Cause Menopause

- Tamoxifen can cause menopause-like symptoms that usually go away when treatment is stopped.
- Aromatase inhibitors are prescribed for women who have already gone through natural menopause, but they can cause recurrent menopausal symptoms.
- Chemotherapy, especially cyclophosphamide, can induce medical menopause. The younger you are, especially if you're under age 40, the more likely your periods are to return once your chemotherapy treatments end. However, you may then experience natural menopause before age 50. You may still ovulate intermittently, so using birth control is an important consideration until it's clear that you're postmenopausal.
- Luteinizing hormone-releasing hormones temporarily shut down the ovaries.
- Bilateral oophorectomy (removal of both ovaries) results in immediate and permanent menopause.

COGNITIVE CHANGES

We all tend to forget things and have difficulty concentrating from time to time. "Chemo brain" is the treatment-related version of forgetfulness, mental fogginess, and cognitive lapses. Symptoms may include periodically being unable to recall details of recent events, forgetting words or where you put things, and finding yourself easily distracted. Cognitive dysfunction can also occur with hormonal, targeted, and immune therapies, but it's more common with chemotherapy, especially cyclophosphamide, doxorubicin, 5-FU, and paclitaxel.

Most women find that these frustrating lapses resolve within 6 to 12 months after treatment, although they seem to last longer in up to 20 percent of chemotherapy patients. You may be more susceptible if you're older, menopausal, have an underlying condition that causes similar issues, or if you're genetically predisposed to cognitive decline. Some experts believe that the psychological stress of a cancer diagnosis and treatment can make cognitive malfunction worse.

Trying to pin down the exact causes of chemo brain is an active area of research. Studies point to a variety of possible factors, including the possibility that chemotherapy limits production of memory cells in the brain or that it degrades areas that direct learning and memory by damaging the protective layer of fats and proteins that surround brain cells. Some studies suggest that certain chemotherapies may reduce levels of dopamine and serotonin, two compounds in the brain that aid cognitive function.

There's no simple, straightforward treatment for chemo brain, although mild to moderate walking, running, dancing, swimming, cycling, or other aerobic exercise can sharpen mental focus. A cognitive therapist can demonstrate techniques that reduce stress, help you relax, and enhance your memory and attention. Some patients report improved concentration and focus when they take Ritalin, a medication that is normally prescribed for attention deficit hyperactivity disorder, or similar drugs that stimulate the central nervous system. Let your doctor know about any changes in your ability to think and concentrate during your treatment. If these problems persist, ask for a referral to a neuropsychologist, who can suggest strategies for cognitive rehabilitation.

Tips for Improving Cognitive Symptoms

- Seek treatment for fatigue, depression, anxiety, and sleep apnea or other sleep problems, which can intensify the effects of chemo brain.
- Ask your doctor to check that your thyroid, vitamin D, and B12 levels are adequate.
- Use visual images to remember names, locations, or other information.
- Keep a notebook handy to make lists, write things down, and keep track of things while you remember them.
- Give your brain a workout: read, play Sudoku, do crossword puzzles, or engage in other activities that may sharpen your thinking skills.
- Request a referral to a cognitive rehabilitation therapist.

FERTILITY ISSUES

Chemotherapy, estrogen-blocking medications, and oophorectomy can diminish, delay, or eliminate your ability to conceive. That can be a tough pill to swallow if you look forward to a future pregnancy. Whether you're certain you want to have children someday or you simply want to reserve the option, your treatment may prompt you to strategize about family planning, even if you would otherwise not be ready to do so.

Other Ways to Become a Parent

If you're able to become pregnant, doctors often recommend waiting at least two years after treatment before trying. Your past breast cancer poses no risk of ill effects to your future babies. If you're unable to become pregnant after treatment, a fertility specialist can provide more information about other ways to become a parent.

If you still have your uterus:
- Donated eggs from another woman can be fertilized with your partner's sperm and implanted into your uterus.
- A donated embryo that is already fertilized (by someone other than your partner) can be implanted into your uterus.

If you become infertile:
- A surrogate—a woman who volunteers to be artificially inseminated with your partner's sperm—can carry the baby to term for you.
- Adoption is always an option to match children who need a loving home with parents who want to raise a child.

As you and your doctor discuss breast cancer treatment options, ask how each one may temporarily or permanently affect your fertility. If you want to preserve the option to have your own biological children (or more of them), a fertility specialist can explain your options before your cancer treatment begins. The most common method of preserving fertility is *in vitro fertilization* (IVF). Some of your eggs can be removed before treatment, fertilized with your partner's sperm in a lab, and then frozen until you're ready to become pregnant. After treatment, the embryos can be implanted in your uterus (if you still have it) and carried to term. Freezing unfertilized eggs is also possible, but it's less often successful. The cost of fertility procedures can be high, and few insurance companies cover them adequately.

IVF is certainly more clinical than the natural method of conceiving, but it's the best alternative to treatment-related infertility. Success depends on your age, reproductive history, the clinic used, and other factors, but improved techniques are becoming more dependable. According to the American Pregnancy Association, success rates for vitro pregnancies are as follows:

- women under age 35: 41 to 43 percent
- women ages 35 to 37: 33 to 36 percent
- women ages 38 to 40: 23 to 27 percent

REDUCED ARM AND SHOULDER MOBILITY

The restorative nature of upper body exercise after breast surgery or radiation therapy can't be overemphasized. Gentle stretching restores your ability to reach your arm up and across your body, as many routine movements require. Not exercising can lead to muscle loss and restricted movement, including "frozen shoulder," a shortening of the muscles that support shoulder joints that reduces range of motion and mobility. A cycle of pain may continue when you don't properly rehabilitate your arm or shoulder after surgery: it hurts, you don't use it, it gets worse.

A daily routine of controlled upper body movements helps to eliminate stiffness and restore range of motion; strengthen chest, arms, and shoulders; and discourage lymphedema. Your surgeon will provide instructions for exercises that you can do at home and let you know when you should begin to do them, usually in three to seven days postoperatively, when your sutures and surgical drains are removed. Running, weightlifting, or more vigorous exercise should be postponed until your body has healed sufficiently and your doctor

Deep Breathing

Deep breathing is also restorative. It strengthens the diaphragm and inter-costal muscles between your ribs while helping you to relax.

1. Lie on your back with your legs straight and your arms relaxed at your sides.
2. Fully expand your chest and stomach as you inhale through your nose as deeply as you can.
3. Hold your breath for three to five seconds.
4. Exhale slowly through your mouth.
5. Repeat this routine four or five times.
6. Do the entire exercise five or six times a day.

gives you the okay. If you have trouble regaining full range of motion, ask your doctor for a referral to a physical therapist who is specially trained in cancer-related rehabilitation. Women who work with physical therapists who are experienced in cancer-related rehabilitation tend to regain strength and range of motion faster than those who work on their own. If you have lymphedema, consult with a certified lymphedema therapist before beginning an exercise program.

LYMPHEDEMA

Removing or radiating lymph nodes creates a lifetime risk for *lymphedema*, chronic swelling in the shoulder, arm, or hand on the side that was treated. Lymphedema symptoms can develop soon after treatment or many years later when a segment of the lymph system becomes damaged and can no longer filter fluids, which then collect in the arm. Doctors can't predict who will or won't develop lymphedema, but the risk is lower after sentinel node biopsy and higher when additional lymph nodes are removed or radiated. The affected arm may feel heavy, tight, or numb. Rings or sleeves that suddenly become too tight may also be signs of lymphedema. In extreme cases, the arm becomes enlarged from shoulder to fingertips (figure 18.3). Prevention is your best defense. Before breast surgery, ask your surgeon about *axillary reverse mapping* to identify and remove lymph nodes that drain the breast, while preserving nodes that drain the arm.

If any of your lymph nodes are removed, be protective of your affected arm. Keep it scrupulously clean to avoid infection and protect it from burns, cuts, insect bites, and other injuries. Have blood pressure readings, injections, and blood samples taken from your unaffected arm. Physicians used to caution women to limit lifting and physical activity involving the affected arm; however, studies show that regular activities and the right type of exercise are beneficial. Ask your doctor about how to reduce your risk of lymphedema and request a referral to a certified lymphedema specialist who can show you which moves can be harmful and which can help. Contact your doctor at the first sign of swelling—even mild swelling—in your arm or hand on the same side as the treated breast.

Managing Lymphedema

We don't have medications to treat lymphedema, and it can't be cured. It's a chronic condition that can be managed in its early stage with compression garments, exercise, and lymphatic massage by a qualified lymphedema therapist and self-massage that you can learn to redirect fluids and reduce swelling.

Some moderate to severe cases can be improved with surgery. *Lymphatic venous anastomosis* connects lymph vessels in the affected area to nearby veins, establishing a bypass for lymphatic drainage. Women who have considerable swelling from advanced lymphedema that no longer responds to traditional compression therapy may benefit from *suction-assisted protein lipectomy*, a specialized kind of liposuction that debulks excess fats from the arm and improves lymphatic drainage. *Vascularized lymph node transfer* for individuals who don't respond to conventional lymphedema treatment replaces lymph nodes that are removed during axillary lymph node dissection with healthy nodes from somewhere else in the body that pick up

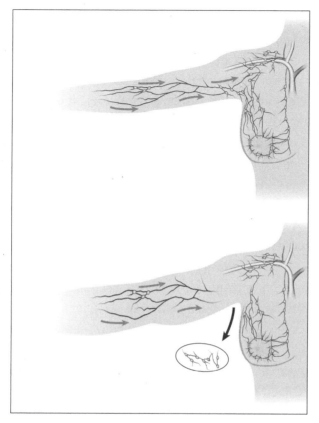

Figure 18.3. Chronic arm lymphedema

the job of draining lymphatic fluids. This sophisticated surgical procedure, which requires special surgical skill and experience and isn't
widely offered, is most often performed in combination with deep
inferior epigastric perforator (DIEP) flap breast reconstruction.

CHRONIC PAIN

There's a big difference between ordinary discomfort as healing
progresses after treatment and persistent pain that remains long
after treatment is over. Lingering discomfort or pain is surprisingly
common after mastectomy or radiation. Finding relief can be frustrating, especially when it affects every movement you make and every

position you try. But you should always seek help for unrelenting pain, because left untreated, it can reduce your functionality and quality of life. In some cases, it can become debilitating. Aside from interfering with your physical, emotional, and psychological well-being, chronic pain hinders your immune system's ability to fight disease and infection. You may need to consult with a pain specialist and go through a trial-and-error process to find a solution that works. Some women experience the following symptoms.

Arthralgia

Women may develop *post-chemotherapy rheumatism*, a syndrome that includes *arthralgia* (joint pain and stiffness) and muscle pain after completing chemotherapy for breast cancer. (Arthralgia is different than arthritis, which is inflammation in the joints.) Symptoms typically affect the fingers, hands, wrists, elbows, shoulders, knees, and ankles.

Arthralgias can also develop quickly as aromatase inhibitors (AIs) reduce estrogen in the body and affect bone health. In studies of breast cancer patients, 20 to 50 percent of women who took aromatase inhibitors developed some type of arthralgia, usually in the first three months of therapy. Experts don't yet know exactly why AIs cause joint symptoms. It may be that a rapid drop in estrogen lowers a woman's pain threshold to conditions that already exist or that reduced estrogen results in high levels of proteins that accelerate bone loss. While over-the-counter and prescribed medications can help, most shouldn't be taken long term, and many shouldn't be used while you're being treated for breast cancer. If you develop treatment-related arthralgia, your doctor may switch you to another aromatase inhibitor to see if that helps. It's important that you keep taking your breast cancer medication as you continue to find ways to relieve your discomfort. Some women find that acupuncture reduces arthralgia pain and improves functionality.

Neuropathy

Neuropathy is a common side effect of chemotherapy, especially from taxane and platinum drugs that can injure or irritate nerves, causing pain, numbness, burning, or pins-and-needles tingling. Many cancer-related neuropathies improve in time. Others last for months or years after treatment. Mild neuropathy can be frustrating; severe neuropathy can affect your ability to perform the simplest actions: walking, getting in and out of chairs or bed, and even breathing normally. Neuropathy that impairs mobility because of numbness in the feet and toes also increases the risk of falling, especially in older women. You're more susceptible to treatment-related neuropathy if you're overweight or obese, diabetic, or you already have neuropathy before you begin treatment. Other conditions can also cause neuropathy, so it's important to determine whether chronic pain is related to breast cancer treatment or an underlying health issue.

Treatment for neuropathy may include massage, anesthetic patches applied to the skin, or acupuncture. Physical therapy and routine exercise, which prompts your body to release endorphins that block pain signals to the brain, can also be beneficial. Walking, bicycling, or swimming, and light weight training can be done safely to relieve pressure in your hips and knees. Try crocheting or knitting to improve painful knuckles. These activities probably won't eliminate your pain, but they can make it more bearable.

Conventional painkillers like ibuprofen or aspirin aren't usually effective for painful neuropathy. It's often treated instead with anticonvulsants or antidepressants that alter chemical signals in the body. Cymbalta, an antidepressant that's also FDA approved to treat chronic musculoskeletal pain, is one option. Other options include the use of a battery-operated *transcutaneous electrical nerve stimulation* (TENS) unit that delivers low-voltage electrical impulses under the skin. Rarely, for patients with severe, intractable pain, an implantable pump can be used to deliver potent pain medicine directly into the spinal fluid. *Cementoplasty*, injections of special medical cement that fill parts of bone destroyed by advanced breast cancer, can strengthen and support bones to relieve pain there. Because the brain is actively involved in how pain is processed and perceived, yoga, neurofeedback, and other mind-body approaches can limit pain by refocusing the brain. They can also help you manage depression, stress, anxiety, and other negative emotions that can increase your pain. Nerveblocking medications or destroying rogue nerves may resolve severe pain that doesn't respond to other treatments.

Postmastectomy pain syndrome is a type of neuropathy that persists three months or more after breast cancer surgery. Lingering discomfort or pain over the chest, axilla, or upper arm is surprisingly common after mastectomy or radiation. For many women this discomfort resolves over 6 to 12 months, but for others it may be ongoing. It's estimated to occur in about half of women after mastectomy, lymph node dissection, or lumpectomy, although it's rarely discussed as a potential risk and is often misdiagnosed as pain that develops as part of the normal healing process. This painful condition is thought to occur when treatment severs or damages the nerves that provide sensation to the chest wall, shoulder, and upper arm, or in the underarm sensory nerves. Symptoms include mild to intense burning, shooting pains, throbbing, or tingling in the arm, shoulder, or chest wall.

A CT scan, x-ray, or MRI can rule out other causes. Treatment may include massage, capsaicin cream, analgesics, nerve-blocking medications, or antidepressants. If postmastectomy pain persists, don't give up on finding relief. You may need to try several approaches before finding one that works well. A *physiatrist*, a doctor who specializes in rehabilitation, can best diagnose the condition and recommend treatment, which often involves a combination of medication and physical therapy.

OSTEOPENIA AND OSTEOPOROSIS

Bones consist of living cells that are constantly replaced by our bodies. By age 35, bones begin to thin as a natural part of the aging process. Chemotherapy, aromatase inhibitors, and luteinizing hormone-releasing hormones that lower estrogen levels often accelerate this bone loss. Suppressing the ovaries with medications that bring on menopause, radiating the ovaries, or removing them has the same negative effect on bone health. These treatments raise the risk of *osteoporosis*, thinning of the bones that increases susceptibility to fractures, and for *osteopenia*, weakening of the bones that is often a precursor to osteoporosis. If you have any of these treatments, it's wise to have periodic bone density tests and, if warranted, medications to minimize bone loss.

You can and should take action to strengthen your bones and slow bone loss. Be sure to get enough calcium and vitamin D from dietary sources or use a supplement to make up the difference (see table 18.1). Regularly walk, jog, or perform other weightbearing exercises to increase bone mass. Limit or avoid alcohol and caffeine—both diminish calcium levels—and don't smoke. Ask your doctor if one of the following bone-strengthening medications is right for you.

- *Bisphosphonates*—including alendrolate, zoledronic acid, bandronate, and others—can improve bone density and are also used to treat women with bone metastases. Denosumab (Prolia or Xgeva) is also used to improve bone density. Treatment with one of these medications may be a good choice if you already have osteoporosis and are taking an aromatase inhibitor.
- Calcitonin is a hormonal nasal spray that improves bone density and reduces bone thinning.
- Teriparatide is a synthetic hormone that helps regulate calcium metabolism and promotes new bone growth.

Table 18.1. National Osteoporosis Foundation Recommendations
for Daily Calcium and Vitamin D Intake for Adults

Age	Calcium (IU)*	Vitamin D (IU)#
≤50	1,000	
≥51	1,200	
<50		400–800
≥50		800–1,000

*Total from diet and supplements.
#Total from sunlight, diet, and supplements.

WEIGHT GAIN AND LOSS

As frustrating as weight gain may be for many women, there are reasons why it commonly occurs with chemotherapy. During treatment, you may feel more lethargic, exercise less, eat poorly, retain fluids, or take prescribed steroids to offset other side effects. All of these factors contribute to added weight. (Although women who are treated with hormonal therapy often blame it for the weight they gain, randomized data don't support this belief.) You may also become heavier if you develop treatment-induced menopause. While gaining a pound or two probably isn't significant, additional weight may affect your overall health. Carrying extra weight is dangerous for your heart and increases the chance of another breast cancer diagnosis, especially after menopause. Gaining more than 5 percent of your weight during or after treatment can raise your risk of a recurrence.

Unlike many other side effects of treatment, weight gain doesn't automatically disappear after treatment. The antidote is diet and exercise. The same weight loss strategies that serve you well when you're healthy are also important while you're being treated: proper proportions of nutritious, balanced meals; fewer fatty snacks; and limited fast foods and restaurant takeout. Ask for a referral to a registered dietician who can customize an eating plan that keeps you healthy and satisfied. Forego dieting and learn how to eat well as you give your body what it needs. Push yourself to be more active. Lose fat and build muscle with aerobic exercise and resistance training.

Although it's more common for patients to gain weight from treatment, some lose weight instead. Chemotherapy can wreak havoc on appetite; it's hard to get excited about foods when your sense of taste and smell are reduced, your appetite is gone, and nothing tastes good. Cancer medications can change how your taste buds respond to different flavors. You may find that your favorite foods are suddenly unbearable or that you enjoy something you previously disliked. Try eating foods that are cool, cold, or at room temperature, which are less likely than warm or hot foods to expose you to unappealing aromas.

If you become underweight, a good rule of thumb is to eat 15 calories per pound of weight: that's about 2,250 calories if you weigh 150 pounds. Add a few hundred additional daily calories if you've lost a significant amount of weight. Work your way through different proteins—lean meats, yogurt, nuts, eggs, and beans—to see what appeals to you and what you can tolerate. Be sure to give your body adequate protein to rebuild and repair muscle fibers and tissue that can be damaged by treatment. Eat several small meals and snacks every two to three hours. If food doesn't appeal to you or it doesn't taste right, try a nutritional meal replacement like Ensure. Ask your doctor if your medication could be causing your weight loss, and if the dose can be adjusted.

CHAPTER 19

Complementary, Integrative, and Alternative Medicine

Strong scientific evidence supports our growing understanding that the mind and the body are intertwined and bridged by emotions and feelings: what we think and feel directly affects our health and well-being, which in turn affect what we think and feel. Taking care of your mind and your spirit can help improve your overall health. Some complementary and alternative therapies may be of benefit, though it is important to discuss these therapies with your medical team.

Historically, a great divide has existed between our traditional medical approach to treating cancer and nonmedical alternatives or unconventional treatments. In the 1980s, for example, cancer patients paid handsomely to receive Laetrile, a compound derived from apricot pits, as an alternative to chemotherapy, despite studies that proved it to be a hoax. Nutraceuticals, high-dose vitamins, oxygenation, ozone, sodium bicarbonate, and other questionable products have since been touted as "miracle cancer cures." Not surprisingly, none of them work. While many therapies outside the realm of standard medicine can make you more comfortable as you go through treatment, others are nothing more than folk medicine or scams. It's important to know the difference.

Standard medical care, sometimes referred to as Western or mainstream medicine, is practiced by health professionals who hold a medical degree, are licensed by their state, and typically follow specific treatment guidelines. Standard medical care depends on treatment decisions that are based on the results of large, rigorously conducted studies that establish the effectiveness and side effects of a particular therapy. "Alternative," "complementary," and "integrative" therapies are nontraditional treatments that can be helpful for some patients. While alternative therapies are unregulated and unproven, many well-respected cancer centers include departments of complementary and integrative medicine.

Complementary medicine can help to reduce the physical and emotional toll of breast cancer diagnosis and treatment. As the name suggests, these therapies supplement medical treatment to ease symptoms and side effects.

Integrative medicine is an overall approach to healing that combines standard medicine and nontraditional therapies, often emphasizing psychosocial, emotional, and spiritual support. Physicians who practice integrative medicine consider how a disease affects your whole person: body, mind, and spirit.

Alternative medicine is any treatment that's meant to substitute for conventional medical treatment, like using high-dose vitamins or special diets to treat breast cancer instead of well-tested surgery, anticancer drugs, or other treatments.

Complementary and alternative medicine (CAM) is an umbrella term that's often used to describe health systems, practices, and products that are intended to improve some aspect of health but aren't part of standard Western medical care. Numerous CAM treatments have their origins in ancient Indian and Asian healing arts that have been used by different cultures for thousands of years before gaining popularity in the United States. These therapies are provided by physical therapists, physician assistants, psychologists, registered nurses, and other health care professionals.

Patient interest in CAM has grown significantly in the past two decades, and quite a bit of research, much of it funded by the National Cancer Institute, shows that although CAM doesn't cure cancer and is not recommended as a first-line therapy, certain options can help provide relief from symptoms and improve overall well-being, even if we don't always understand exactly why. An estimated 40 to 80 percent of women with breast cancer use some type of complementary or alternative therapy.

Most CAM products and services are unregulated, and practitioners don't always need a license or certification, so it's important to choose options carefully. The National Center for Complementary and Alternative Medicine (www.nccih.nih.gov) provides study results on various CAM therapies and information on licensing and certification of CAM practitioners. If you're currently undergoing treatment for breast cancer and are considering any type of CAM, first talk to your doctor, who can provide additional information about which therapies can be beneficial or interfere with your treatment. Health insurance increasingly covers the cost of some CAM services that are considered medically necessary, so it's a good idea to ask for a written referral from your physician.

LEVERAGING THE MIND-BODY CONNECTION

Scientific evidence supports the premise that the mind and the body are intertwined and bridged by emotions and feelings: what we think and feel directly affects our health and well-being. In fact, an entire scientific field is devoted to this concept: it's called *psychoneuroimmunology*, the study of the interactions between our nervous system, immune system, and thought. *Mind-body therapies* tap into the brain's capacity to influence bodily functions. These therapies include hypnotherapy, meditation, imagery, visualization, prayer, and many others. Once considered by Westernized cultures to be unworthy of serious consideration, the power of the mind-body connection is undeniable, proven, and has taken a place in the toolbox of Western medicine. Mind-body techniques won't cure breast cancer, but they can help you get through treatment, give you a calmer outlook, and help you feel better.

Yoga

Unlike many other CAM therapies, the benefits of *yoga* are well studied. Regularly practicing the low-impact positions and controlled breathing builds strength and flexibility. Whether done at home or in a class, yoga provides physical and emotional benefits. Some studies show that breast cancer patients who practice yoga report reduced fatigue, pain, worry, and anxiety. An analysis of 13 studies of women with menopause symptoms who practiced yoga also found that it reduced hot flashes and other physical and psychological symptoms at least as well as other types of exercise. Not all poses are possible for a body in pain, however, and after surgery, some could even be harmful until you're fully healed. A well-trained instructor who has experience dealing with cancer patients can demonstrate proper alignment and adjust your movements. If you decide to give yoga a try, consider hatha yoga, which focuses on breathing, gentle smooth movement, and relaxation. More athletic forms of yoga should be delayed after breast surgery until you've healed and your doctor gives you the okay to begin.

Mindful Meditation

Mindful meditation, the most common type of meditation practiced in the West, is good medicine that quiets the body as it relaxes the mind. You needn't stand on your head, twist your body into a pretzel, or practice for years to enjoy its benefits. Using controlled breathing and concentration, mindfulness techniques focus your attention less on sensations (like pain) and thoughts (like worry, sadness, or fear), and more on being attentive to the present, so that you become more aware and more serene. Many studies show it to be moderately effective for pain relief, although how it works is unclear. Brain imaging studies show that mindfulness also boosts the body's immune mechanisms. It can take a while to get the hang of tuning out the thoughts that constantly fill our heads, but it's well worth the effort. Start with

5-minute daily sessions and then gradually increase to 30 minutes or more. Even a few minutes of meditation are beneficial. Numerous smartphone apps, including Headspace, Calm, and others, can be a good place to start.

1. Sit straight but comfortably in a quiet place.
2. Focus on your breath as you inhale and exhale.
3. Return your attention to your breath when your mind wanders.

Guided Imagery

If you've ever awakened with the memory of a particular dream and wondered how your brain could conjure up such fantastical thoughts, you understand the principle behind *guided imagery*. It's a type of self-induced hypnotic state triggered by the use of mental images to achieve deep relaxation. During a guided imagery session, you control your breathing and relax your muscles as you listen to live or recorded direction that helps you visualize and mentally experience the sounds, smells, and view of a particularly soothing scene. Your brain picks up these positive cues and takes over. You fall into a deeply relaxed state that allows you to mentally travel and use imagery to control your pain, nausea, or other symptoms. You might visualize floating on a lake that absorbs all your pain or imagine a visit to your brain's control center, where you turn knobs or flick switches to dial down your symptoms.

Cognitive Behavioral Therapy

Cognitive behavioral therapy is a special type of mental health counseling that helps you to understand how your thoughts and feelings influence your behavior. It helps you to think about negative aspects of your life—relationships, health, fear, and anxiety about cancer outcomes—in a more positive way. If you feel anxious and fearful every time you get infused with chemotherapy, for example, cognitive behavioral therapy can help you view the experience differently: "I can't control the fact that I need chemotherapy, but I know that I can get through it and will be better for it" instead of "I'm afraid of what chemo will do to me and I wish I didn't have to go through it."

Hypnosis

Although it may sound like hocus pocus, clinical hypnosis is a state of intense concentration that allows you to focus on resolving a specific problem. Hypnosis tunes out the conscious mind so that the subconscious can be directed to a specific problem. The benefits of hypnosis have been studied for breast cancer–related pain, anxiety, fatigue, insomnia, and even hot flashes with good results, and several cancer centers and hospitals now have clinical hypnosis therapists on staff. During a hypnotic state, you're relaxed, comfortable, fully awake, and aware of your surroundings. Sessions are conducted by a certified clinical hypnotherapist, who leads you to a state of relaxation before instilling therapeutic statements that suggest relief from symptoms.

Humor

The thought of laughing during times when you struggle may be the furthest thing from your mind, yet laughter is one way to cope with the intense emotions that often accompany cancer. Several studies show that laughter releases chemicals in the brain that relax muscles and produce pleasurable feelings. It also boosts the immune system, which is especially important if you're recovering from surgery, chemotherapy, or radiation. You can laugh just about anywhere, of course, without any special equipment, and it's free of charge. If your favorite comedy doesn't tickle your funny bone, try a laughter yoga class or follow along with a laughter yoga video on YouTube.

ENERGY-BASED THERAPIES

Some CAM therapies are based on the premise that maintaining a balanced flow of the body's vital energy promotes health and well-being. Ancient healing arts refer to this essential life force by different names: it's "qi" (pronounced *chee*) in traditional Chinese medicine and "prana" in Hinduism. Cultural beliefs dictate that this life energy flows to bodily organs along pathways called meridians: a constant flow of qi promotes a healthy mind and body, while illness and pain develop when one's qi becomes unbalanced or disrupted. Several types of CAM are based on restoring an individual's qi balance to address health issues, including relief from certain side effects.

Acupuncture

Acupuncture practitioners insert multiple hair-thin needles in special positions just beneath the skin for 15 to 30 minutes to stimulate specific meridians. Some practitioners send a small electrical signal through the needles or heat the needle tips to further stimulate the body's self-healing mechanisms. Western practitioners hypothesize that acupuncture works by stimulating specific nerves, which signals the brain to release endorphins that decrease pain signals and stimulate production of proteins that reduce inflammation.

Depending on the condition being treated, some people experience immediate relief after one or two sessions, although several treatments are usually necessary. Acupuncture is used for a variety of ailments, including some side effects of cancer treatment. It's been shown to improve treatment-related nausea, fatigue, hot flashes, and pain, including joint pain from taking an aromatase inhibitor. Most states require acupuncturists to be professionally certified or licensed, so check with your state licensing agency to ensure that a practitioner is appropriately credentialed. If you've had lymph nodes removed, avoid having acupuncture in the affected arm to reduce the risk of lymphedema.

Acupressure

Traditional Chinese *acupressure* and *shiatsu*, its Japanese counterpart, stimulate acupuncture points with gentle pressure from the fingers, knuckles, palms, elbows, or feet—it's acupuncture without needles. While acupressure hasn't been studied as extensively as acupuncture, research does show that wrist acupressure relieves chemotherapy-based nausea and vomiting, and patients often report that it can also relieve stress and pain. Several sessions may be needed for the best result. You should avoid acupressure in the area of your breast cancer or if you have bone metastases.

Reiki, Tai Chi, and Qi Gong

Reiki practitioners place their hands lightly on the body or just above the skin for several minutes in positions that are near "energy centers" of the body. This is said to redirect energy flow to improve a person's sense of well-being. Limited research on the benefits of Reiki have been inconclusive. There is more research behind *tai chi,* which is often called "moving mediation," and *qi gong,* which is composed of movements that evolved from martial arts. The characteristic slow and purposeful movements that blend together into what appears to be a peaceful dance are performed with a focus on breathing to manipulate energy. Tai chi is especially helpful for individuals with bone or joint pain, for whom the slightest movement is often difficult.

MASSAGE

If you've ever had a hand, foot, or whole-body massage, you know that the soothing touch of well-trained hands not only feels good but can also promote a greater sense of well-being. That's because massage releases endorphins that promote calm and peaceful feelings. Whether massage is given superficially or deep into muscle tissue, it's one way to temporarily banish anxiety, stress, worry, and soothe fatigued muscles. Oncology massage therapists, who understand how cancer and treatment affect the body, provide specialized massage that can reduce nausea, lessen pain and anxiety, and help you sleep better. If you're worried that massage may stimulate your breast cancer cells or "spread" them around your body, no evidence supports that myth.

Look for a licensed massage therapist who is trained and experienced working with breast cancer patients, and always tell your therapist that you're being treated for breast cancer. If your doctor doesn't know of anyone nearby, inquire at your local hospital or cancer center to see if they have massage therapists on staff.

Talk with your oncologist before beginning any massage therapy, especially if you're undergoing surgery or other treatment. Ask about any restrictions you may need to be aware of before having a massage, including:

- *If you're recovering from breast surgery*: You'll need to lie on your back during a massage until your doctor tells you that your chest has healed enough to lie on your stomach.
- *If you're being treated with chemotherapy*: Ask for a light massage rather than a deep or strong massage, which could cause bruising due to your potentially lowered blood platelet count.
- *If you're being treated with radiation*: Your massage therapist should avoid touching or applying any oils, creams, or lotions to the sensitive skin in the treatment area, and should be careful not to touch the markings your radiation technician placed on your breast.
- *If some or all of your lymph nodes have been removed*: Your therapist should avoid your affected underarm or use only a light touch.
- *If you have lymphedema in your arm*: Your massage therapist should avoid the affected arm and underarm, other than manual lymphatic drainage performed by a certified lymphedema massage therapist.

AROMATHERAPY

Aromatherapy uses essential plant oils from flowers, herbs, or trees to improve physical, mental, and spiritual well-being. Inhaled or massaged into the skin, aromatherapy has been used to improve mood and to reduce anxiety for thousands of years. Oils may be used with other complementary treatments, such as massage or acupuncture, or accompany standard medical treatments to manage symptoms caused by cancer or cancer treatment.

Numerous studies of aromatherapy have been conducted with cancer patients. Some studies have found aromatherapy to be as effective as cognitive behavioral therapy and preferred by patients for emotional distress. Overall, inhaling essential oils, especially lavender oil, appears to temporarily reduce anxiety, depression, and nausea and to improve sleep. Ginger aromatherapy appears to have little effect on chemotherapy-induced nausea and vomiting, but it may improve appetite in some women. It's relatively inexpensive and can be worthwhile to see if it helps your symptoms. Aromatherapy is generally considered safe, as long as you're not allergic to the oil, and safety testing on essential oils has found few side effects.

MUSIC AND ART THERAPIES

If you enjoy music, you already know that it can be therapeutic and can quickly transport you to a happy mental place. Used since ancient times to affect and heal the human spirit, *music therapy* as a formal discipline emerged in the United States in the late 1940s to address physical and psychological symptoms. Sessions are tailored to meet a patient's individual needs and abilities and can involve listening to, writing, performing, or discussing music and lyrics, guided by a trained therapist. A review of 52 clinical trials involving more than 3,700 cancer patients concluded that music produces beneficial physical and psychological effects, improving anxiety, pain, fatigue, and quality of life. Trials have also found that listening to live or recorded music significantly reduces anxiety and distress in breast cancer patients before surgery and radiation therapy.

Art therapy is a way of coping with emotional conflicts, reducing stress, and expressing unspoken or unconscious concerns about breast cancer. You needn't be especially artistic or produce a masterpiece to benefit. Conducted one-on-one or in a group, sessions are conducted by a therapist who encourages you to express your emotions through painting, drawing, sculpting, or other types of artwork, followed by discussion of your feelings about the art you've created.

MEDICAL MARIJUANA AND CBD

Marijuana (cannabis) has been used for medicinal purposes throughout history. It contains over 100 chemical substances, including more than 60 active ingredients known as cannabinoids. Most research has focused on two cannabinoids: tetrohydrocannabinol (THC), a compound that produces euphoric effects, and cannabidiol (CBD), a component that improves sleep and reduces inflammation but doesn't produce the "high" of THC.

A National Academies of Sciences, Engineering, and Medicine report based on the findings of marijuana health research concluded that evidence conclusively shows that cannabis or cannabinoids improve chemotherapy-induced nausea and vomiting and chronic pain. A growing number of chemotherapy patients agree. Dronabinol (Marinol, Syndros), a synthetic THC, and Nabilone (Cesamet), a synthetic cannabinoid, are FDA approved for severe treatment-related nausea and vomiting that do not improve with other medications. Possible side effects of both drugs include drowsiness, confusion, memory loss, headache, insomnia, a feeling of euphoria, and other effects related to marijuana. Both drugs may be covered by health insurance when prescribed by a physician.

Even though medical marijuana is legal in many states, it remains illegal under federal law. The 2018 Farm Bill, however, legalized hemp products, including those that contain CBD, that are grown by

---

ASCO Endorsements

The American Society of Cancer Oncologists endorses the following evidence-based methods of managing symptoms and side effects of conventional treatment, as long as they don't replace conventional therapies.

- Music therapy, meditation, stress management, and yoga are recommended for anxiety and stress reduction.
- Meditation, relaxation, yoga, massage, and music therapy are recommended for depression and mood disorders.
- Meditation and yoga are recommended to improve overall quality of life.
- Acupressure and acupuncture are recommended for reducing chemotherapy-induced nausea and vomiting.

---

licensed growers and don't contain more than .3 percent of THC—they may calm anxiety, reduce inflammation, or soothe joint pain, but they won't get you high. The CBD industry is worth billions of dollars, and it's just getting started. The product line includes CBD-infused lotions, candies, oils, tinctures, and many other products. Studies haven't yet verified just how helpful these products might be, but they have found that the contents of CBD products, like so many other unregulated supplements, don't always contain the ingredients that are listed on the label.

DIETARY SUPPLEMENTS

More than 50,000 drinks, pills, and powders are marketed in the United States as having health benefits. From dandelions to deer antler velvet, these supplements promise everything from weight loss and improved brain function to curing cancer. Hopeful consumers spend in excess of $30 billion annually on dietary supplements, even though promising sales claims are mostly unproven. Supplements can be purchased on the Internet or in stores without prescription or professional guidance. It can be difficult to reliably identify the composition, purity, and safety of these products, which aren't regulated by the FDA.

Nutritional supplements don't prevent or cure cancer, and for most adults, they provide no benefit. Certain dietary supplements are essential for people who have vitamin and mineral deficiencies, macular degeneration, and some other medical conditions. Your oncologist may prescribe calcium and vitamin D supplements if you're taking hormonal therapy that can weaken your bones, for example, or recommend a multivitamin or mineral supplement if your cancer prevents you from easily absorbing nutrients from food. Many of these supplements can interfere or interact dangerously with your cancer treatment, so never take any without discussing them with your oncologist. The federal Office of Dietary Supplements is an excellent source for information about what works and what doesn't, what's safe, and what still needs to be studied.

Garlic. In numerous studies, people who routinely eat garlic have been found to be less likely to develop certain common cancers. While this doesn't necessarily prove cause and effect, it does seem promising. Even more promising is that, in a lab environment, isolated compounds found in garlic have successfully stopped breast cancer cells from growing, possibly because it boosts immune system response. There's no proof, however, that this occurs in people who ingest garlic. If you're treated with docetaxel, be aware that some research shows that garlic may keep it from being properly metabolized by the body. Talk to your doctor about whether you should avoid garlic during treatment.

Herbs. Some women report that ginger used alone or with anti-nausea drugs eases nausea and vomiting from chemotherapy. One study found that consuming a high-protein ginger drink twice a day significantly reduced chemotherapy-related nausea and reduced the need for antinausea medication. Some herbs are known to interfere with treatment and should be avoided. Echinacea, curcumin, valerian root, and St. John's wort, which some people use for depression, can hinder the effect of chemotherapy. Aloe vera juice acts as a laxative, which may reduce the amount of chemo drugs in the intestines. Ginkgo biloba, an herb that is said to improve memory and cognitive dysfunction, has estrogenic properties; some experts are concerned that it may raise the risk of recurrence. Be sure to talk with your oncologist before you take (or continue to take) this or any herb.

Green tea. Green, black, and white teas come from the same plant, but they're processed in different ways. Black tea is fermented, while green and white teas, which have more cancer-fighting antioxidants, are steamed, heated, and then dried. Green tea enhances mental alertness, primarily because of its caffeine content. It contains an abundance of epigallocatechin gallate, a potent polyphenol that reduces inflammation. This anti-inflammatory effect may be why green tea is linked with a reduced risk for diabetes, cardiovascular disease, and other health conditions in which inflammation plays a role. Study results of the effect of green tea on breast cancer have been mixed. Some research shows that it may reduce the risk of recurrence in women who have early-stage breast cancer, but more study is needed before researchers can say that this is a reliable outcome and determine how much green tea needs to be consumed to gain this benefit. Large amounts of green tea may interfere with the activity of chemotherapy drugs.

Vitamins and Minerals

Vitamins are essential, and health problems develop when we don't get enough of them in the right amounts. While they help the body defend against diseases, vitamins alone don't prevent or cure cancer, and some may interfere with treatment.

Vitamin C is a powerful antioxidant found in fruits and vegetables. It's needed for healthy skin, bone, connective tissues, and blood vessels. It also helps the body absorb iron, and in adequate amounts, it helps to decrease total and low-density lipoprotein (LDL) cholesterol (the "bad" kind) and triglycerides. Vitamin C may also help to protect against a variety of cancers by combating free radicals that cause cellular damage. Scientists are studying whether high doses of vitamin C given intravenously can decrease treatment side effects or improve the effectiveness of chemotherapy and radiation.

Vitamin D is one of the most studied supplements for cancer prevention and treatment, due to a growing understanding of how it affects cell development. It's important for bone heath, particularly if you're postmenopausal and take an aromatase inhibitor. Vitamin D can accumulate in the body, so exceeding the recommended daily amount isn't advised without medical supervision.

Vitamin E supports immune function and eye health, discourages inflammation, and decreases the risk of coronary heart disease. Two studies that followed women for seven or more years found that taking 300 to 400 IU of vitamin E daily was not protective against any type of cancer. Vitamin E dietary supplements, especially in high doses, might interact with chemotherapy and radiation therapy.

Folate (vitamin B) is found in leafy vegetables, fruits, beans, meats, and other foods. Many processed foods, including cereals, breads, flour, and baked goods are fortified with folic acid, the synthetic version of folate. Folate is especially important for pregnant women to prevent miscarriage and birth defects. Even though folate supplements haven't been shown to reduce breast cancer risk, health care professionals sometimes recommend them at standard doses.

Glutamine, a nonessential amino acid, protects nerves in the hands, feet, and digestive tract. It may reduce potential damage from chemotherapy, especially from taxane drugs. Some cancer patients have a glutamine deficiency, although researchers don't know why. This is another area that needs further study, but a 2016 review of research found that supplementing with glutamine reduced chemo-induced peripheral neuropathy. Glutamine is a key nutrient for breast tumors, which use more of this substance than healthy cells because cancer cells divide more rapidly. In a laboratory setting, reducing the uptake of glutamine by breast cancer cells slowed or stopped tumor growth.

Tips for Selecting a Complementary Health Practitioner

- Ask your doctor for the names of reputable local practitioners.
- Verify a practitioner's training, certification, and other credentials with your state's licensing agency (if your state requires licensing).
- Choose a practitioner who has experience dealing with breast cancer.
- Ask whether the practitioner is willing to communicate and cooperate with your health care team.
- Let your health care team know which practitioners and therapies you're considering before you begin.
- Ask your health insurer whether a particular complementary therapy and a specific practitioner are covered.

CHAPTER 20

Meeting the Emotional Challenges of Breast Cancer

Newly diagnosed women often experience a variety of emotions, including shock, upset, and even panic, but also often a sense of determination and hope. This mix of emotions may seem unhealthy to someone who hasn't dealt with a cancer diagnosis, but it's a common reaction to something as shocking and unexpected as breast cancer.

Health care providers often speak to patients about the physical impacts of treatment, but not as much about the psychological and emotional burden that many patients experience. No matter where you are in the breast cancer experience—newly diagnosed, in treatment, or living as a survivor—emotional roadblocks can threaten your quality of life and outlook.

Coping with breast cancer is anything but easy, even if it isn't the first serious problem you've had to face. It's a deeply personal experience that can invoke feelings that tax your emotional resilience and your physical strength. Women are often diagnosed with breast cancer at a time in their lives when they have many deep and important relationships and responsibilities. Parenting during and through cancer can be challenging, both physically and emotionally, particularly with the worry about possibly dying from the disease. Work and career roles and relationships may also change during treatment and then change again when treatment is completed, adding to the confusion and upheaval a diagnosis often brings. Everyone's journey is different, and even two women with the same diagnosis may react differently. Some

352

are emotionally strong through their cancer journey, while others find it difficult to regain a sense of personal balance and control.

ACKNOWLEDGING YOUR EMOTIONS

Newly diagnosed women often experience a variety of emotions that may seem unhealthy to someone who hasn't dealt with a diagnosis, but there is no wrong way to react to learning you have breast cancer. It's not always easy to be positive, and some days will be better than others. Emotional setbacks can occur if your tumor doesn't respond to treatment as expected, you lose your hair, or a medication side effect hijacks your day.

You can't change your diagnosis, but you can control how you react to it and your overall outlook going forward. Patients often say that diagnosis and treatment leave them feeling helpless, and that they fear that their lives will never again be as they were before diagnosis. This level of angst is a type of emotional paralysis that suppresses motivation to get up, move around, think positively, and pursue the very therapies that will improve your condition and make your life better.

Intense emotions are a natural response to a health crisis. Like physical side effects, they may be temporary, and they'll likely become easier to deal with as other life events begin to require more of your attention. If they persist, however, they need to be addressed so that they don't become chronic or continue to impact your well-being. Acknowledging and talking about how you feel are meaningful steps toward putting yourself emotionally back on track. If you're unable to speak honestly about your situation with family or friends, consider sharing your feelings with a social worker or counselor. If negative emotions remain unresolved and consume too much of your thoughts, a mental health professional can help you move beyond them.

After the shock of a traumatic event, including the loss of a loved one or a cancer diagnosis, many people experience five stages of emotional response—denial, anger, bargaining, depression, and acceptance. Not everyone experiences all of these feelings or goes through them in the same order.

Denial

Disbelief is often the first thing women feel when they hear that they have breast cancer. It's a basic coping mechanism for dealing with news that's difficult to accept. Your first thought may be that your diagnosis is a mistake—maybe the lab mixed up your results with someone else's?—or that breast cancer just can't be happening to you. At this stage, you may be too numb to feel anything for a while. Extreme denial has a more negative effect if you don't want to know anything about your treatment or prognosis and choose to ignore it as much as possible.

Anger

Once the reality of your diagnosis sets in, it's not unusual to feel angry that your body has betrayed you or how it's about to disrupt your life and perhaps your work. You may feel that you've been treated unfairly and ask yourself, "Why me?" or "What have I done to deserve this?" Fearing that you can't do anything to make your diagnosis just go away, you might also feel frustrated, irritable, or even hostile toward others. As odd as it may sound, some women say that they find themselves feeling angry and jealous of women who don't have breast cancer. Talking with friends and family or one of your doctor's previous breast cancer patients can help you acknowledge your anger and overcome it. If you can't seem to control your anger or it doesn't go away, ask your doctor for a referral to a counselor or therapist who can help you.

Bargaining

In the bargaining stage, it's common to develop a case of the "if onlys." If only you would have exercised more or eaten fewer processed foods, or tried to lead a better life, then maybe you wouldn't be deal- ing with breast cancer. If your tumor was found at a later stage, you may wonder how your treatment and prognosis would have been dif- ferent if you were diagnosed earlier. These thoughts are unanswer- able, and there is no benefit to lingering on them. Patients often try to offset their fears by bargaining with God or the universe by promising to change their lifestyle or be a better person if only they can get through treatment and go on to a life without cancer. Some women promise to think only positive thoughts in exchange for recovery or hope that doing good deeds will positively affect their healing.

Depression

At some point after a diagnosis, most people experience temporary sadness, and some fall into depression. While sadness is an under- standable and even healthy reaction to breast cancer, depression is distinctly different. Sadness is a coping mechanism that's triggered by something that is disappointing, hurtful, or difficult. It's a focused emotion: you feel sad that you'll lose your hair or your breast, for ex- ample. Depression is a more serious problem. It's a chemical and bi- ological imbalance in the brain that you can't simply shake off or "get over," and it doesn't get better without treatment. A cancer diagnosis can trigger some degree of post-traumatic stress disorder (PTSD), a type of depression that's caused by a trauma, like being victimized by crime, or by a terrifying event, such as September 11.

Up to 30 percent of breast cancer patients report feeling de- pressed at some point. Usually, this is *reactive depression* that devel- ops in the first three months after diagnosis. It's a temporary malaise that isn't the same as clinical depression, although it shares many of the same symptoms: fatigue, loss of appetite, and an overall sense of emptiness. As a result, you don't feel like you can make decisions or move forward. Reactive depression is brought on by a specific stress- ful experience or event, like the loss of a loved one or the end of a re- lationship, and usually lasts a few weeks to a few months. Depression that continues is more serious. It can affect the decisions you need to make about your treatment, slow your recovery, and increase your risk of dying.

The good news is that depression improves when it's treated with psychotherapy. One-on-one, with your spouse or partner, or in a group, psychotherapy is a proven method of helping people resolve the feelings that undermine their health and happiness. Psycho-oncologists—doctors, nurse practitioners, and psychologists who are specially trained to offer psychiatric and emotional support to cancer patients—can help you and your family deal with unhealthy and disruptive emotions and resolve troubling issues. You may need extra help if you were depressed before your diagnosis.

Therapy may include counseling, relaxation techniques, hypnosis, or cognitive therapy to change negative thought patterns that sustain depression. An experienced therapist can explain whether you might also benefit from antidepressant medication to correct any chemical deficiencies in your brain that cause mood swings, a lack of feeling, or other emotions that are associated with depression. It may take several weeks to see a difference, but for many people, these interventions bring about life-changing improvement. Learning self-help techniques can also improve your symptoms and help to prevent a

Signs of Depression

Let your health care team know if you develop any symptoms of depression that last most of the day, nearly every day, so that you can get help as soon as possible.

- Mood swings
- A disinterest in most things around you
- A noticeable loss of pleasure from normal activities
- Sleeping much more or less than usual
- Fatigue or loss of energy
- Feelings of worthlessness or inappropriate guilt
- A decreased ability to think or concentrate
- Thoughts of death or suicide

relapse. One example is to learn and practice strategies that replace negative thoughts ("My breast cancer will never get better") with positive affirmations ("Today, I'm going to take steps to improve my situation").

Acceptance

The last stage in the emotional spectrum is acceptance of your diagnosis. Depending on your outlook and attitude, it may come to you quickly or you may need time to adapt to the reality of having breast cancer, even if you had a premonition that your biopsy would be positive or that you were prepared for the worst. Acceptance is an important step, because only then can you move beyond the emotional restrictions that negative feelings cause. No one feels happy about their diagnosis, but accepting it makes way for a calmness that you need to consider real options. This is especially critical because treatment choices are complex. While you may not completely release all of your feelings of grief and sadness, when you accept your circumstances, you'll have these emotions under control so that you can make better decisions about what's best for you.

A PLAN FOR SELF-HELP

With a little planning, you can take efforts to counteract negative feelings and feel emotionally stronger.

- *Do your homework.* One of the most productive actions you can take to replace the uneasiness of not knowing what's ahead is learning about your condition. Knowledge truly is power. It will help you make better decisions, and it's the best mental antidote to the mystery and fright that a new diagnosis can bring.
- *Find purpose every day, if only in small things.* Try not to give in to the urge to remain inactive and dwell on the downsides of

your circumstances. To the extent your treatment allows, do what you typically do. Play with your kids, run your business, live your life.

- *Take a break from being a patient.* Too often, cancer becomes so overwhelming that it seems to push out all thoughts of normal life. It's important to find ways to disarm the power you may think breast cancer holds over you. Make time to read, garden, or take part in whatever emotionally satisfying activities you enjoy that aren't related to treatment or breast cancer. Stick to your ordinary, precancer routine as much as possible; do whatever feels right to give yourself a break from being a patient.

- *Give your brain a rest.* Establish a daily quiet time, when you can direct your mind away from worry, fear, and anxiety. Try daily meditation, yoga, or tai chi to calm the noise in your mind.

The Power of Faith and Spirituality

Many patients find comfort in their faith or spirituality, which can be a source of strength during diagnosis, treatment, recovery, and beyond. Going through the rigors of breast cancer is difficult, and it can challenge your beliefs and test your faith. Whether you are religious or not, we're all spiritual beings; the comfort, peace, and significance we find in life are as essential to our well-being as physical and emotional balance. Spirituality is a state of mind that can't be seen or measured. It defines the truths that we live by, which may or may not be based in religious theory. Studies show that people who have a deep religious or spiritual belief system tend to have stronger coping skills during treatment and are more peaceful at the end of their lives. You may find that strength in a religious service or as you meditate at home. What's important isn't where you find this peace and path forward, but that you find it.

A belief system that helps you make sense out of the experiences of life is important to your well-being. Spiritual distress can begin if life becomes very different from the way you thought it would be or should be. Looking back on their breast cancer experience, many survivors say that it inspired them to redefine their values and goals and to find new meaning in their lives. Talking with a loved one, clergyperson, or hospital chaplain can be helpful as you go through this process.

Listen to uplifting or soothing music. Try to laugh at something every day. It relieves tension, and it's not possible to feel sad or anxious while you're giggling or guffawing.

- *Write about what you feel.* Writing is a cathartic outlet for emotions, and at times it can be easier than talking face-to-face. Whether you journal, blog, or write poetry, seeing the words on paper or on your computer screen is like having a conversation with yourself. Try writing a letter to your body, your breasts, or yourself, letting your thoughts flow freely and uncensored. If you have trouble getting started, begin by asking yourself what you're afraid of. Answer honestly, and then ask yourself what you should do about it.

- *Maintain your social network.* Fear and negative feelings that spiral out of control often cause isolation. The worse you feel, the less you want to get up, get dressed, or speak with others. While there will undoubtedly be times when you don't feel like talking about what you're going through, it's important to stay connected with life outside of treatment. Keep up relationships outside the family to remind yourself that friendship and support are powerful medicine. Socialize with friends to nurture your spirit and stay focused.

- *Recognize when you need professional help.* Feelings shape our reactions to virtually everything that we experience in life. Everyone has ups and downs, and emotions that reflect those experiences. We see a doctor when we're sick, and we take our car to a mechanic when it's not running right. Yet many of us feel embarrassed when we need an emotional tune-up. Needing professional help isn't a sign of weakness, no more than going to the dentist when you have a toothache or seeking help for a migraine. If negative thoughts persist and become more than a temporary funk, the value of a mental health professional can't be overestimated.

THE VALUE OF A SUPPORT GROUP

It can be difficult to deal with the emotions breast cancer causes, especially if you feel isolated and alone. Sometimes the comfort and support you need comes from others who have firsthand knowledge of what you're going through. A breast cancer support group is a safe environment where you can openly talk about your experiences and receive caring support in return, and that can be a welcome relief. Participants are patients or survivors who appreciate and understand what you're going through because they've walked in your shoes. Breast cancer patients often say that the solidarity of their support group gives them strength and a more hopeful perspective. Participating in a group may also encourage you to talk about concerns or issues that are too difficult to share with family or friends. The compassionate camaraderie can help you to feel more empowered and more in control, wherever you are in your breast cancer journey. Support groups that welcome family members may also be beneficial for your spouse and children. These groups focus on family concerns, such as role changes, relationship changes, financial worries, and how to support you through treatment.

Getting the Most from a Support Group

- If you prefer a group that meets in person, check with your doctor or nurse, local hospital, other patients, or the nearest American Cancer Society office for information.
- If you live in a remote area or you don't feel comfortable participating in person, search online for a support group.
- Join a group that is well matched to your circumstances—women who have triple-negative, metastatic, or BRCA-related breast cancer, for example, or singles who have been diagnosed.
- It's important to find a group that's a good fit. If you don't feel comfortable with one, try another.
- Participate routinely to get the most from the experience.

The Power of Gratitude

Cultivating a grateful attitude is a powerful motivator that can lead to life transformations. Gratitude shifts your focus from what your life lacks to what you already have. It makes you feel satisfied, and that's a prescription for good mental health. Behavioral research shows that people who are grateful tend to be more resilient, cope better, and are generally happier than others who have a negative view of themselves and the world. Many women say that experiencing breast cancer and treatment increases their overall sense of gratitude. Certainly, there will be times when you don't feel thankful that you've lost your hair or you're having another day of nausea, but thinking negatively for too long can be emotionally risky, because the more you do so, the harder it is to "snap out of it."

CHAPTER 21

Family Matters during and after Breast Cancer

Breast cancer is like an unwanted guest that moves in, affecting everyone in the house. With this in mind, it can be helpful to tell your family members about your plan of care, and to let them know specifically how they can best support you through this journey.

A diagnosis of breast cancer affects not only you, but your loved ones as well. Although the people who love and care for you won't have your treatment or suffer your side effects, seeing you uncomfortable, confused, or in pain will affect them. Some psychologists consider family members to be "secondary patients" who may need just as much support as you will as you go through breast cancer together. In fact, the National Coalition for Cancer Survivorship includes family members in their definition of cancer survivors.

YOUR CHILDREN

Every parent who is diagnosed with cancer wonders if they should tell their children, and how they should do it. While parental instinct may tell us to shield our children from bad news, experts recommend talking to your children about your diagnosis and treatment, because in the absence of information, they often perceive that something is wrong and may become worried if they think that it's their fault or that an illness is worse than it actually is.

Generally, it's important to share information about a breast cancer diagnosis in a timely and honest manner. Your demeanor influences your kids' reactions: if they see that you're okay, they'll be okay. Think about what you'll say before having the conversation with your children, and be sure that you and your partner are on the same page. Children process information differently. Some ask lots of questions, while others are mostly disinterested. Tailor your explanation to each child's personality and level of understanding. It's also okay to share information in a "metered" manner over several days or weeks that gives children time to absorb and process what you tell them.

Don't be afraid to say "cancer." Most children have heard the word before. Describe it simply and honestly, using age-appropriate terms to explain concepts that help kids conceptualize and understand. Discuss your diagnosis openly, but keep it simple for little ones, giving them only the details they need to understand. If you're explaining surgery, for example, you might say that your doctor is going to take out stuff called cancer so that it won't make you sick or something along those lines. If you'll be hospitalized for a few days, expect to be sick from treatment, or you'll lose your hair, explain why this will happen.

Older kids and teens will want to know more. Let them know it's okay to be scared, and encourage them to voice their concerns and talk freely. It might be the first time that your roles are reversed as your older children accompany you to appointments and find ways to keep you amused and entertained. Answer your child's questions and address their concerns; ignoring their fears can make the situation seem scary. If you don't know the answer, just say, "I don't know. I'll find out and then we can talk about it together."

It's important to maintain your children's sense of security. Explain how your treatment and recovery will affect their lives, and who will take care of them if you'll be in the hospital or will be unable to care for them. Let youngsters know that "Aunt Kim will take you to soccer practice" or "Dad will make your lunch every morning." With older children and teens, describe how your treatment side effects may affect them: "I'm going to be very sleepy for a few days" or "I'll need help around the house for a while." Arrange to keep their routines as normal as possible. Children know when something is wrong, even if they don't know what it is, and they want to be reassured that they aren't at fault and that their world will remain as unchanged as possible.

YOUR SPOUSE OR PARTNER

Breast cancer can certainly test the bond between two people. It can strengthen the closeness and trust you share with your partner or further weaken an already fragile relationship. Partners of breast cancer patients face difficult challenges of their own. They may need to take on more parenting duties and household responsibilities while they're also trying to cope with their own worry and fear about your situation. Financial concerns can develop if you're unable to work or if your partner must work longer hours to make up for declining income. If your partner needs to reduce work hours to care for you, that may further reduce family income and increase fiscal burdens and pressure.

Emotional distance can develop if your partner seems to be unsympathetic toward what you're going through, resents the impact breast cancer has on the normal household routine, or when he or she feels unsure of how to deal with the situation. Partners frequently feel threatened by issues they cannot control or fix. Sometimes, despite their love and good intentions, they don't know what to do or say in a way that is supportive. This can be especially frustrating for you, especially when you just want them to listen to your concerns and support you emotionally. Your partner's own confusion and fear—will he or she lose you?—may drive behavior that undermines your relationship. Make it clear that you hope your partner will be there for you and that the two of you will get through this life-changing experience together. Commit to approaching issues openly and honestly when you're overwhelmed or when the family becomes affected by your treatment and recovery.

Communication is critical in all relationships, particularly those that are already strained. Talking about the issues you face and how you feel can sometimes be uncomfortable, but avoiding discussion of the situation and the problems it may create only makes a bad predicament worse.

Sex and Intimacy

One topic your medical team may not address is how breast cancer and treatment might affect your intimate relationship with your spouse or partner. Medical school doesn't teach doctors how to discuss these issues, and your physician may be unaware of helpful resources to recommend. "Bedroom" issues often remain undiscussed and unresolved. Most oncologists don't talk about how treatment can affect sexuality and intimacy, and women often don't feel comfortable broaching the subject with their doctors.

You may be perfectly comfortable in your body and effortlessly slip back into the closeness and intimacy you experienced before your diagnosis. But for some women, it's not that easy. After months of treatment, physical pleasure may be the last thing on your mind, especially if it's physically painful, you feel emotionally uncomfortable, or you just can't seem to get in or stay in the mood. This can be a frustrating change for you and your partner, especially while you're coping with additional emotional and practical issues. Women sometimes report that they can't help thinking about cancer and treatment during sex, which is a "turn-off" that spoils the mood.

Treatment-related menopausal symptoms can quickly deflate your libido while reducing your natural lubrication, leaving you with vaginal dryness that makes intercourse painful or impossible. If you've lost one or both breasts, you may feel less confident and less feminine than before and worry about how your partner sees you. If you've had a bilateral mastectomy, lost breast sensation takes some getting used to, especially if your breasts were important to your lovemaking before. If you've had breast reconstruction, you may be disappointed with the way your new breasts look or the lack of feeling in your new breast. Don't assume that you're undesirable if your partner doesn't initiate intimacy or makes a point of staying away from your breasts. He (or she) may be afraid of hurting you or making you feel pressured, and may be reluctant to push intimacy when you're tired or stressed and obviously not in the mood, especially if you're emotionally distant.

Getting Back in the Game

It can take time, effort, and patience to rekindle your intimacy and get your love life back on track. This is a difficult issue to discuss, and may be one that you and your spouse are too embarrassed or too uncomfortable to verbalize. A lot depends on your level of intimacy before your diagnosis and your willingness now to talk and resolve these issues. Sharing the experience is important to your relationship and will make things easier for both of you. Express your feelings, and encourage your partner to do the same.

Intimacy is more than just sex. It's touching, trusting, sharing, and caring deeply. It helps to keep an open mind about ways to feel sexual pleasure and redefine how you go about it. If your precancer intimacy routine isn't possible or no longer works, experiment with new ways to reinvigorate your sex life. Ask your doctor about vaginal lubricants. If you feel awkward or embarrassed in your postmastectomy body, wear lingerie or turn off the lights until you become more comfortable in your own skin. It's important to explain how you feel and what you want. Explore new possibilities and new erogenous zones together. Direct your partner's attention to the areas where you feel touch, instead of where you don't.

If you're otherwise healthy and untroubled but have no interest in sex, talk to your doctor about medication that can minimally boost your libido. Flibanserin (Addyi) and bremelanotide (Vyleesi) are medications that treat a tired libido, what is officially known as *hypoactive sexual desire disorder*. Neither medication directly affects your sexual experience. They work on substances in the brain that somewhat increase sexual desire for some women.

Dating after Breast Cancer

Dating after cancer can be stressful and confusing. When do you discuss your cancer, and how much of the details of your health history should you share? When you're ready to begin looking for your special someone, there are no hard and fast rules about when and what to say. Just rely on your instinct to know when the time is right. If you're comfortable with the other person, you'll know when that is and when it isn't. If you and your date are discussing a relative's cancer diagnosis, that may be a logical time to share your own experience. In other cases, it may not come up until it becomes clear that your relationship is heading to the bedroom. Let your own comfort with the topic and how you feel about the other person dictate when and how much you share. That might be on your first date or later in your relationship. Two websites that can help you connect with other cancer survivors who are looking for meaningful companionship are www.romanceonly.com (love without intercourse) and cancermatch.com. You determine your own level of anonymity and privacy on both sites.

Remember that your brain is the most powerful sexual organ you have. You're still very much a woman, but it may take a while for you to believe it. These issues can be resolved as long as the two of you are willing to discuss and share the experience. It's not a question of whether you can regain a meaningful love life, but rather how you go about it. If you need help to regain your prior intimacy, talk to your health care team. If necessary, consult with a psychoanalyst who specializes in cancer-related intimacy issues.

THE FAMILY

Family dynamics are often complex, and a family's balance and harmony amid cancer diagnosis and treatment can be difficult, even in a close-knit household. Breast cancer is like an unwanted guest that moves in, affecting everyone in the house. With this in mind, it can be helpful to tell your family members about your plan of care, and to let them know specifically how they can best support you through this journey. Dysfunctional symptoms can develop when breast cancer becomes the family's new focus and seems to overshadow everything else. Family members may feel a loss of control if they can't make your cancer go away or return the household to its normal routine and positive environment. It helps to maintain the household's pre-cancer schedule as much as possible and recruit help from friends and neighbors as needed.

Cancer and the treatments it requires can introduce a complex array of lifestyle changes and emotional responses, which can be difficult for family members to handle. But it can also be an opportunity to role model to your children how adults can face adversity in a way that strengthens family unity and improves the way you deal with difficult issues. Families that ordinarily engage in open, honest discussion will have a less difficult time, especially if everyone feels free to voice their opinions about the situation. You needn't overtalk the situation, but without open dialogue, family members may become emotionally disconnected, perpetuating discord in the household. Taking a few proactive steps will help to create an environment at home that encourages discussion so that problems can be discussed and resolved.

- Encourage discussion about issues that arise, so that the family can resolve them before they become a bigger problem. Communication between family members is key to keeping family relationships healthy.
- Respect that family members will have different styles of communication and ways of coping with difficult situations.
- Ask for help to maintain the household's rhythm and order. Discuss what your family can expect while you recover from surgery, radiation, or chemotherapy or deal with treatment side effects. Make decisions together about how this can best work. Together, discuss what things might change and how everyone can move forward without feeling unhappy or put upon.
- Explain that roles may change. Your treatment and recovery may require a shift in roles, and other family members may need to take on some or all of your daily responsibilities if

your treatment or recovery keep you from fulfilling all of your normal household duties. Your spouse or partner may need to do the grocery shopping or drive the kids to school. Your children may have more responsibilities around the house and yard; older kids may need to take on babysitting for younger siblings or preparing meals. These changes represent an upheaval in the household's normal routine and can be difficult for some family members to get used to. You may eventually want to resume many, most, or all of your previous responsibilities, including making decisions that were made by your spouse or partner during your treatment. This too can be stressful and challenging, and talking about it may help.

- Ask for patience. Let your family know that you'll look to them for support when you're frustrated, depressed, or in pain. Reassure them that the effects of your treatment may affect them, but that eventually things will return to normal.
- Don't assume that everyone's okay. Talk with your spouse about periodically checking in with each family member to see how they're coping emotionally and physically.
- Think through how your family relationships may change again when your treatment and initial recovery are completed and you are moving back toward normal or a "new normal."

CHAPTER 22

Insurance and Money Matters during Breast Cancer Treatment

The cost of treating and curing breast cancer can be overwhelming, and some patients are left with large out-of-pocket costs. Being prepared for these costs and planning for them can reduce financial stress and anxiety that can otherwise blindside you later on.

If you have health insurance that pays for all of the medical care you need, you're fortunate. Treating cancer can be expensive, even when insurance covers many of the expenses. The amount you pay for deductibles, co-pays, and transportation and lodging (if you travel for your treatment or breast reconstruction) can quickly accumulate to unexpectedly high amounts, especially if you have recurrent or metastatic breast cancer that involves ongoing treatment. This "financial toxicity" can be devastating, especially if you need time off and you've already used all of your paid vacation time or sick leave at your job or you become too sick to work and pay your bills.

Patients are paying more for their health care as employers continue to pass rising health care costs to employees. If you have an 80/20 plan, for example, where your insurer pays 80 percent of medical costs, the 20 percent that you're responsible for may quickly add up to tens of thousands of dollars for doctor visits, surgeries, hospitalization, medications, and outpatient treatments. (Traditional Medicare is an 80/20 plan, unless you have supplemental coverage that pays all or part of the 20 percent except for your co-pay.) As an example,

370

if the overall cost of your breast cancer treatment was $100,000, your health plan would pay $80,000 while you would be responsible for $20,000. Additional medical interventions that are necessary to treat side effects or other unforeseen complications that may develop can also contribute to your medical expenses. Some plans include "catastrophic coverage" that provides additional payment when your own out-of-pocket expenses exceed a certain amount.

Keep a Paper Trail

Maintaining accurate, organized records is important when you need to pay medical bills, file a claim with your insurance company, or file for financial assistance. It's also a necessity for itemizing medical deductions on your federal and state tax returns. Carefully organize all bills, receipts, records, and documents related to your breast cancer treatment (table 22.1). Keep copies of all written correspondence and a call log of your conversations with your insurance company, noting the date, time, details of the discussion, and name of the employee with whom you spoke.

Table 22.1. Retaining Your Medical Records, Bills, and Payments

Records Related to Your Medical Treatment	Records Involving Your Health Insurer
Admission and discharge paperwork from hospitals or treatment facilities	Confirmation of preauthorizations
Medical reports and test results from all lab work, biopsies, and diagnostic procedures	Notes on conversations with customer representatives
Medical bills from all health care providers	Claims filed and claims paid
Canceled checks or credit card payment receipts for all out-of-pocket expenses you paid	Claim denials, appeals, and all related correspondence
Receipts related to meals, lodging, travel, and other related miscellaneous expenses that you paid	Payments, including reimbursements with explanation of benefits

Before your treatment begins, understand what your health insurance plan covers and what you'll be required to pay. Find out if it requires you to use certain "in-network" providers or hospitals for your treatment that minimize the amount you pay. Ask the billing specialist in your oncologist's office to provide the billing codes for the procedures you'll have. Then contact your insurance company and verify whether or not they'll be covered, if you need preauthorizations, and how much you'll be responsible for paying. If you find that your health coverage doesn't cover enough of your medical costs, you might consider switching to a plan that will provide more coverage, even though you may pay higher premiums. (You'll need to wait until the annual open enrollment period to change plans.)

APPEALING A CLAIM DENIAL

Being notified that your health insurance claim has been denied can leave you feeling angry and helpless. You have a legal right to appeal any insurance denial, and in fact it's a good idea to do so, because many claim denials are overturned when they're appealed. The process involves writing a letter requesting that your insurer reconsider its decision. Appealing a denial requires a bit of investigation on your part and can be time consuming and frustrating, but in many cases, it's well worth the effort. Here's how to go about it.

- *Understand why your claim was denied.* Your health insurer must provide you with a written description of its refusal. Usually this is the "Explanation of Benefits" (EOB) form that explains how the company arrived at its decision. Common reasons include "benefit not provided" (your plan doesn't provide the treatment or service in question), "not medically necessary" (the insurer doesn't consider the treatment or service necessary for your continued health), and "out of network" (medical services were provided by a health care professional who isn't a part of your insurer's network of approved providers). If you're still not clear why your claim was denied, call the company and ask.

Laws That Protect Your Health Insurance Rights

- The Health Insurance Portability and Accountability Act of 1996 ensures the privacy and security of your medical information.
- The Affordable Care Act extends coverage to millions of uninsured Americans. The law includes premium subsidies and cost-sharing subsidies designed to reduce the costs of coverage for Americans who qualify. It prohibits health insurers from imposing lifetime dollar limits on annual caps, limiting essential benefits, or excluding individuals or canceling their policies because of a preexisting health condition, including breast cancer. It also protects your right to appeal a denial.
- The Women's Health and Cancer Rights Act requires group health plans that cover mastectomy to also pay for breast prostheses (with a doctor's prescription) and all stages of breast reconstruction, including surgery to the opposite breast to achieve a symmetrical appearance and treatment for any related complications. Insurers must provide coverage consistent with your existing plan benefits, with the same deductibles and co-payment. (Some plans provided by the government and religious organizations are exempt.)
- The Family and Medical Leave Act requires employers with 50 or more workers to provide up to 12 weeks of unpaid, job-protected leave with continued group health insurance benefits under the same terms and conditions you have when you're on the job. You can take all 12 weeks at once or break the time into smaller increments, such as three separate periods of four weeks each. You're eligible if you're unable to perform the essential functions of your job due to a health condition or if you need to care for a spouse or a legal same-sex partner, child, or parent who has a serious health condition.
- The Consolidated Omnibus Budget and Reconciliation Act (COBRA) allows you to temporarily stay in your employer's insurance plan for up to 18 months if you stop working, change jobs, or reduce the number of hours you work. If you're covered by your spouse's plan, you can still get up to three years' coverage if you divorce or your spouse dies. Plans provided by the federal government and churches are exempt. Employers with fewer than 20 employees are also exempt, although some states require COBRA coverage for businesses with fewer than 20 employees.

- *Investigate.* Check an up-to-date copy of your benefits handbook, sometimes called "Evidence of Coverage," to determine whether the service in question is covered. (It's a good idea to do this before you receive any medical service.) Notify your insurance carrier if the benefit is listed as covered but has been denied.

- *Identify mistakes.* Read the Evidence of Coverage and the Explanation of Benefits carefully, looking for errors. Denials often result from an incorrect insurance identification number, the wrong medical code, or some other administrative error. If a simple administrative error has been made, notify your insurance company. If your doctor's office made the error, ask that a corrected invoice be submitted.

- *Focus on the reason for denial.* Contact your insurance company to request a copy of the medical opinion on which your denial is based; this should be the focus of your request for reconsideration. Request a case manager, who will become familiar with your case. Any further contact with your insurance company about the denial or appeal can be made directly to her.

- *Build your case.* Gather all the information you have about the issue. Be clear and factual about why your procedure or treatment should be covered, and include supporting documentation. Ask your doctor to write a detailed letter on your behalf, explaining why the treatment or service was medically necessary. Include published statements from the American Cancer Society or other national breast cancer organizations, national treatment guidelines (www.nccn.org), and studies from peer-reviewed publications (www.pubmed.gov is a good resource) that justify your argument. Although you may be upset or frustrated, be as clear and as succinct as possible as you describe your case.

- *Resubmit your claim.* Gather the materials you need to resubmit your claim. Include a copy of the denial letter and any documentation that supports your rationale. Write a cover letter that contains your insurance policy number, your appeals claim number, and a request for a "physician review," meaning that your appeal will be reviewed by a doctor who specializes in the service denied. Also, state clearly that you're requesting reconsideration of the denial. Follow your plan's appeal procedure exactly, submitting all paperwork on time to meet required deadlines. If your policy states that you have 30 days to appeal a decision, be sure that the insurance company receives your request within that time frame.

- *Contact the Patient Advocate Foundation (www.patientadvocate .org).* Representatives of this nonprofit organization will help you develop your appeal or act as a liaison with the insurer on your behalf and handle your appeal at no charge.

If you have health coverage through your employer, the appeal process generally has two levels. Appeals are first decided by a claims reviewer and signed off by a medical professional; a denial is least likely to be overturned at this level. The second appeal is considered by a review panel that includes at least one physician in the same specialty your appeal involves—an oncologist or a plastic surgeon, for example. If you get health insurance coverage from your employer, ask your company's human resources department if your plan is self-funded, meaning that your employer has a say in which claims are paid or denied. If your plan is self-funded and your appeal is denied, ask your HR department to reconsider the denial or file an appeal at the state level (the website of your state's department of insurance will have instructions for doing this).

FINDING HELP IF YOU'RE UNINSURED OR UNDERINSURED

If you're uninsured when you're diagnosed, you may still be able to get coverage through the Health Insurance Marketplace (www .healthcare.gov), a resource that will direct you to a federal- or state-operated health insurance exchange where you can compare, research, and purchase an affordable plan. Most states offer a "guaranteed issue" individual health plan that you can enroll in regardless of your health, age, gender, or other factors that might predict your use of health services. Some states subsidize reduced-cost health insurance for low-income residents. Your treatment can begin as soon as your coverage takes effect.

Medicare health insurance, which is funded by the federal government through the Social Security Administration, is provided for US citizens and legal residents age 65 and over who have worked at least 10 years. You may also be eligible if you're permanently disabled and received disability benefits for at least two years. Medicaid pays for medical care for individuals who have income and assets below a certain level. Although Medicaid is a federal program, each state sets its own eligibility rules and administers the program.

The Disability Rights Legal Center (www.thedrlc.org) provides information and assistance related to health insurance and legal issues for people with cancer and/or disabilities. This nonprofit organization can clarify issues about maintaining employment throughout your treatment, accessing health care and government benefits, taking medical leave, and estate planning.

Reduced Cost Services

If you can't afford your medical bills, you have several options. Many hospitals and health care providers contract with the state or federal government to provide services at lower costs to people who qualify. Talk to your doctor's billing specialist or hospital administration about getting a discount or ask if you can pay the Medicare rate, which is usually lower than the amount that is charged to individuals. Federal law requires nonprofit hospitals to provide financial assistance to qualified low-income patients who can't repay their medical bills. States may require for-profit hospitals to offer one of these programs, and many other hospitals do so voluntarily. Another option is to establish a payment plan to accommodate your limited finances.

Other Sources of Financial Assistance

If you can't afford the out-of-pocket costs of your health care, you may be eligible for financial aid programs. An oncology social worker or a representative of the American Cancer Society can explain the benefits and eligibility requirements of various programs that offer these special plans. Numerous nonprofit organizations, including the Patient Access Network Foundation (www.panfoundation.org), can help. The National Breast and Cervical Cancer Early Detection Program of the US Centers for Disease Control (www.cdc.gov), for example, provides low-income, uninsured, and underinsured women with breast (and cervical) cancer screening and diagnostics.

- If you're unable to work because of your breast cancer, you may qualify for Social Security Disability Income. The Social Security Administration (www.ssa.gov) can determine your eligibility and how much you might receive based on how much you've already paid into Social Security.
- Long-term disability insurance, if provided by your employer, can replace a portion of your salary if you must miss work for an extended period.
- The Cancer Financial Assistance Coalition (www.cancerfac.org) maintains an online database of national organizations that help financially burdened cancer patients. The Pink Fund (www .pinkfund.org), for instance, provides short-term financial aid to breast cancer patients during treatment and recovery.
- CareCredit (www.carecredit.com) offers payment plans for medical services.
- If you have a retirement plan with your employer, you may qualify for the hardship provision that allows you to prematurely withdraw a portion of the funds.
- If you have life insurance, a provision of your policy may allow you to prematurely withdraw funds if you have a chronic or life-threatening medical condition or if you're unable to care for yourself. Restrictions and qualifications vary, and you may

be required to pay extra premiums or leave a reduced benefit for your beneficiary. It's a good idea to have documentation from your doctor attesting to your condition to avoid tax issues.

- If you own your own home, converting a portion of the equity—the difference between the home's value and the amount you still owe—into cash may be another alternative. A financial advisor can explain the advantages and disadvantages of a home equity loan, a cash-out refinance, or a reverse mortgage to determine whether one of these alternatives makes good financial sense for your circumstances.

Important Health Insurance Terms

- *Out-of-pocket costs* are the total amount you pay for medical care that isn't covered by your health insurance.
- A *premium* is the fee that you pay monthly, quarterly, or yearly for your health insurance.
- A *co-payment* is the amount you pay each time you receive care; the amount depends on the terms of your health care policy.
- A *deductible* is the amount you must pay before your health plan begins to cover the cost of your health care. You may be responsible for the first $1,500 dollars, for instance, before your health plan then begins to pay.
- *Co-insurance* is the percentage of health care costs you pay after you've paid your deductible. If you have a $100 bill for health services, for instance, you're responsible for the entire amount if you haven't yet met your required deductible. If your policy has an 80/20 provision, your insurer will pay $80, and you're responsible for the remaining $20.
- *Health insurance marketplaces* (or exchanges) run by the federal government and some states help people and businesses shop for, compare, and buy affordable health insurance.
- *In-network* providers are health care professionals or facilities that are contracted with your health care insurer.
- *Out-of-network* providers are health care professionals or facilities that aren't contracted with your plan and may cost you more than network providers.

Help Paying for Prescription Medications

If your health insurance doesn't cover a prescribed medication and you can't afford it, ask your doctor if a generic version of the medication or an alternate medication that is covered will work for you instead. Many pharmaceutical companies have programs to help people get the medicine they need at a reduced cost or no charge. Contact the drug manufacturer's patient assistance program to see if you're eligible. Partnership for Prescription Assistance (medicineassistance tool.org) can help you find the patient assistance programs of pharmaceutical companies.

Medicare's Extra Help program (www.ssa.gov) helps to cover the costs of monthly premiums, annual deductibles, and prescription co-payments related to a Medicare prescription drug plan. To be eligible, you must already be a Medicare recipient, have limited resources and income, and reside in one of the 50 states or the District of Columbia.

PART FIVE

Moving On

CHAPTER 23

Supportive Care and Symptom Management for Women with Metastatic Breast Cancer

No matter what your diagnosis and prognosis are or what treatment you're having, something can always be done to improve your quality of life as a patient.

Living with a serious illness can affect every part of daily life, but palliative care and hospice care are two important approaches that can help. These two very special supportive services share some similarities and yet are distinctly different. Your doctor can provide information about both services in your area.

PALLIATIVE CARE

Although it's often confused with hospice, which is end-of-life care, *palliative care* is specialized medical attention for people living with a serious illness, including breast cancer. Palliative care doesn't attempt to cure your underlying disease, replace your treatment, or prolong your life. Rather, it focuses on improving your emotional, psychological, and physical symptoms to make life easier for you and your family as you go through treatment. No matter what your diagnosis is, what treatment you're having, or what your prognosis is, something can always be done to improve the quality of your life as a patient.

You can and should seek palliative care soon after your diagnosis. It can be beneficial whether you're diagnosed with early-stage breast cancer and need help to get optimal relief from treatment side effects or you're coping with emotional and physical symptoms associated with advanced breast cancer. As your health care team continues to treat your breast cancer, your palliative team works to relieve your side effects—pain, anxiety, nausea, loss of appetite, trouble sleeping, and other problems—that develop as a result of surgery, chemotherapy, or other treatments. This specialized care is especially helpful for metastatic disease, and it can make your life a lot easier as you go through different therapies. Even when your treatment stops working or you decide to no longer accept treatment, the palliative focus can not only improve the way you feel, but it can also give you the highest possible quality of life. Some research even suggests that this type of compassionate care increases survival. The American Society of Clinical Oncology recommends palliative care for everyone with advanced cancer within eight weeks of diagnosis.

Palliative care can be provided to you in a hospital, a nursing home, an outpatient palliative care clinic, or in the comfort of your own home. Useful from diagnosis throughout treatment, palliative care encompasses a wide range of therapies and services, including:

- Treatment to control your pain and other uncomfortable side effects.
- Input to your personalized care plan.
- Coordination of your palliative care with the doctors who provide your breast cancer treatment.
- Assistance making difficult medical decisions.
- Practical help navigating the health insurance system and completing insurance forms.
- Emotional and spiritual support for you and your family.
- Recommendations for resources that can assist in decisions about treatment, financial concerns, and grief counseling, if needed.

- Help completing your advance directives so that your family and physicians are aware of the kind of end-of-life care you want to receive.

Your Palliative Care Team

Before your palliative support begins, you and your family will meet with members of your multidisciplinary palliative care team to identify your goals for care and what you need. Your team will work with you, your family, and your other doctors to ensure that you receive the medical, social, emotional, and practical support that you need. One team member will stay in close touch with you—in most cases, this is the nurse—and you'll meet with other members of the team as needed.

Your palliative team may include:
- a doctor who specializes in palliative care
- a nurse
- a social worker
- physical or speech therapists
- a dietician or nutritionist
- household aides
- a member of the clergy

Paying for Palliative Care

Health insurance normally covers some palliative services that are provided by doctors and nurses, but it doesn't always pay for non-medical services, like a household aid who helps with meals. Some plans may also cover the cost of a nutritionist, social worker, or other specialized services. Your health insurance company or your palliative care team can determine what your coverage includes. Your long-term health care policy, if you have one, may also include hospice benefits.

Medicare Part B (optional coverage that you pay into) pays for visits from doctors, nurse practitioners, and social workers, and it may also cover some treatments and medications that provide palliative care, although Medicare doesn't use the term "palliative." Your palliative care provider will bill Medicare for services provided, but you should ask about the co-pays or fees you'll be asked to pay; request a fee schedule from the palliative provider before you agree to receive services. Medicaid may also cover some palliative care treatments and medications, depending in which state you live. Your state Medicaid office can provide more information.

HOSPICE CARE

You can transition from palliative care to *hospice care* if your doctor estimates your life expectancy to be six months or less. At this point, you understand that treatment is no longer able to cure or slow the progression of your breast cancer, but this doesn't mean that all treatment is necessarily discontinued. While you may no longer have chemotherapy or other treatments, you may continue to be treated for high blood pressure, heart disease, diabetes, or other medical conditions other than breast cancer.

Hospice care provides comfort and care for terminally ill individuals during the final stages of life (table 23.1). The goal of this compassionate care isn't to treat your disease or help you to die, but to provide comfort and care in your final months, while counseling and supporting your family and caregivers and respecting your personal, cultural, and spiritual priorities. Generally, people and their families at this stage need physical comfort, mental and emotional support, spiritual encouragement, and help with practical tasks. Hospice provides care in all four areas.

All hospice programs must meet state requirements to be licensed and continue to provide care. They must also comply with federal regulations to obtain approval for Medicare reimbursement, including initial certification and routine inspection to ensure that they meet regulatory standards.

Table 23.1. How Palliative Care and Hospice Care Differ

Palliative Care	Hospice
Anyone with a serious disease	Anyone with a life expectancy of six months or less
Doesn't depend on prognosis	Depends on prognosis
Provided at any stage of illness	Provided when life expectancy is six months or less
Doesn't need physician's certification	Requires physician's certification of life expectancy
Curative treatment continues	Curative treatment stops
May start at diagnosis	Starts when end of life is near
Covered by some health care plans	Covered by many health care plans
Continues depending on the terms of your health care coverage	Continues as long as you meet eligibility requirements

Your hospice team manages your discomfort, pain, breathing difficulties, and other symptoms to keep you as comfortable as possible while your day-to-day care is provided by family and friends. Although most people at this stage prefer to remain in their own homes, care can also be given in a hospice facility. Your hospice team will provide numerous invaluable services, including:

- Managing your pain and symptoms to keep you comfortable.
- Providing medications, medical supplies, and equipment.
- Coaching your family on the best way to care for you.
- Arranging for special therapies as needed, including speech and physical therapy.
- Taking over your care temporarily to give your caregivers a respite.
- Arranging for short-term inpatient care if your symptoms are too difficult to manage at home.
- Providing emotional support to you and your family.
- Offering grief support to surviving loved ones and friends.

Getting Started

If your doctor suggests that you consider hospice care, it doesn't necessarily mean that death is imminent. But it's important to begin hospice care as soon as it becomes necessary, to take full advantage of the help it provides. Experts recommend learning about hospice care, discussing it with your family, and making decisions about it long before you actually need it. Any discussion about end-of-life care can be difficult and uncomfortable to discuss, but it's best for you to share your wishes with your family or loved ones before you need hospice.

If you and your family directly request services from a hospice care company, the hospice staff will contact your physician to determine whether a referral is appropriate, or you can ask your doctor to initiate a referral to a hospice service on your behalf. Before your care begins, you'll receive a visit from the hospice nurse, who will verify that you meet eligibility guidelines and review the services that hospice will provide for you. Your services can begin soon after you sign the necessary consent forms. It may take a day or two for your hospice care to begin, but it can be escalated if you urgently need it sooner.

Upon entering hospice care, you'll be asked to designate your primary caregiver, who will work with the hospice team to develop a care plan that meets your needs and personal preferences. Usually, this is your spouse or partner, but it can be another family member or a trusted friend. If you stay in your own home, your caregiver is usually the one who is responsible for providing most of your physical care and who will work with your hospice team to make decisions on your behalf. Before hospice care begins, your primary caregiver will need to coordinate the level of your care between your insurance carrier and the hospice team to decide which services will be most beneficial to you and to what extent they are covered by your health insurance.

One or more team members visit regularly, and they remain available at any time of the day or night. Home health attendants can help with housekeeping, cooking, personal care, and grooming, if needed.

Hospice volunteers can also provide companionship or provide practical services like grocery shopping or delivering medications. You'll also have access to social workers and chaplains who can provide emotional, social, and spiritual support. Counseling and grief support for your loved ones is another important and compassionate part of hospice that is usually offered for at least one year.

Your Hospice Care Team

Hospice care is performed by a core team that includes a doctor who specializes in pain management, a nurse, and a medical social worker. Because these individuals work in people's homes, they are well trained to listen, understand what you need, protect your privacy and confidentiality, and work with your family. Your hospice team will work closely with your primary care physician to coordinate your care. Your team may include several hospice specialists, including:

- a doctor who specializes in pain management
- a nurse
- speech, physical, and occupational therapists, if needed
- a medical social worker
- home health aides
- a member of the clergy or other spiritual counselor

Paying for Hospice

If you plan to have hospice care, contact your health insurer to see what coverage is included in your policy. Medicare provides comprehensive coverage of hospice if your doctor believes you have less than six months to live if your breast cancer takes its usual course. You pay no deductible for hospice services, but you may be required to make a co-payment for prescriptions. If you stop treatment but your doctor thinks that it's too soon for Medicare to cover hospice care, you may need a lot of help with daily living before Medicare will start paying for hospice. Medicare provides two 90-day periods of hospice care followed by an unlimited number of 60-day periods. If your condition improves or stabilizes so that you no longer meet eligibility or need hospice, you'll be discharged from the program. In that case, your Medicare benefits revert to the same coverage you had before you entered hospice. You must also withdraw from hospice if you enter a clinical trial, but if need be, you can be recertified and re-enroll in hospice at any future time without penalty or extra cost as long as you remain medically eligible. Medicare will continue to pay for your hospice care as long as your doctor continues to certify that death is near.

Medicaid coverage is similar in most states. The cost and delivery of a hospital bed, wheelchair, walker, oxygen, or other medical equipment you may need are also included. If your health care policy doesn't cover hospice services, or you aren't insured and can't afford it, your local hospice provider can give you information about special programs that reduce or cover the cost for some patients.

Meaningful Thoughts

Despite all of the advances in medicine, the diligent efforts of medical practitioners, and all of the hopes, prayers, love, and sacrifice of patients and their families, many women die from breast cancer each year. It can be easy for other people to tell a woman with advanced breast cancer that it's important to live each day to the fullest, but that is often difficult to do. In *The Four Things That Matter Most: A Book about Living*, author Dr. Ira Byock writes that our lives are like a book. You may know that you're approaching the end, but you never know when you're on the last chapter. He encourages all of us to fill our remaining chapters with meaningful people, deeds, and words, and to remember four things that are important to say to others as time grows shorter: "Please forgive me, I forgive you, thank you, and I love you."

TIPS FOR LIVING WITH METASTATIC BREAST CANCER

- Join a metastatic cancer support group, either in person or online. Giving and receiving support to and from others who understand your concerns can be invaluable.
- Make a short list of what really matters to you and how you want to spend your time. Travel to your dream location, write that book you've always had in your mind, or pursue other passions, if you're able.
- Focus your attention and spend your time on people and issues that bring you happiness and add to your quality of life. Live one day at a time, focusing on what and who you enjoy. Play with your grandchildren, spend more time with your spouse, visit with friends, or volunteer somewhere that gives you purpose, makes you happy, and brings you peace.
- Speak openly and honestly about your feelings with loved ones. Tell them what you want them to know while you have the chance. Resolve or let go of family squabbles.
- Create or update your will and other important legal documents, including an *advance health directive*, sometimes called a "living will," which informs your doctors of the care you do or don't want when you're unable to tell them yourself. A *do-not-resuscitate order* that stays in your medical file is also part of an advance directive. This form instructs hospital staff not to revive you if your heart stops or if you stop breathing. Another legal form is a *durable power of attorney*, which empowers someone you trust to make health care decisions for you when you're unable to do so. Provide notarized copies of these documents for your family, your estate trustee, and your attorney.
- Talk to your loved ones about your wishes regarding services after your death. Let them know if you prefer a nonreligious service or a traditional funeral according to your faith, such as a burial or cremation and a memorial service or celebration of life.

- It's not easy, but try to find a way to accept what is and release yourself from the fear you may feel. Facing his own terminal cancer, Stanford neurosurgeon Paul Kalanithi said, "In some ways, having a terminal illness makes you no different from anyone else: everyone dies. You have to find the balance—neither being overwhelmed by impending death nor completely ignoring it." He also advised, "Stop skipping dessert."

CHAPTER 24

Living Well beyond Cancer

HEALTHY BREAST CANCER SURVIVORSHIP

Living with fear and uncertainty compromises your physical well-being and your ability to enjoy life and to make plans for the future. Living with hope is empowering. Breast cancer survivors sometimes find that they are more resilient than they knew, and they may even experience meaningful personal growth from having undergone their unwanted experience with breast cancer.

Finally, breast cancer and treatment are behind you and you're a member of the cancer survivors' club. You may feel a wonderful sense of relief and closure. At the same time, you may feel sad and maybe anxious that you'll no longer have the frequent interactions and constant monitoring of your health care team, particularly if you've built a strong bond with them.

Adjusting to life after breast cancer can take time, and although the crisis that you've lived with for so many months may be over, you might feel lost in the abrupt transition from patient to non-patient. You may need several months to fully regain a healthy level of energy and sense of well-being, especially if you're still dealing with treatment side effects. As you get back to life without breast cancer, you'll gradually have more and more days when it doesn't occupy most of your thoughts. Give yourself credit for getting through your diagnosis and treatment. Be vigilant about your health, and take good care of yourself. Above all, enjoy life.

Life won't necessarily be exactly as it was before, however, because the experience will likely have changed your perspective. Despite the hardships, breast cancer can be a life-changing gift that forces you to look at life in a different way. You have the power to determine what that change will be. It may involve holding on to things that are familiar or opening yourself to new ideas; you may reassess your priorities and make positive changes in your life. Breast cancer may have shown you an inner strength that you didn't know you had and a newfound self-confidence and motivation to make the most of every day. This is the "new normal" that survivors often describe. Some survivors also talk about "post-traumatic growth syndrome," which describes this personal growth during or after the challenge of cancer.

THE SEASONS OF SURVIVORSHIP

In 1985, Dr. Fitzhugh Mullen wrote "The Seasons of Survival," an article about the phases of his own journey through cancer. Although the model he described has changed over time, it still describes that for most cancer survivors today, diagnosis and primary treatment often comprise a relatively short period of time that is followed by many years of living cancer free.

The seasons of survival for most breast cancer survivors include:

- Acute survivorship is the time of diagnosis and treatment that may include surgery, radiation, chemotherapy, or hormonal therapy.
- Extended survivorship is a period of surveillance and observation with planned visits to your breast cancer team after initial treatment. This is often referred to as a five-year period.
- Permanent survivorship describes the years when women typically think less about their diagnosis and when breast cancer becomes part of their past medical history. Most women in this phase typically do not report ongoing symptoms related to their treatment, but some report what are known as "late and long-term side effects," and some may develop a second cancer.

> **Susan's Story**
>
> The overall effect that all this had on me, quite frankly, was depressing. You take a step back, and you realize how vulnerable you are. You feel very, very vulnerable. It took the wind out of my sails, and I couldn't just go on with life as if a change hadn't occurred. It definitely had a deep effect on me. It took me a while to redefine myself and to get to know myself again. If I had it all to do over again, I would. Would it be difficult? Yes. You just push yourself. I think ultimately it makes you a stronger person, and it makes you realize that you can do things that you never thought you'd be able to do, and that you could make decisions that you never thought you would have to make. It pushes you to a new level of maturity, and without a doubt it just makes you a more compassionate person.

- Chronic survivorship describes the experience of women who live with breast cancer as a chronic disease that is being treated with the hormone therapies, chemotherapy, or targeted therapies described in this book.

OVERCOMING UNCERTAINTY ABOUT THE FUTURE

Whether you're a "glass half full" or a "glass half empty" type of person, you may feel anxious and uncertain about breast cancer returning. As you move into your life beyond breast cancer, certain things may trigger unease. You may worry that every follow-up scan and test may find a new tumor. Media stories about breast cancer, the anniversary of your diagnosis, or hearing about someone else who has been diagnosed may also make you feel vulnerable, while every headache, cough, or ache that develops may seem ominous. It's important to understand the signs of recurrence, as described in chapters 14 and 15, so that you can alert your physician as soon as possible if any of them occur. Remember that many of these symptoms can be caused by other conditions as well. Although recurrence is always a possibility, most survivors never need breast cancer treatment again.

Identifying these emotional triggers and talking about them can help you preemptively address them and minimize the effect they have on your life. Share your fears with your family. Talk in person or online with members of your support group, who can give you the benefit of their experience. Discuss your worries with your health care team, and be honest about what you don't understand or what you fear. Just having the conversation can make a positive difference, but they can't help you if you're not vocal about issues that concern you.

Having a Survivorship Care Plan (described later in this chapter) that clearly describes your follow-up monitoring and care can help you feel less vulnerable, enabling you to focus on the present and avoid worrying about things that may never happen. Living with hope is empowering. Living with fear and uncertainty compromises your physical well-being and your ability to enjoy life and to make plans for the future. Realize that you've done everything that can be done to beat your breast cancer, so that you can now focus on living your life and enjoying each day. If you can't seem to shake your fear that breast cancer will return, speak to a therapist about cognitive behavioral therapy, which can help reduce your anxiety and replace negative thought patterns with positive ones.

Wanda's Story

Before that fateful night when my surgeon called with the biopsy results confirming breast cancer, my life was proceeding smoothly. Recently promoted, I was preoccupied with my career, serving on community boards, teaching Sunday school, and being a wife, mother, daughter, sister, aunt, friend, and colleague. You never think of getting breast cancer yourself, so you don't prepare. The first thing I remember thinking was, "How long do I have to live?" My heart was dropping out of my chest. I was filled with negative thoughts and negative feelings. How would I tell my parents and my son, who had just started at the Naval Academy? It would be too hard for them to hear this. And my husband—we had just celebrated our 27th anniversary—how would he handle it? Would he ever touch me again? It was such a sinking, hurt feeling. I also thought, "Oh, my God, I have these wild, crazy cells inside me and I could be dead tomorrow. They're probably going to cut both breasts off." I don't even know what my surgeon's words were, I just remember my feelings about what he was saying: "You could have a lumpectomy, but some people want a mastectomy. We have to do something quickly." I went to another surgeon and a medical oncologist for second and third opinions. I read more, got on the Internet, and looked at statistics—statistics never look good for cancer people. You know, you have a 10 percent chance of whatever. I can't live with statistics. I really can't.

I decided I was going to settle down into this. Whatever comes is what I was going to accept. But I needed time to get there. I didn't want to feel rushed. My oncologist spent so much time with me, I felt guilty. He was so nice, so wonderful, and I felt so affirmed by him. He talked to me, and he drew charts and breasts. He walked me through the chemotherapy process that he recommended. I decided on lumpectomy and radiation followed by chemotherapy. That was interesting. My hair fell out. On Fridays, I felt sick as a dog. On Tuesdays and Thursdays, I felt okay enough to teach. I surrounded myself with positive things. I read about cancer, but also about holistic and spiritual kinds of things, about being at peace. I also made lifestyle and career changes. I got off every board I was on. It was too stressful, so I took my life down a notch. I'm thankful for being able to settle in with this, because now I'm more at peace. I'm just going to enjoy what I have each day. Despite it being cancer, my diagnosis was a gift.

MOVING IN THE RIGHT DIRECTION

Taking charge of your health is the best thing you can do for your overall mental and physical well-being. Studies suggest that maintaining a healthy lifestyle has a more significant impact on longevity than intensely screening for recurrence.

Give Your Body the Nutrition It Needs

Eating nutritionally balanced meals is something you can do to improve your overall health, no matter your age. If you're not sure where to begin or how to revamp otherwise less-than-healthy eating habits, visit www.choosemyplate.gov or consult with a nutritionist who can help you create an easy-to-follow plan. Many informative books are available, but avoid the ones that promote fad diets.

- Choose a primarily plant-based diet that includes a variety of fruits, vegetables, whole grains, beans, legumes, nuts, seeds, and lean protein.
- Eat mostly whole foods, rather than prepackaged, processed, or fast foods.
- Limit your intake of meat and other animal products, which are high in saturated fats.
- Avoid or limit sugary sodas and presweetened beverages.
- Consume healthy fats, including avocado, olive, canola, and sunflower oils, but do so in moderation, because all oils are high in calories. Limit use of coconut and palm oils, which are highly saturated.
- Enjoy fatty fish (salmon, anchovies, sardines, trout, and others) twice weekly.
- Keep snacking to a minimum. When you do snack, have fresh fruit or vegetables, a handful of nuts, or low-fat yogurt instead of cookies or chips.
- Season foods with herbs and spices. Limit salt and salty foods.
- Avoid drinking alcohol or limit consumption to one glass or less per day.
- Read nutrition and ingredient labels, and make good choices.

Maintain a Healthy Weight

Whether you were slim or heavy before your diagnosis, you may have gained weight as a result of being treated with chemotherapy, steroids, or hormonal therapies. Being overweight or obese not only affects your overall health but also increases the likelihood of having a recurrence. You're more likely to gain weight if you become postmenopausal within a year of your diagnosis.

Nearly two-thirds of women who are treated with chemotherapy gain weight. This may be surprising, considering that the stereotypical image of patients who take chemo is that they're extremely thin. Weight gain during chemotherapy depends on how long you take the medication and the level of steroids that you need to decrease the risk of an allergic reaction or to minimize nausea and other side effects. On average, women gain 5 to 6 pounds while on chemotherapy, compared to no weight gain in women who are treated with surgery alone or tamoxifen. Added pounds may also result from high-calorie comfort foods that you may have indulged in during your treatment and less physical activity if you were fatigued or felt ill much of the time. You may also weigh more now if your treatment brought on early menopause.

Losing weight can take time, and it isn't always easy. Experts recommend healthy eating and regular physical activity to lose one or two pounds per week. Avoid fad diets that promise rapid weight loss; research shows that you're more likely to keep weight off when you lose it slowly and steadily. The "Controlling Your Weight" tips in chapter 4 will help get you started in the right direction.

Pay It Forward

As a breast cancer survivor, you have the benefit of hindsight that newly diagnosed women don't have. If you're inclined to share what you've learned, you can help other women who face the same issues that are now behind you. Whether you spend an occasional hour or get involved full-time, the opportunities to help someone through the journey are endless.

- Volunteer at your local breast cancer organization, treatment center, or hospital.
- Get involved with one of the many online breast cancer support organizations.
- Let your oncologist, plastic surgeon, or radiologist know that you're happy to act as a patient resource for newly diagnosed women.
- Participate in breast cancer awareness events.
- Learn to become a breast cancer advocate.
- Help out in a support group.
- Donate or participate in breast cancer fundraising.

Stay Physically Active

Exercise is beneficial for both mind and body. Staying active reduces fatigue, helps to manage your weight, and produces endorphins that make you feel better. It's especially critical for breast cancer survivors, because it not only decreases the risk of a recurrence but also reduces the chance of cardiovascular disease, the primary cause of death in women over 50.

Always check with your doctor before starting an exercise program. Although physical activity generally improves overall immune system response, it may not be recommended if your immune system is suppressed from medication or other reasons. Exercise can also be of benefit if you have lymphedema. A certified lymphedema therapist can show you how to gradually increase your upper body strength without increasing fluids in your arm.

- If you're not used to being active, begin with a 10-minute daily walk and gradually increase your time and distance. Use a pedometer to motivate yourself to get at least 10,000 steps a day.
- Strive for 150 minutes of moderate exercise or 75 minutes of vigorous activity each week, and include strength training at least two to three days per week.
- Incorporate exercise into your daily activities. Park away from your destination and then walk to it. Take the stairs instead of the elevator. Stretch or use a stationary bike while you watch television.
- Schedule an exercise interval when you plan your other daily activities.
- Exercise with a friend or a group to stay motivated.
- Change up your exercise routine periodically, so that your muscles don't get used to what you do. Swim, walk, dance, or join a yoga or Pilates class.
- If you feel fatigued, try scheduling exercise at a time during the day when your energy level is at its highest.

Debbie's Story

My husband felt a lump in my left breast when I was 33. My doctor said that I had fibrocystic breasts and not to worry. When I requested a mammogram, he said that my breasts were too firm and nothing would show up. I accepted his advice and went on with my life. Over time, my breast became more and more painful, and the lump grew. I was tired much of the time, and again I went to my doctor to see if I was anemic. The doctor told me that anyone with my schedule would be exhausted—I had a 4-year-old, worked full-time, and went to graduate school part-time.

Over the next three years, my breast became increasingly painful; it kept me awake at night. It began to dimple, and my nipple inverted. The lump continued to grow. Then I saw an OB/GYN and had a mammogram. As I undraped my breast, I knew immediately by the look on the technician's face that I had cancer. Although she didn't say anything, she couldn't hide her shock. Things began to move quickly. I had a biopsy the next week. The surgeon found a tumor the size of a racquetball that appeared to be cancer. The sample was sent to the lab, and the results went to the oncologist. Then the doctor confirmed my suspicion. I can't say I was surprised at my diagnosis. Cancer ran in my family, but no one had been diagnosed with breast cancer.

I regretted so many things and wished that I could go back in time and change. I was angry with myself for spending so much precious time at work and graduate school instead of with my son. He was so young to have to go through this trauma. My worry about him was excruciating, and I felt so guilty. At my next appointment with the oncologist, he explained that my cancer cells had estrogen receptors, and that was a good thing. He suggested chemotherapy to shrink the tumor before surgery and then mastectomy. I didn't have to imagine the effectiveness of the chemo because the results were obvious. The tumor grew smaller and smaller over several months; my breast seemed to deflate. Seeing proof that the cancer was being destroyed allowed me to maintain my positive attitude. I worried less and wasn't as frustrated by the side effects. When the tumor was barely palpable, I stopped chemo to build up my immune system for surgery. I had a mastectomy and my lymph nodes were removed; none of them tested positive. I never imagined such good news. One month after surgery, I restarted chemo and then had radiation, which ended soon after.

Thirteen years later, I am free from cancer. I am truly blessed, and I'm grateful to so many people who supported me during my treatment.

Don't Smoke, Vape, or Chew Tobacco

Tobacco in any form, including secondhand smoke, carries dangerous carcinogens. According to the US Surgeon General, "Smoking cessation represents the single most important step that smokers can take to enhance the length and quality of their lives." Continuing to smoke after your diagnosis can have dire consequences: your risk of dying from breast or other cancers, respiratory disease, or cardiovascular disease is greater than the risk of survivors who have never been smokers. Overcoming a tobacco addiction can be difficult, but it's never too late to realize the benefits of quitting. Talk to your doctor or contact the American Lung Association (www.lung.org) if you need help.

Get Enough Sleep

More and more research shows that getting enough quality sleep is vital for mental health, physical health, and quality of life. Sleep is the interval when the body repairs the heart and blood vessels and when the brain forms new pathways. Sleep disturbances—trouble getting to sleep or staying asleep—interfere with the body's ability to complete these and other critical maintenance functions that keep us healthy.

Insomnia (trouble getting to sleep) is twice as common among breast cancer patients and survivors as it is in the general population. Stress, anxiety, side effects of medications, and other health conditions can keep you awake. This is problematic because, in addition to feeling tired and experiencing reduced concentration and memory, losing sleep can decrease the effectiveness of your immune system against disease. That can be particularly worrisome if your immune system has already been compromised by chemotherapy or other treatment. Some studies have found that reduced sleep may be a risk factor for developing breast cancer, and that not getting the recommended seven to eight hours of daily sleep may affect survival after diagnosis.

Try the following tips to make it easier to fall asleep and stay asleep:

- Open your curtains or go outside to get some exposure to natural light every day.
- Exercise regularly, but not within two or three hours before bedtime.
- Nap for no more than 20 to 30 minutes, and never in the late afternoon or evening.
- Avoid alcohol and caffeine, especially in the evening.
- Go to bed at about the same time each night.
- Avoid tobacco products; nicotine is a stimulant.
- Avoid using electronic and mobile devices two to three hours before bedtime. They emit blue light that reduces melatonin, a hormone that makes you sleepy.
- If you can't get to sleep, get up and do something relaxing until you feel sleepy again.

FOLLOW-UP CARE

You may be free of breast cancer, but you'll still need follow-up care once your treatment has ended. Follow-up care is important to manage any persistent treatment side effects and to treat any long-term or late side effects that develop, including lymphedema, thickening of the lung (fibrosis) from radiation therapy, or heart problems from chemotherapy or from anti-HER2 trastuzumab. National guidelines recommend that you continue to be monitored by your oncologist for at least three years after your primary treatment (table 24.1). All other care related to your overall health, such as overall health care and routine health screening, transition back to your primary care physician.

Follow-up visits to your doctor also increase the chance of detecting any recurrence early on and screen for other cancers. Routine lab tests and imaging aren't generally recommended to screen for recurrence because they often reflect false positive results and they don't improve survival outcomes or quality of life in women who don't have symptoms. Regular mammography is recommended if you still have your natural breast(s).

Compared to someone who has never had breast cancer, if you're a breast cancer survivor, you have a higher risk for another diagnosis in either breast. You also have elevated risk for colon, uterine, ovarian, thyroid, melanoma, and other cancers. So, in addition to screening

Table 24.1. Recommended Follow-Up Care after Breast Cancer Treatment

Care	When	Which Survivors?
Breast self-exam	Monthly	All with remaining breast tissue
History and physical exam	Every 3–6 months for three years, every 6–12 months for the next two years, then annually	All
Mammogram	• Baseline 6–12 months after breast-conserving therapy, then annually • Annually of remaining breast after unilateral mastectomy • None required after bilateral mastectomy or on a reconstructed breast	All
Breast MRI	Annually	High risk only*
Bone density test	Baseline after treatment, then every two years	Postmenopausal survivors who take an aromatase inhibitor, and premenopausal survivors who take tamoxifen or a GnRH agonist, or had treatment-related early menopause
Pelvic exam	Annually	All
Gynecologic exam	Annually	Postmenopausal survivors who take tamoxifen

for a breast cancer recurrence, it's important that you're routinely screened for these cancers as well. You may need additional or more frequent testing and follow-up if you're at high risk.

Your Survivorship Care Plan

Everyone who completes cancer treatment should have a Survivorship Care Plan that details their diagnosis and treatment and outlines long-term follow-up care. Ideally, your doctor should prepare and discuss this report when your treatment ends. Ask for it if your doctor doesn't provide it, or use the American Society of Clinical Oncology's easy-to-use online tool (www.cancer.net), and ask your physician to complete it.

A Survivorship Care Plan summarizes your diagnosis and treatment and outlines information that is critical for your long-term care, including:

- The type of breast cancer you had and the biological characteristics of the tumor.
- The breast cancer treatments you received and any potential long-term effects.
- The screenings and therapies that you had for physical, psychological, or other issues and conditions related to your breast cancer treatment.
- Information about any treatment that you continue to receive, such as tamoxifen or an aromatase inhibitor.
- Details regarding the frequency and type of follow-up care you should receive.
- Contact information for your health care team and the physician who will coordinate and provide your ongoing care.

Sample Survivorship Care Plan

HEALTH CARE PROVIDERS
Primary Care Provider:
Surgeon:
Medical Oncologist:
Radiation Oncologist:
Other Providers:

TREATMENT SUMMARY	
Diagnosis	
Cancer Type/Subtype: Left/Right/Both Breasts Receptors: ☐ Estrogen positive ☐ Progesterone positive ☐ HER2 positive	Year of Diagnosis: Stage: ☐ I ☐ II ☐ III
Treatment Completed	
Surgery: ☐ Yes ☐ No	Year of Surgery:
Surgical Procedure/Findings:	
Breast Cancer Surgery: ☐ Lumpectomy ☐ Total Mastectomy ☐ Modified Radical Mastectomy ☐ Radical Mastectomy Lymph Node Removal: ☐ Sentinel Biopsy ☐ Axillary Dissection: no. of nodes removed:	

Radiation: ☐ Yes ☐ No	Body Area Irradiated:	Year Completed:

Systemic Therapy: ☐ Yes ☐ No ☐ Before Surgery ☐ After Surgery	
Systemic Medications	Year Completed
☐ 5-Fluorouracil	
☐ Carboplatin	
☐ Cyclophosphamide	
☐ Docetaxel	
☐ Doxorubicin	
☐ Paclitaxel	

☐ Pertuzumab	
☐ Trastuzumab	
☐ Other	

Persistent Symptoms or Side Effects at Completion of Treatment:

Fatigue: ☐ No   ☐ Yes   Numbness: ☐ No   ☐ Yes

Menopausal Symptoms: ☐ No   ☐ Yes   Pain: ☐ No   ☐ Yes

Psychosocial/Depression: ☐ No   ☐ Yes   Other (enter type(s)):

Ongoing Treatment

Medication	Planned Duration	Possible Side Effects
☐ Tamoxifen		Hot flashes, vaginal discharge (common), endometrial cancer, serious blood clots, eye problems (all very rare). Other rare side effects may occur.
☐ Aromatase Inhibitors		Hot flashes, joint/muscle aches, vaginal dryness, bone loss (common); hair thinning (rare). Other rare side effects may occur.
☐ GnRH Agonist		Hot flashes, vaginal dryness (common). Other rare side effects may occur.
Other:		

Familial Cancer Risk Assessment

Breast and/or Ovarian Cancer in 1st or 2nd Degree Relatives: ☐ Yes   ☐ No

Received Genetic Counseling: ☐ Yes   ☐ No   Genetic Testing: ☐ Yes   ☐ No

Genetic Test Results:

Cancer Surveillance or Other Recommended Tests

Coordinating Provider	Test	Frequency
	Mammogram	Annually
	MRI breast	As indicated by provider
	Pap/pelvic exam	As indicated by provider
	Colonoscopy	As indicated by provider
	Bone density	Every two years if on an aromatase inhibitor or as indicated by your provider

(continued)

Speak with your doctors or nurses if you experience any of the issues below or have any concerns.

☐ Anxiety or depression	☐ Insurance	☐ Sexual functioning
☐ Emotional and mental health	☐ Memory or concentration loss	☐ Stopping smoking
☐ Fatigue	☐ Parenting	☐ Weight changes
☐ Fertility	☐ Physical functioning	☐ Other
☐ Financial advice or assistance	☐ School/work	

Lifestyle/behaviors can affect your ongoing health, including the risk for a new or recurrent breast cancer:

☐ Alcohol use	☐ Physical activity	☐ Other
☐ Diet	☐ Sunscreen use	
☐ Manage your medications	☐ Tobacco use/cessation	
☐ Manage your other illnesses	☐ Weight management (loss/gain)	

Other comments:

Prepared by: Delivered on:

Source: Adapted from the American Society of Clinical Oncology's Cancer Survivorship Plan

Resources

Breast Cancer

American Cancer Society (www.cancer.org)

BreastCancer.org (www.breastcancer.org)

Bright Pink (www.brightpink.org)

Metastatic Breast Cancer Network (www.mbcn.org)

National Cancer Institute (www.cancer.gov)

Susan G. Komen Breast Cancer Foundation (www.komen.org)

Triple-Negative Breast Cancer Foundation (www.tnbcfoundation.org)

Young Survival Coalition (www.youngsurvival.org)

Breast Cancer Genetics and Risk

Confronting Hereditary Breast and Ovarian Cancer, by Sue Friedman, DVM, Rebecca Sutphen, MD, and Kathy Steligo (Baltimore: Johns Hopkins University Press, 2012)

Facing Our Risk of Cancer Empowered (www.facingourrisk.org)

Informed Medical Decisions (www.informeddna.com)

National Society of Genetic Counselors (www.nsgc.org)

Coping

Cancer Club (www.cancerclub.com)

Family Caregiver Alliance (www.caregiver.org)

Kids Konnected (www.kidskonnected.org)

Laughter Yoga (www.laughteryoga.org)

National Alliance of Caregiving (www.caregiving.org)

National Hospice and Palliative Care Organization (www.nhpco.org)

National Lymphedema Network (www.lymphnet.org)

Insurance and Financial Issues

Cancer Care (www.cancercare.org)

Insurance Information Institute (www.iii.org)

Medicare (www.medicare.gov)

Patient Advocate Foundation (www.patientadvocate.org)

United Breast Cancer Foundation (www.ubcf.info)

Women's Health and Cancer Rights Act (www.dol.gov/ebsa
/publications/whcra.html)

Mastectomy and Breast Reconstruction

American Society of Plastic Surgeons (www.plasticsurgery.org)

BreastFree (www.breastfree.org)

The Breast Reconstruction Guidebook, 4th ed., by Kathy Steligo
(Baltimore: Johns Hopkins University Press, 2017)

Reach to Recovery (www.cancer.org/treatment/supportprograms
services/reach-to-recovery)

Recovery and Survival

Cancer Survivors Network (http://csn.cancer.org/forum)

LiveStrong (www.livestrong.org)

Living Beyond Breast Cancer (www.lbbc.org)

National Coalition for Cancer Survivorship (www.canceradvocacy.org)

National Lymphedema Network (www.lymphnet.org)

Glossary

Absolute risk. The chance of something happening, like developing a certain disease, within a specific time period.

Accelerated partial-breast irradiation (APBI). Radiation therapy that delivers higher doses to the lumpectomy site (rather than the whole breast) over a shorter period of time than traditional radiation therapy.

Acellular dermal matrix (ADM). Sterilized donor skin used to replace missing tissue.

Acupressure. A form of alternative massage that stimulates acupuncture points with gentle pressure from the fingers, knuckles, palms, elbows, or feet.

Acupuncture. A form of alternative medicine that improves certain conditions by inserting thin needles into the body to stimulate and rebalance energy points.

Adjuvant therapy. Treatment given after surgery.

Advanced breast cancer. Cancer that has spread beyond the breast to other parts of the body.

Advance health directive. A document that informs your doctors of the care you do or don't want when you're unable to tell them yourself.

Alpha-linolenic acid. A type of omega-3 fat.

Alternative medicine. Unproven therapies that are meant to substitute for conventional medical treatment.

Androgen. A primarily male hormone that women have in limited quantities.

Antiemetic. A drug used to prevent or reduce nausea.

Antioxidant. A substance that protects cells from damage.

Areola. The circle of darkened skin around the nipple.

Aromatase inhibitor (AI). A drug that blocks the production of estrogen.

Aromatherapy. The use of essential oils to produce a sense of well-being.

Arthralgia. Conditions that cause joint pain and stiffness.

Art therapy. Guided sessions of painting, drawing, sculpting, or other artistic endeavors that reduce stress.

Atypical hyperplasia. Dividing cells that have an abnormal shape or unusual internal features.

Autologous tissue flap. Skin, fat, tissue, and sometimes muscle that is moved from one area of the body to another to replace missing tissue.

Axillary lymph node dissection (ALND). Surgical removal of lymph nodes in the underarm to remove cancer cells.

Axillary lymph nodes. Lymph nodes in the underarm.

Axillary reverse mapping. A procedure to evaluate patterns of lymph fluid drainage.

Benign. Not cancerous.

Bilateral breast cancer. Cancer that simultaneously occurs in both breasts.

Bilateral mastectomy. Surgical removal of both breasts.

Bilateral salpingo-oophorectomy (BSO). Surgery to remove the ovaries and fallopian tubes.

Biopsy. A procedure that removes a sample of cells, fluid, or tissue to check for disease.

Biosimilar. A copycat drug that has almost the same safety, purity, and effectiveness of the medication that it mimics.

Bisphosphonates. Medications that strengthen bone.

Brachytherapy. A type of internal radiation therapy that places the radiation source close to the tumor.

Breast cancer. Uncontrolled growth of abnormal breast cells.

BReast CAncer genes 1 and 2 (BRCA1 and BRCA2). Genes that help cells repair DNA damage. When mutated, these genes significantly increase the risk of developing breast, ovarian, and other cancers.

Breast-conserving surgery (lumpectomy). Surgical removal of a cancerous lump and some healthy surrounding tissue.

Breast-conserving therapy (BCT). Surgical removal of a cancerous lump and some healthy surrounding tissue, followed by radiation.

Breast implant. A device filled with saline or silicone gel that replaces missing breast tissue.

Breast implant–associated anaplastic large cell lymphoma (BIA-ALCL). A rare type of non-Hodgkin lymphoma.

Breast lymphoma. An abnormal malignancy in the lymph system of the breast.

Breast prosthesis. A temporary breast form that can be worn to provide shape and symmetry after the breast is removed.

Breast reconstruction. Procedures that use an implant or a patient's own tissue to restore breast shape and volume after mastectomy.

Breast sarcoma. Tumors that begin in the fat, blood vessels, nerves, and other soft tissues of the breast.

Breast self-exam (BSE). Examination of your own breasts to check for irregularities.

Breast surgeon. A general surgeon who specializes in surgical procedures of breast.

Breast ultrasound. Technology that uses high-frequency sound waves to create images of the breast interior.

Calcification. A deposit of calcium in the tissue that may indicate a malignancy.

Cancer. Abnormal and uncontrolled cell growth.

Cancer of unknown primary (CUP). A cancer that has an unknown origin.

Cancer syndrome. Multiple cancers that may develop as a result of having a genetic mutation.

Capsular contracture. Tightening of the scar capsule surrounding an implant.

Carcinogen. Something that can damage healthy tissue and cause cancer.

CDK4/6 inhibitor. A class of drugs that target cyclin-dependent kinase enzymes to prevent cancer cells from multiplying.

Cementoplasty. Injections of special medical cement that strengthen and support damaged bone.

Chemoprevention. Drugs that reduce the risk of developing cancer.

Chemotherapy. Drugs that destroy cancer cells.

Chromosome. The part of a cell that carries all of an organism's genetic information and instruction.

Claus model. A computerized program that estimates a person's risk of invasive breast cancer during the next 10 years.

Clear margin. A border of tissue around a malignant tumor that is free of cancer cells.

Clinical breast exam (CBE). An examination of the breasts by a health professional.

Clinical complete response. No evidence of disease shown by physical examination, blood tests, or imaging scans after treatment.

Clinical trial. A study that tests the safety and effectiveness of a new treatment or procedure in humans.

Close margin. An area of tissue around a malignant tumor that contains nearby cancer cells.

Cognitive behavioral therapy. Counseling that provides an understanding of how your thoughts and feelings influence your behavior.

Co-insurance. The percentage of health care costs you pay after you've paid your deductible.

Cold cap. A cap that applies cold temperatures to the head during chemotherapy to prevent or reduce hair loss.

Combination chemotherapy. More than one type of chemotherapy given at the same time.

Comedo necrosis. An area of dead cancer cells.

Complementary medicine. Treatments that are used with standard treatments.

Complete pathological response. No evidence of disease in a tissue sample after treatment.

Computed tomography (CT or CAT) scan. An x-ray that produces sectional images of the body.

Contralateral prophylactic mastectomy (CPM). Preventive removal of the healthy breast opposite of the breast that is treated for cancer.

Co-payment (co-pay). A fixed amount that you're required to pay for medical services or prescriptions.

Core needle biopsy. Removal with a needle of a small plug of tissue from a lump or mass.

Costochondritis. Inflammation that develops in the connective tissue between a rib and the breastbone.

Cowden syndrome. An inherited predisposition to breast and other cancers caused by a mutation in the PTEN gene.

Cribiform. Low- to medium-grade cells that look and behave like normal cells.

Cyberchondria. A term used by psychologists to describe heightened anxiety from being exposed to too much online information.

Cytotoxic. Toxic to living cells.

Deductible. The out-of-pocket amount you must pay for medical expenses or prescriptions before your health insurance coverage begins.

Deep inspiration breath hold (respiratory gating). A breathing procedure that helps to protect the heart from radiation to the breast or chest.

Delayed-immediate reconstruction. Placement of a tissue expander after a skin-sparing mastectomy to preserve breast shape and facilitate reconstruction if postmastectomy radiation is needed.

Delayed reconstruction. A separate procedure to re-create a breast sometime after mastectomy is performed.

Delayed wound healing. A wound that is slow to heal.

Dense breasts. Breasts that have more glandular tissue than fat.

Deoxyribonucleic acid (DNA). Molecules within cells that carry inherited genetic information.

Diagnostic mammogram. An x-ray of the breast used to provide additional information about an unusual or suspicious area.

Digital mammography. Technology that produces computerized images of the breast.

Direct-to-implant reconstruction. A surgical procedure that places a full-sized implant immediately after mastectomy.

Distant metastasis. Cancer that spreads from its origin to other parts of the body.

Distant recurrence. Cancer that returns somewhere in the body other than the original site.

Do-not-resuscitate order. A document that instructs hospital staff not to revive you if your heart stops or if you stop breathing.

Duct. The part of the breast that delivers milk to the nipple.

Ductal carcinoma in situ (DCIS). Early-stage, noninvasive cancer that begins in the breast ducts.

Ductal lavage. A method of collecting cells from the milk ducts in the breast.

Durable power of attorney. A document that empowers someone you trust to make health care decisions for you when you're unable to do so.

Dyspareunia. Vaginal dryness and irritation that make intercourse painful.

Epidemiological studies. Research that identifies patterns of disease among large groups of people.

Estrogen. A primary female hormone.

Estrogen receptor negative. Cancer cells that do not need estrogen to grow.

Estrogen receptor positive. Cancer cells that need estrogen to grow.

Excisional biopsy. Surgery to remove an entire lump of suspicious tissue.

External beam radiation therapy. Radiation that treats cancer with high-energy x-rays.

False negative. A test that fails to find cancer.

False positive. A test result that detects cancer when none is present.

Fat grafting. A procedure to liposuction fat, purify it, and then inject it into specific areas of the body to improve cosmetic defects.

Fibroadenoma. A benign tumor in the breast.

Fibrocystic breasts. Benign changes in breast tissue.

Fibrosis. Painful scarring of tissue.

Fine needle aspiration. A type of biopsy that withdraws cells from a lump or a mass with a thin, hollow needle and a syringe.

Free radicals. Toxic molecules that damage DNA.

Gadolinium. A contrast dye that is sometimes used with magnetic resonance imaging.

Gail model. A computerized program that estimates a person's risk of invasive breast cancer during the next five years.

GammaPod. A type of radiation therapy developed specifically to treat early-stage breast cancer.

Gene. Bits of DNA inside chromosomes that issue cellular instructions.

Gene editing. The ability to make changes in a gene.

Generic drug. A medication that is a copy of a brand-name drug, with the same dosage, side effects, strength, safety, administration, and use as its brand-name counterpart.

Genetic counselor. A health professional who is trained to interpret patterns in a family's medical history and estimate an individual's risk for disease.

Genetic mutations. Benign or malignant changes in genes.

Genetics. The study of inherited traits and diseases.

Genetic testing. Testing of a person's blood or saliva for the presence of a genetic mutation.

Genomic test. A study that predicts the aggressiveness of a tumor.

Grade. Classification of a cancer based on how abnormal cells look and how quickly they're growing.

Guided imagery. A type of self-induced hypnotic state triggered by the use of mental images to achieve deep relaxation.

Health insurance marketplace. A resource for comparing and buying health insurance.

Hematoma. Blood that leaks from a blood vessel under the skin.

Hereditary breast and ovarian cancer (HBOC) syndrome. An inherited predisposition to breast, ovarian, and other cancers caused by a genetic mutation.

Hereditary breast cancer. Breast cancer caused by an inherited genetic abnormality.

Hormone receptor. A protein on the surface of cells that attaches to a hormone.

Hormone therapy. Treatment that blocks production or reduces the level of hormones in the body.

Hospice care. Specialized care for people with life-limiting illnesses.

Hot flash. A sudden, uncomfortable feeling of heat.

Human epidermal growth factor 2 (HER2). A protein that signals cells to grow.

Hyperplasia. Increased cellular growth.

Hypoactive sexual desire disorder. A lack or absence of sexual desire.

Hypofractionated whole-breast radiation. Radiation therapy that delivers slightly higher doses per day during fewer sessions than traditional radiation therapy.

Image-guided biopsy. A sampling of cells or tissue that is performed with imaging technology.

Immediate breast reconstruction. Surgery to re-create a breast that is performed at the same time as a mastectomy.

Immunotherapy. Therapy that stimulates the immune system to fight disease.

Incisional biopsy. Surgery that removes a small portion of a suspicious lump or mass of tissue.

Inflammatory breast cancer (IBC). Cancer cells that accumulate in the lymph vessels beneath the breast skin.

In-network. Medical providers and facilities that are contracted with a particular health insurance company to accept predetermined fees for services.

Integrative medicine. Treatment that combines standard Westernized medicine and complementary therapies.

Intensity-modulated radiation therapy (IMRT). A type of three-dimensional radiation therapy that uses computer-generated images to target the tumor from multiple angles.

Internal radiation therapy (brachytherapy). A type of internal radiation therapy that places the radiation source close to the tumor.

Interstitial radiation. A type of internal radiation therapy given through multiple catheters.

Intervention study. Research to identify behaviors that can improve health.

Intraoperative radiation therapy (IORT). Partial breast radiation given during surgery.

Invasive breast cancer. Cancer that has spread beyond its origin in the breast.

Invasive (infiltrating) ductal carcinoma. Cancer that develops in the ducts of the breast and spreads to surrounding breast tissue.

Invasive (infiltrating) lobular carcinoma (ILC). Cancer that develops in the lobules of the breast and spreads to surrounding breast tissue.

In vitro fertilization. A procedure that removes eggs from a woman's ovary, combines them with sperm outside the body, and either implants the resulting embryos into her uterus or freezes them for future use.

Lesion. An abnormal change or damage to tissue.

Li-Fraumeni syndrome (LFS). An inherited predisposition to breast and other cancers caused by a mutation in the TP53 gene.

Linear accelerator. A machine that delivers a prescribed dose of radiation.

Lobular carcinoma in situ (LCIS). A condition of abnormal cells that are confined to the lobules of the breast.

Lobular neoplasia. Irregular cells that form in the lobules of the breast.

Lobule. The part of the breast that produces milk.

Locally advanced breast cancer. Breast cancer that has spread to the breast skin, chest wall, or lymph nodes in the underarm, but no further.

Local recurrence. Cancer that returns at the original site or in the surgery scar.

Local therapy. Treatment that focuses on the area of the tumor.

Locoregional recurrence. A recurrence found in the treated breast and nearby lymph nodes.

Lumpectomy. Surgery to remove a breast tumor and a small amount of surrounding tissue.

Lymphatic venous anastomosis. Surgery to improve lymphatic drainage.

Lymphedema. A chronic accumulation of lymph fluid in the arm or leg that develops when lymph vessels or lymph nodes are damaged or removed.

Lymph fluid. Colorless fluid that transports cellular debris throughout the lymph system.

Lymph nodes. Small glands that are part of the immune system and filter impurities in the body.

Lymphocytes. White blood cells that are a part of the immune system.

Lymph system. A network of small glands connected by lymphatic vessels that filter impurities in the body.

Lynch syndrome. An inherited predisposition to breast and other cancers.

Macrocalcifications. Calcium deposits that develop from benign breast conditions or aging.

Magnetic resonance imaging (MRI). A technology that uses magnets and radio waves to produce three-dimensional images of the body's interior.

Malignant. Cancerous.

Mammalian target of rapamycin (mTOR) pathway inhibitors. A class of drugs that target the mTOR pathway to slow cancer growth.

Mammogram. An x-ray that detects breast tissue abnormalities.

Mammography. A technology that uses x-rays to produce images of breast tissue.

Margin (surgical). The rim of tissue removed around a cancerous lump.

Mastectomy. Surgical removal of the breast.

Mastitis. An infection that develops when milk ducts in the breast become blocked during nursing.

Medical oncologist. A doctor who specializes in treating cancer.

Medullary carcinoma. A type of breast cancer that resembles the gray tissue of the brain stem.

Menopausal hormone therapy (MHT). Supplemental hormones given to balance low levels of the same natural hormones.

Metaplastic carcinoma. A rare type of invasive breast cancer.

Metastasis. Cancer that has spread beyond its original location to other parts of the body.

Metastatic breast cancer (MBC). Cancer that has spread from the breast to distant points in the body.

Microcalcifications. Minute calcium deposits in the breast that may be harmless but can signal the start of breast cancer.

Microinvasion. Cells that begin to break through the ducts and enter the soft tissue of the breast.

Microsurgeon. A surgeon who is specially trained to perform procedures under magnification.

Mind-body therapies. Practices that use the brain's capacity to influence bodily functions.

Mindful meditation. The practice of paying attention to the present moment.

Modified radical mastectomy. Surgical removal of breast tissue, skin, some or all of the underarm lymph nodes, and the lining over the chest muscle.

Moist reaction. Peeling of the skin underneath the breast that can be caused by radiation.

Molecular breast imaging (MBI). A breast imaging technology that uses a radioactive tracer to highlight cancer cells.

Monoclonal antibody. A medication that targets a specific molecular characteristic, like HER2, of a tumor.

Monosaturated fats. Healthy fats found in avocados, nuts, and nut oils.

Mucin. A component of mucus.

Mucinous carcinoma. A rare subtype of invasive breast cancer.

Multifocal breast cancer. Cancer found in more than one area of the breast.

Multigene panel testing. A genetic test that simultaneously checks for mutations in several different genes.

Music therapy. Guided sessions of listening to, writing, performing, or discussing music and lyrics that reduce anxiety and stress.

Mutation. An abnormality that develops in a gene.

Necrosis. Tissue that has died.

Neoadjuvant therapy. Treatment given before surgery.

Neuropathy. Pain caused by damaged nerves.

New primary cancer. A new and unrelated cancer that develops in the area of the initial diagnosis.

Night sweats. Hot flashes that occur during sleep.

Nipple reconstruction. A surgical procedure that re-creates new nipples after mastectomy.

Nipple-sparing mastectomy. Surgical removal of the breast tissue that preserves most breast skin, including the nipple.

No mutation detected. A genetic test result that shows no evidence of a known mutation in the genes that were scanned.

Noninvasive breast cancer. Cancer that doesn't spread beyond its origin in the breast.

Nucleus. The genetic control center inside all cells.

Observational study. Research that follows the same group of people over time to determine how their health changes.

Oncogene. A gene that regulates normal cellular growth and division.

Oncoplastic surgeon. A breast surgeon with plastic surgery training who can reshape the remaining breast tissue after a lumpectomy.

Oncoplastic surgery. A surgical procedure that removes diseased tissue and rearranges remaining tissue for cosmetic improvement.

Oophorectomy. Surgical removal of the ovaries.

Osteopenia. Weakening of the bones.

Osteoporosis. Thinning of the bones.

Out-of-network. Medical providers who aren't contracted to accept predetermined fees for services with a particular health insurance company.

Out-of-pocket cost. The total amount you pay for medical services not covered by your health insurance.

Outpatient procedure. A procedure that doesn't require an overnight hospital stay.

Ovarian suppression. Medication, surgery, or radiation to stop production of estrogen.

Paget's disease. An uncommon and aggressive form of breast cancer that develops in the ducts at the base of the nipple and then spreads into the nipple and the areola.

Palliative care. Medical care that supplements treatment by improving emotional, psychological, and physical symptoms.

Papillary carcinoma. A rare type of cancer that develops in fingerlike projections.

PARP inhibitor. A drug that targets the poly ADP ribose polymerase (PARP) enzyme in cancer cells.

Partial-breast radiation. Radiation treatment that targets only the tumor bed and some surrounding tissue.

Partial mastectomy. Surgery to remove a part of the breast.

Partial response/remission. A decrease in the size of a tumor or the extent of cancer in the body.

Pathological complete response. Cancer that disappears in response to treatment.

Pathologist. A physician who determines whether cancerous cells are present in tissue samples.

Pathology. The study of the cause and molecular nature of diseases.

Pathology report. A pathologist's clinical description of sample cells and tissue.

Peau d'orange. Dimpling of the breast skin that resembles an orange peel.

Pedicled tissue flap. Skin, fat, and muscle that remains connected to its original blood supply and is tunneled under the skin from the donor site to the chest to re-create a new breast.

Pedigree. A diagram of a family's medical history.

Perforator flap. A surgical procedure that uses skin and fat to re-create a breast.

Perimenopause. The transition from a woman's childbearing years to menopause.

Perinatologist. An obstetrician who specializes in complicated pregnancies.

Peripheral neuropathy. Numbness, tingling, or pain in the hands or feet.

Personalized medicine. Treatment that is customized for an individual patient.

Phyllodes tumor. A fast-growing type of breast cancer.

Physiatrist. A doctor who specializes in rehabilitation.

Phytonutrient. A naturally occurring beneficial substance found in fruits and vegetables.

PI3K inhibitors. A class of drugs that target the PIK3CA gene to slow cancer growth.

Placebo. A "fake" substance or treatment that has no therapeutic effect.

Plastic surgeon. A doctor who specializes in cosmetic or reconstructive surgery.

Platelet. A small blood particle involved in blood clotting.

Polyunsaturated fats. Healthy fats found in fish, plants, and nuts.

Positive margin. Cancer cells that are found in border tissue that surrounds a biopsy sample.

Post-chemotherapy rheumatism. A painful side effect of some chemotherapies that deforms joints and reduces bone mass.

Postmastectomy pain syndrome. Chronic pain in the chest that persists after recovery from mastectomy.

Precancerous. An abnormality that can evolve into cancer.

Premium. A fee paid for health insurance.

Prevention study. Research that looks for better ways to prevent a disease in people who have never had it or to prevent the disease from returning.

Previvor. Someone who is predisposed to a disease but hasn't been diagnosed.

Primary treatment. The first treatment given.

Progesterone. An essential hormone.

Progesterone receptor negative. Cancer cells that don't need progesterone to grow.

Progesterone receptor positive. Cancer cells that need progesterone to grow.

Prognosis. The long-term outlook for someone after diagnosis.

Prophylactic bilateral mastectomy (PBM). Surgical removal of both breasts to reduce the risk of developing breast cancer.

Proton therapy. Radiation delivered with positively charged energy particles.

Psychoneuroimmunology. The study of the interactions between our nervous system, immune system, and thought.

Psychostimulants. Medications that increase energy levels by stimulating the mind and body.

Qi gong. A type of moving meditation that includes deep breathing and slow movements.

Quadrantectomy. Breast cancer surgery that removes a tumor and about a quarter of the breast.

Radiation oncologist. A doctor who specializes in treating cancer with radiation.

Radiation pneumonitis. Inflammation of the lung that can develop from radiation therapy.

Radiation therapist. A medical professional who operates machines that deliver radiation.

Radiation therapy. Treatment with high-energy x-rays or radioactive seeds that destroy cancer cells and reduce the risk of recurrence.

Radical mastectomy. Surgery that removes the breast tissue, nipple, areola, chest muscles and the overlying lining, and underarm lymph nodes.

Reactive depression. A type of clinical depression that develops in response to a specific event.

Receptor. A protein on the surface of cells that binds to a specific substance and affects some type of cellular activity.

Recurrence. Cancer that returns after treatment.

Re-excision. A subsequent surgery to remove additional tissue.

Regional recurrence. Cancer that returns in the lymph nodes near the area of the original tumor.

Reiki. An alternative approach to reduce stress and promote healing by redirecting a person's energy flow.

Relative risk. A measure of risk of something happening in one group of people compared to the risk of the same event in another group.

Remission. A decrease or disappearance of the signs and symptoms of cancer.

Restaging studies. Tests that are performed to determine the extent of a metastatic cancer.

Revision surgery. A surgical procedure to improve the results of an earlier operation.

Risk factor. Something that increases or decreases the likelihood of disease.

Saline. A sterile saltwater solution used to fill tissue expanders and some breast implants.

Saturated fats. Unhealthy fats found in animal products and some tropical oils.

Scalp cooling. A method of preventing or reducing hair loss from chemotherapy.

Screening mammogram. An x-ray that searches for unusual or abnormal areas in the breast tissue.

Seed localization. Placement of a small radioactive seed to mark the location of a tumor.

Selective estrogen receptor modulators (SERMs). Drugs that block the effect of estrogen on breast tissue.

Sentinel lymph node. The first lymph node that cancer will reach if it progresses beyond the breast.

Sentinel lymph node biopsy (SLNB). A surgical procedure that removes one to three lymph nodes nearest the breast so that they can be examined for cancer cells.

Seroma. Excess fluid that collects under the skin.

Shiatsu. A type of alternative massage that stimulates acupuncture points with gentle pressure from the fingers, knuckles, palms, elbows, or feet.

Silicone. A synthetic gel used to fill some implants.

Skin-sparing mastectomy. Surgical removal of the breast tissue that preserves most of the breast skin.

Sporadic. Not hereditary.

Stable disease. Cancer that doesn't grow or shrink.

Staging. A description of the extent of a cancer.

Stereotactic core biopsy. A sampling of breast cells that uses a computer analysis of x-rays taken from two different angles to pinpoint a breast abnormality.

Suction-assisted protein lipectomy. A procedure that removes excess fat from lymphatic limbs.

Surgical oncologist. A physician who specializes in cancer surgery.

Systemic therapy. Treatment given throughout the entire body through the bloodstream.

Tai chi. An ancient Chinese exercise that involves a series of slow, gentle movements and deep breathing.

Targeted drug or therapy. Treatment other than chemotherapy that targets a specific molecular substance that drives the growth of cancer cells.

Textured breast implants. Breast implants that have a roughed exterior and adhere to tissue.

Thermography. Technology that measures the temperature of the breast skin to detect breast cancer.

Three-dimensional conformal radiation therapy. A type of radiation that conforms to the shape of a tumor.

Three-dimensional nipple tattoo. A tattoo that simulates the presence of a nipple on a reconstructed breast.

Tissue expander. A temporary saline implant that gradually stretches skin and/or muscle to make room for an implant.

Tissue expansion. A procedure that stretches skin to enable reconstruction.

Tomosynthesis (3-D mammography). Advanced mammography that takes images of the breast from different angles.

Total mastectomy. Removal of the breast tissue, skin, and nipple to prevent or treat cancer.

Transcutaneous electrical nerve stimulation (TENS). Low-voltage electrical impulses that are delivered under the skin to relieve pain.

Triple-negative breast cancer (TNBC). A breast cancer that lacks receptors for estrogen, progesterone, and HER2.

Tubular carcinoma. Breast cancer tumors that look like small tubes under a microscope.

Tumor marker. A substance that circulates in the blood and indicates the possible presence of cancer.

Tumor promoter gene. A gene that accelerates abnormal cellular activity.

Tumor suppressor gene. A gene that stops or slows cellular growth and repairs damaged DNA.

Tyrer-Cuzick model. A computerized program that calculates the risk of having an inherited mutation in a gene other than BRCA1 or BRCA2.

Ultrasound. A technology that uses high-frequency sound waves to produce computer images of the inside of the body.

Unilateral mastectomy. Surgical removal of one breast.

Usual hyperplasia. An excessive number of normal-looking cells that don't affect breast cancer risk.

Vaginismus. An involuntary tightening of the vaginal muscles that makes penetration impossible.

Variant of uncertain significance. A genetic test result that detects an unclear change in a gene.

Vascularized lymph node transfer. A surgical procedure that replaces removed or damaged lymph nodes with a person's own healthy lymph nodes.

Watchful waiting. Delaying treatment for a disease or condition until such time as symptoms appear or it becomes worse.

Whole-breast radiation. Radiation treatment that targets the entire breast.

Wire localization. A presurgical procedure that marks an area of abnormal tissue with a fine wire.

Women's Health and Cancer Rights Act. Federal legislation that requires health insurance companies that pay for mastectomy to also pay for prostheses and breast reconstruction.

Yoga. An ancient physical and spiritual discipline for uniting the mind and body.

Index

inflammatory breast cancer, 29, 162, 297–99, 300

Institutional Review Board (IRB), 288–89

integrative medicine, 337

Internet, 131–34

intervention studies, 289

intraductal breast cancer, 297

invasive breast cancer, 27–31, 65, 162, 203, 210, 306; prevention, 27, 67; recurrence, 27, 255; treating, 304–7; uncommon, 305–7

invasive ductal carcinoma, 29, 30, 204, 306, 310

in vitro fertilization, 325–26

ixabepilone (Ixempra), 272, 274

Johns Hopkins University, 78–79

Kalanithi, Paul, 392

Kegel exercises, 321

King, Mary-Claire, 74

Klinefelter syndrome, 31, 310

Laetrile, 336

lapatinib (Tykerb), 281

letrozole (Femara), 222, 226, 275–76, 278, 279

leukemia, 9, 182, 235

leuprolide (Lupron), 222, 229–30, 278, 302

lifestyle changes. *See* risk factor reduction strategies

Li-Fraumeni syndrome, 74–75, 156

linear accelerators, 168–69

lobular carcinoma, 300; invasive, 29; in situ, 25–27, 47

lobular neoplasia, 25–26, 38

locally advanced breast cancer, 299–300

local therapy. *See* surgical treatment

Look Good Feel Better, 317

Love, Susan, 97

lumpectomy, 26–27, 143, 159, 242–43, 248, 255, 306, 307; cancer recurrence after, 147, 164, 201, 251, 255–56, 257; for ductal carcinoma in situ, 203, 205, 206–7, 210; mastectomy *vs.*,

152–55, 183, 247; postmastectomy pain syndrome and, 332; during pregnancy, 303–4; quadrantectomy, 144; re-excision, 144. *See also* breast-conserving therapy

lumpectomy with radiation, 144, 146, 160, 169, 170, 171, 184, 305; cancer recurrence after, 147, 152; for ductal carcinoma in situ, 111.46, 203, 205, 206, 207–8, 210, 211–12; intraoperative, 176–77; for invasive breast cancer, 210

luteinizing hormone-releasing hormones, 227, 323, 333

lymphatic drainage, manual, 344

lymphatic venous anastomosis, 328

lymphedema, 158, 160–61, 180, 327–29, 342, 344, 403

lymphedema specialists, 400

lymph node dissection, 158, 332, 344; axillary, 158, 159, 160–62, 216, 258, 299, 303–4, 328–29; postmastectomy pain syndrome and, 332; sentinel node biopsy, 158–60, 162–63, 203, 216, 303–4, 306–7, 327

lymph nodes, 157–58; axillary reverse mapping, 328; cancer spread to, 115, 116, 117, 164, 258, 298, 299, 300, 306–7; enlargement, 20, 21

lymphocytes, 245

lymphomas, 9, 307–8; anaplastic large-cell, 190–91, 308

Lynch syndrome, 75

magnetic resonance imaging (MRI), 27, 99–101, 104, 156, 161–62, 258, 265, 266, 299, 300, 332; comparison with mammography and ultrasound, 100–102, 101–2; of dense breasts, 98

mammalian targets of rapamycin (mTOR), 279, 282

mammography, 19–20, 87, 93–97, 104, 161–62; after radiation therapy, 163; baseline, 20; in breast cancer survivors, 404; choosing a facility, 93; comparison with ultrasound and MRI, 101–2; controversy, 98–99; of